'This is a comprehensive book on Bowen Therapy, written by passionate Bowen instructors and practitioners. A must, not only for Bowen therapists, but for everyone who wants to know more about Bowen: the scientific community, the general public, women, athletes, and people who unfortunately are suffering and searching for a solution.'

– Louise Tremblay, iBowen and AIMTC (International Academy of Contemporary Therapeutic Methods) Founder and Director, Bowen and Niromathé International Instructor and author of The Little Bowen Book

by the same authors

A Multidisciplinary Approach to Managing Ehlers-Danlos (Type III) – Hypermobility Syndrome
Working with the Chronic Complex Patient
Isobel Knight
With contributions from Professor Howard Bird, Dr Alan J. Hakim,
Rosemary Keer, Dr Andrew Lucas, Dr Jane Simmonds and John Wilks
Foreword by Professor Rodney Grahame
ISBN 978 1 84819 080 1
eISBN 978 0 85701 055 1

A Guide to Living with Ehlers-Danlos Sydrome (Hypermobility Type)
Bending without Breaking
2nd edition
Isobel Knight
Foreword by Dr Alan Hakim
ISBN 978 1 84819 231 7
eISBN 978 0 85701 180 0

of related interest

Body Intelligence
Creating a New Environment
2nd edition
Ged Sumner
ISBN 978 1 84819 026 9
eISBN 978 0 85701 011 7

Freeing Emotions and Energy through Myofascial Release
Noah Karrasch
Foreword by C. Norman Shealy
ISBN 978 1 84819 085 6
eISBN 978 0 85701 065 0

The Mystery of Pain
Douglas Nelson
ISBN 978 1 84819 152 5
eISBN 978 0 85701 116 9

Using the
Bowen
Technique

to Address Complex and Common Conditions

John Wilks and Isobel Knight

with contributions from Kelly Clancy and others

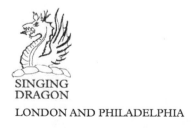

SINGING
DRAGON

LONDON AND PHILADELPHIA

Figures 1.1, 5.1, 5.2, 5.3, 8.1, 11.1, 13.1 reproduced with permission from Martin Gordon.
Figures 10.1 and 10.2 reproduced with permission from Karel Aerssens, Bowen Netherlands.
Figure 15.1 from McDermott n.d. reproduced with permission from Shane McDermott.
Figures 15.2, 15.3, 15.4 and 15.5 reproduced with permission from Art of Contemporary Yoga Ltd.
Figure 15.9 and Box 15.1 reproduced with permission from the Hypermobility Syndromes Association.

First published in 2015
by Singing Dragon
an imprint of Jessica Kingsley Publishers
73 Collier Street
London N1 9BE, UK
and
400 Market Street, Suite 400
Philadelphia, PA 19106, USA

www.singingdragon.com

Library of Congress Cataloging in Publication Data
Wilks, John, 1955-
  Using the Bowen technique to address complex and common conditions / John Wilks and Isobel Knight.
    pages cm
  Includes bibliographical references and index.
  ISBN 978-1-84819-167-9 (alk. paper)
  1. Massage therapy. 2. Fasciae (Anatomy) I. Knight, Isobel, 1974- II. Title.
  RM721.W536 2015
  615.8'22--dc23

                              2014025337

British Library Cataloguing in Publication Data
A CIP catalogue record for this book is available from the British Library

ISBN 978 1 84819 167 9
eISBN 978 0 85701 129 9

Printed and bound in Great Britain

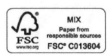

This book is dedicated to the memory of Fergal O'Daly (1948–2014), a wonderful friend, Bowen practitioner, osteopath and healer

Contents

Disclaimer

The contents of this book are for information only and are not intended as a substitute for appropriate medical attention. The authors and publishers admit no liability for any consequences arising from following any advice contained in this book. If you have any concerns about your health or medication, always consult your doctor.

Preface

The aim of this book is to expand our knowledge and application of this relatively new technique. When compared to most other therapies such as osteopathy, chiropractic or acupuncture, Bowen is still very young, with a lack of consensus about how it works and why. Now that Bowen is becoming much more accepted into mainstream medicine, we hope this book will go some way to changing that.

Most of the material in the book is aimed at increasing our understanding of this extraordinary technique. It explores some concepts and ideas based on recent research, with the intention of making us better practitioners, able to apply the principles of Bowen with greater efficiency and precision. Both of us have found bringing recent research about fascia and pain into the treatment room to be absolutely invaluable in terms of getting better results and being able to target treatments more effectively.

The book is also aimed at the general public and we hope it will go some way to increasing our understanding of the marvellously complex body that we inhabit and are dependent upon for our functioning and wellbeing.

There are certain concepts discussed extensively in this book. Some of them may be familiar to the reader and some not. As this book is only designed to be an overview of the technique, it is impossible to go into a deep explanation of some of these terms. We have tried to avoid doing this, particularly where there are already good, accessible books on the subject. Ideas for further reading on each of these topics will be found in the body of the text and in the bibliography at the end of the book.

The following concepts are referred to in the book because they are so essential to understanding the way Bowen operates. Some of these may be familiar and some not, but they would all benefit from further reading:

- The autonomic nervous system and its component parts, the sympathetic and parasympathetic nervous systems, are poorly understood by the general public, but Bowen has very specific ways of affecting these systems which are crucial to our efficient functioning and even happiness.

- Fascia is discussed in detail in the book, but more reading and research on this topic would always be useful. Our understanding of this important and ubiquitous connective tissue has expanded incrementally over the last 20 years and is really the foundation of what Bowen is and how it affects the body. Hence you will notice it is discussed in almost every chapter.

- Tensegrity is a term borrowed from sculpture and architecture to explain the exquisite tensional relationships in the body, which maintain both our posture and relationship to gravity. When applied to the body, the word often used is *biotensegrity*.

- Receptors (mostly intra-fascial receptors) live everywhere in the body in different densities with a myriad of different functions. Bowen moves affect these sensitive neurons in a variety of specific ways that influence our immune system, posture, perception of pain, etc.

- The vagus nerve, probably the most important part of our autonomic nervous system, is affected by Bowen in various procedures with specific effects. Some university researchers have spent their lives studying the vagus, but only now are new concepts and understanding of how deeply this nerve affects our health and functioning beginning to be discovered.

- The concept of how early experience affects our physical, emotional and psychological wellbeing. There are several examples of this in the book but, for further reading, books by Peter Levine (1997) and Babette Rothschild (2000) can be immensely helpful and healing. For the more technically minded, papers by Bessel van der Kolk (2014) and Allan Schore (2003) are invaluable.

Most of these ideas are explained as best as we can in the book and specific medical terms and conditions are also explained as they occur in order to make them understandable to someone without a medical background. Having said that, many concepts to do with the functioning of the human body are not easy to explain, and it would be counter-productive to over-simplify things which are necessarily complex. Hence, some sections are not an easy read and may well benefit from revisiting a few times to understand the intricacies of how Bowen affects certain processes in the body.

A book this size can never cover all the aspects of Bowen but we have tried to represent the broad scope of Bowen as it applies to everyday healthcare. Practitioners throughout the world all tend to have their own specialities, but it is enlightening to hear first-hand from people applying it on a daily basis in very different fields, from palliative care to rehabilitation after injury, from chronic pain to the sports field. You will notice that the book also contains references to other therapies that can support Bowen work. Bowen was never intended to be a cure-all for everything and it is essential for any Bowen practitioner to have a network of other health professionals to refer to where appropriate. There is always the active involvement of the client in recovery and this may mean referral to an exercise or dietary specialist.

This book intentionally aims to expand our understanding of the Bowen Technique by looking at the mechanisms by which the technique works, and looking at related therapies which can enhance our understanding of the technique. There are chapters on research and how Bowen can help certain conditions that are difficult to treat using conventional medicine. These include conditions such as fibromyalgia, chronic fatigue, lower back pain, frozen shoulder, tennis elbow and carpal tunnel syndrome. There are also sections on dance, pregnancy, assessment, using Bowen in getting people back to work, in palliative care, dance and in sport. Approaches that can support Bowen work are also discussed, including homoeopathy, nutrition and accurate assessment.

At the end of most chapters there is a series of case studies, which help bring some of the more technical aspects of the work to life. These have been generously offered by Bowen practitioners throughout the world and have been intentionally selected to represent the wide variety of ways that Bowen is practised and the kind of conditions it helps address. These case studies were chosen to show the complex application of Bowen and some of the responses people have. All of these testimonials were given with clients' permissions but their identities and some of their personal details have been changed. We hope this book will provide a useful tool not just for Bowen practitioners but all health professionals who are looking to expand their understanding of complex conditions and multidisciplinary approaches to common diseases.

The mammoth task of writing this book has been enormously aided by the generous help of our numerous contributors throughout the world. There are autobiographies of the main authors at the end of the book and for each of the case studies the names of the practitioners and their locations are credited.

This book would not have been possible without the supremely generous help of the editors, Lisa Clark of Jessica Kingsley and Dr Georgina Wilks. We have been very lucky to have had a large number of contributors bringing their individual areas of expertise to the book: Kelly Clancy, Michael Quinlivan, Alastair McLoughlin, Alastair Rattray, Dr Carolyn Goh, John Coleman, Sandra Gustafson, Michael Morris, Joanne Avison, Sharon Levin, Titus Foster, Lina Clerke, Charlotte Meerman, Ann Winter, Rosemary MacAllister, Jean Hanlin, Nickatie DiMarco, Jo Wortley, Jean Nortje, Paula Esson, Anne Schubert, Margaret Spicer, Dr Tim Robinson, Andrew Johnson, Alexia Monroe, Maggie Chambers, Vicki Mechner and many others. Without them, we would not have been able to cover the wide scope of Bowen practice it so deserves. We would also like to express our sincere thanks to the pioneers of this work – Tom Bowen, of course, but also Ossie and Elaine Rentsch, without whom this wonderful work would not have seen the light of day. Other writers and teachers such as Louise Tremblay, Manfred Zainzinger, Isy Saunders,

Julian Baker and Gene Dobkin also deserve our sincere thanks for relentlessly promoting this work when it was not only unknown but little understood.

Thanks also to Bowen practitioners throughout the world who have contributed ideas and stories that have helped bring this book to life.

References

van der Kolk, B. (2014) *The Body Keeps the Score: Mind, Brain and Body in the Transformation of Trauma.* London: Allen Lane.

Levine, P. (1997) *Waking the Tiger: Healing Trauma – The Innate Capacity to Transform Overwhelming Experiences.* Berkeley, CA: North Atlantic Books.

Rothschild, B. (2000) *The Body Remembers: The Psychophysiology of Trauma and Trauma Treatment.* New York: W.W. Norton.

Schore, A.N. (2003) *Affect Regulation and the Repair of the Self* (1st edition). New York: W.W. Norton.

Introduction

It was six men of Indostan
To learning much inclined,
Who went to see the Elephant
(Though all of them were blind),
That each by observation
Might satisfy his mind.

The *First* approached the Elephant,
And happening to fall
Against his broad and sturdy side,
At once began to bawl:
'God bless me! – but the Elephant
Is very like a wall!'

The *Second*, feeling of the tusk,
Cried: 'Ho! – what have we here
So very round and smooth and sharp?
To me 'tis mighty clear
This wonder of an Elephant
Is very like a spear!'

The *Third* approached the animal,
And happening to take
The squirming trunk within his hands,
Thus boldly up and spake:
'I see,' quoth he, 'the Elephant
Is very like a snake!'

The *Fourth* reached out his eager hand,
And felt about the knee.
'What most this wondrous beast is like
Is mighty plain,' quoth he;

''Tis clear enough the Elephant
Is very like a tree!'

The *Fifth*, who chanced to touch the ear,
Said: 'E'en the blindest man
Can tell what this resembles most;
Deny the fact who can,
This marvel of an Elephant
Is very like a fan!'

The *Sixth* no sooner had begun
About the beast to grope,
Than, seizing on the swinging tail
That fell within his scope,
'I see,' quoth he, 'the Elephant
Is very like a rope!'

And so these men of Indostan
Disputed loud and long,
Each in his own opinion
Exceeding stiff and strong,
Though each was partly in the right,
And all were in the wrong!

John Godfrey Saxe, *The Blind Men and the Elephant* (1872)

So it is with the Bowen Technique. Depending on which therapist you talk to, Bowen is sometimes described in terms of anatomical relationships in the connective tissue; some will explain that it works on an energetic level, some say it affects the sensory and motor feedback loops, some talk about its effect on the lymphatic system, others about how it affects the fascial network and still others about the meridians and chakra system (e.g. the nadis or subtle nerve channels of the ayurvedic system of medicine).

The truth is that, as the above poem points out, all these are true but none are singularly so. This probably also explains the extraordinarily powerful effect of the Bowen treatment on patients, as it undoubtedly affects the body on multiple levels at the same time.

Part of the confusion has arisen because Tom Bowen was not a good communicator, particularly when it came to explaining what he was doing. According to Romney Smeeton, a student of Bowen, he did not 'teach' anyone, but just allowed a small number of people to observe him at work and ask questions. He was also working mostly with acute clients as were most of his students or 'boys', as he used to call them. As the technique was taught to a wider audience, though, it became clear that Bowen's approach also had a powerful effect on the chronically ill, the terminally ill and the hypersensitive client as well. Treating these types of client needed a different approach – a lighter touch, longer treatment plans and longer treatments – something that was also part of Bowen's way of working with children with disabilities. This legacy has resulted in a large number of therapists working very successfully in this way today.

Development of the Bowen Technique

In 2001 Vicki Mechner wrote:

> Thomas Ambrose Bowen was born in Australia on 18 April 1916. An ardent sports fan, he spent countless hours watching the masseurs at local football games in Geelong, Victoria. He began massaging footballers' injuries, and then studied informally with Ernie Saunders, a legendary 'manipulator' in a suburb of nearby Melbourne. Bowen studied anatomy texts and developed his distinctive technique through continual experimentation, mainly by treating the bad backs of his colleagues at the factory where he worked.
>
> By the early 1950s, his wife, Jessie, had been hospitalized several times with severe asthma. Bowen developed a soft-tissue manipulation procedure for it. The combination of this procedure and the restricted diet he developed kept her asthma under control thereafter. In 1957 he began treating people in the evening at the home of friends Stan and Rene Horwood. Bowen soon gave up his day job and rented office space, with Rene as his office manager. He called himself an osteopath, a title that was not regulated in Australia at that time.
>
> Bowen's uncanny assessment skills enabled him to address the root cause of patients' problems with very few moves. With an assistant in each treatment room to get patients ready, he worked at a prodigious rate. By 1973 he had a very large practice.
>
> As his reputation spread, many health professionals wanted to learn his technique. Only six did so to his satisfaction. One soft-tissue therapist, four chiropractors and one osteopath completed two to three years of weekly individual study with Bowen. After several weeks or months of following him from room to room and watching him work, each was allowed to work on patients under Bowen's close supervision. They incorporated his technique into their own practices. Even after Bowen considered them ready, they continued to visit him regularly to learn his latest refinements.
>
> Bowen wouldn't accept payment for treating children, football players, pregnant women and poor or physically disabled people. When Bowen lost a leg to diabetes in 1980, three of his students ran his clinic until he resumed work at his former pace, although from a wheelchair.
>
> After Bowen's death in 1982, Kevin Ryan (the osteopath) kept the clinic running for two months. He and Romney Smeeton (one of the chiropractors) continued the free Saturdays for the disabled for another 12 years. They and

chiropractor Keith Davis still practice Bowen's technique in their busy clinics. Of the other chiropractors, Kevin Neave retired in 1989, and Nigel Love died in 1999. Oswald Rentsch (the massage therapist) opened a Bowen Technique clinic with his wife, Elaine, in 1976; they have taught seminars in their interpretation of the technique since 1986. Ryan teaches occasional workshops to Bowen practitioners and, since 1998, has taught a 26-contact-hour Bowen course to osteopathy students at a university in Melbourne. Rene Horwood, who, in addition to running Bowen's business, helped him develop some of his procedures, passed away at 93 in September 2001.

Bowtech

Oswald Rentsch ('Ossie' to all who know him) undertook the study of massage in 1959 with the goal of easing his wife Elaine's unremitting pain. A childhood neck injury had damaged her spine severely, and she fully expected to become an invalid. Fifteen years later, still searching for relief for Elaine's suffering, Ossie began a weekly commute two hours each way to study with Tom Bowen.

Elaine soon became Bowen's patient. She recalls her first visit: 'When he touched my neck, he said, "It will take six months to get this right." But even after the one treatment, I could feel energy moving in my neck.' Elaine's health gradually returned. She continued accompanying Ossie to the clinic, where she sometimes assisted Bowen's patients and observed his treatments. In 1976, with Bowen's advice and blessings, Ossie and Elaine opened a clinic in Hamilton that was modeled after his.

'At Tom's suggestion, we didn't advertise,' recalls Ossie. 'By the end of six months we were booked solid. Many professionals came to watch us work, and they kept asking us to teach, saying, "If you don't teach this, Bowen's work will disappear." Finally, a fellow in Perth got a group together and we went there to teach.'

Through the Bowen Therapy Academy of Australia, the Rentschs have taught 'Bowtech,' as they call their interpretation of Tom Bowen's technique, to tens of thousands of practitioners throughout the world. They began training instructors in 1994.

One of the issues that many experienced teachers have is that it is easy for practitioners to adopt the 'procedural' way that Bowen is taught without using their palpation and assessment skills to adapt the work to suit each client individually. The fact is that many practitioners get extraordinary results from applying the 'recipe-type' approach to the work (rather like one-size-fits-all) which means that is easy for a practitioner who is new to bodywork to apply Bowen formulaically and get remarkable results. Changes in posture, wellbeing, sleep patterns and emotional health are very common after applying the 'recipe' of what are called the Basic Relaxation Moves (or what was originally taught as pages 1, 2 and 3 in the early manuals).

For the therapist, there is something quite magical about observing the results of something so simple and yet something so inexplicable. Applying these gentle moves to the body in a predetermined sequence just doesn't seem to add up to the profound effect on clients. This, in itself, understandably gives rise to a reluctance on the part of the therapist to change the 'recipe' or tinker too much with what they have been taught for fear of watering down the results. However, for many clients this procedural approach is not enough and we need to go deeper to find the origin of their problem and work on it. Without finding the origin of a problem, we are unlikely to get long-standing changes and the problem will keep recurring. This is the essence of the role of the therapist, but it must be borne in mind that the root cause of someone's problem might be physical (and not obviously connected to their symptoms), emotional or something they are doing in their everyday life that is exacerbating their condition. This is why this book concentrates on emphasizing ways of supporting clients through appropriate exercise, diet and adjusting environmental factors. This might be a question of changing something as simple as not carrying a wallet in their back pocket (you would be surprised how many clients complaining of sciatic pain do this and don't make the connection!) to looking at deeper emotional issues contributing to their condition (which may need referral to someone qualified to work in this area).

The big issue that has made it more difficult to move forward with developing the Bowen Technique is the lack of understanding and consensus of how Bowen works. There has been a lot of interest recently about Tom Bowen's interest in the meridians of Traditional Chinese Medicine (TCM) and shiatsu in particular. Romney Smeeton, who worked closely with Tom, relates that in 1978 Bowen handed him a shiatsu book and said, 'That's the whole basis of this work, lad.' Certainly Ernie Saunders, Tom's mentor, travelled widely to the USA, South Africa and the UK and was exposed to the theories of acupuncture and shiatsu and undoubtedly shared these with his colleagues on his return. It is interesting that well over 90 per cent of all Bowen moves are performed over known acupuncture points, but practitioners point out that Bowen seems to have a different effect to traditional acupuncture. Many clients will have had acupuncture treatments that they have not responded to, but do respond with Bowen and vice versa, so there are clearly other mechanisms going on. However, there is a clear link between acupuncture points and places in the body where the deep and superficial fascia connect that was researched many years ago. This is discussed later in this book.

There is no doubt that Tom Bowen discovered something extraordinary with his way of working and it is also clear that there is so much more to discover. It also seems likely that he didn't fully understand the depth of this work. Certainly his knowledge of anatomy and physiology was poor, at least in the sense of being able to name structures in the body, although his thirst for knowledge did extend to visiting the local abattoir to inspect the fresh cadavers, thereby obtaining a deep understanding of functional anatomy, particularly in relationship to the fascia, which is the fundamental tissue that we work on in Bowen.

In the sense of being able to 'read the body' and assess where areas of restriction were, he was legendary, but much of this was probably on a level that he couldn't explain or just didn't want to. From my experience, there is something about when a practitioner really 'sees' the origins of someone's problem which can be highly complex and involve physical and emotional aspects at the same time, it can often be too complex and too limiting to explain to someone else. This is possibly why he apparently used to turn off his hearing aid, maybe also partly because when he needed to concentrate intensely he didn't want to be distracted. Don't forget that he was incredibly busy, seeing several people at once, and wouldn't have had time to explain in any detail to those who were shadowing him in his work.

One other important thing to understand is that the origins of this work were primarily in treating sports people and acute situations (both Tom Bowen and Ernie Saunders worked extensively with football teams), so Tom's way of working short treatments (some commentators estimate that his clients can't have been on the couch more than about ten minutes) is not necessarily ideal for all practitioners and clients today.

The following chapter looks at some of the mechanisms that the Bowen Technique employs and how our understanding has developed to enable the practitioner to address a wide variety of symptoms.

1

How Bowen Works

The soul of man, with all the streams of pure living water, seems to dwell in the fascia of his body.

A.T. Still, MD (1899)

As we discussed in the Introduction, Bowen is unusual in that it affects the tissues of the body (particularly what we call the connective tissues – muscles, tendons, ligaments and fascia) in a variety of ways simultaneously. The effect of a Bowen treatment is not limited to relaxing tight muscles or increasing hydration in the tissues, but it can also be used to increase tonus in the core muscles, contractile strength within the fascia and to initiate a lowering of sympathetic tone in the autonomic nervous system, thereby affecting what is called the hypothalamic-pituitary-adrenal axis (the HPA axis; see Chapter 9 for more details).

Fascia

The Bowen Technique has a very specific effect on fascia, which is the tissue that surrounds organs, muscles and muscle fibres, and creates a network in the body. Primarily, Bowen moves are made directly on muscles (although some moves are also performed on tendons, ligaments, joints and nerves), but because all these structures are surrounded by a network of fascia it is inevitable that whatever structure is activated, the fascia that surrounds it (and is integral to it) is affected at the same time, albeit with slightly different physiological effects.

Fascia and connective tissue have varied roles in the body. For example, one of fascia's crucial functions in efficient movement is its property of recoil, which is dependent on good hydration (an important effect of Bowen work). This can be seen clearly in the denser sheet-like areas of fascia such as the thoracolumbar aponeurosis, which is the starting point for a lot of Bowen work. One reason that Bowen insisted on beginning a treatment at this point in the body was partly as an assessment tool for the therapist to ascertain any asymmetrical tightness in the erector spinae muscles (in other words, if the body was compensating for some postural imbalance resulting in either tightness or increased muscle bulk on one side). He talked about these two moves (one on the left and one on the right over the erector spinae muscles and thoracolumbar aponeurosis level with L4) as 'putting the stoppers in', something that apparently Ernie Saunders taught him and similarly insisted on. Anatomically, it also makes sense to start a treatment here as it is directly over one of the attachment sites of the dural membranes at L3 and L4. The dura form a very strong relationship in the body (which W.G. Sutherland described as a reciprocal tension in the dural membranes – see below) between the key attachment sites, which are:

- coccyx
- sacrum (at S2)
- lumbars (at L3 and L4)
- top of the neck (at C2 and C3)
- the base of the skull at the foramen magnum of the occiput
- within the skull at the temporal bones, the sphenoid and the ethmoid (sometimes called the third eye).

Interestingly, the areas of the body Tom Bowen was keen on working directly correlate to these dural attachment sites, perhaps because he realized that they have a strong reciprocal effect on posture. Whether he picked this information up intuitively, by talking to colleagues or by reading textbooks we shall never know, but what is clear is that there are many parallels in understanding with osteopathic, chiropractic and craniosacral principles. In chiropractic the relationships between the lumbar and cervical regions are termed Lovett Brothers, something that is a key principle of Sacro Occipital Technique (SOT) first proposed by Major Bertrand DeJarnette, a chiropractor, osteopath and engineer, in 1924.

Cranial osteopathy was fairly well established by the time Bowen started in practice, as it had been developed by William Sutherland, a pupil of Dr Still, the originator of osteopathy, in the early 1900s. Much of the language of cranial osteopathy came from two diverse sources – the Old Testament and the automobile (which was becoming all the rage when Sutherland was developing his ideas). Terms such as 'gear shifts' and 'ignition' were used to explain mechanical processes in the body (such as the mechanical relationships created by tension in the dural membranes or between the various bones of the skull) whereas the more florid language of the Old Testament, such as the cerebrospinal fluid as being an expression of the 'Breath of Life', was reserved to express the beauty and depth of the work and the notion that there was some higher organizing force that practitioners were encouraging their clients bodies to become aligned to.

As with much in Bowen, the use of the terminology is somewhat vague about what Bowen actually meant by 'stoppers' and there are many commentators who have their own take on what they do and why they are important. Graham Pennington talks about how the location of the bottom stoppers exactly corresponds to an acupoint called QiHaiShu (Sea of Qi), which he describes as having been used for thousands of years for the treatment of low back pain and which has the potential to strengthen the back and the knees. Bowen's own rather cursory explanation was that if you work on specific areas of the body without first doing the stoppers, then the person would feel dizzy. This is certainly borne out in practice and can be seen occurring after working the coccyx and neck work (taught in the Bowtech specialized procedures) without putting the stoppers in first. Clients are advised not to drive after this as it can make them feel quite disorientated.

Interestingly, the sensation of losing your ability to orient to your surroundings is a classic response of the autonomic nervous system, specifically the parasympathetic system, which is stimulated during a Bowen treatment (see the mechanisms for how this works below). Getting a client into a more parasympathetic state is crucial for healing to take place, as it is very difficult for the body to repair if it is caught in a sympathetic (fight or flight) response. Other manifestations of a parasympathetic state are the client feeling cold, clammy and getting a gurgling tummy, a frequent cause of embarrassment to many clients as they are lying on the couch. This is not just a placebo response to lying down – animals such as horses also show a strong parasympathetic response after even the first few moves of a Bowen treatment, when they dribble, urinate and often go to sleep. Luckily, not many human clients display exactly the same responses (although babies often do).

The function of the stoppers, then, seems to be multiple:

- They start the process of allowing the body to relax by lowering the body's sympathetic tone (see their effect on the Ruffini receptors described below).

- They have a therapeutic effect on the lumbar fascia by encouraging hydration and a lowering of sensory nerve firing.

- They have a relaxing effect on the whole paraspinal muscles (not just locally).

- They get the body prepared by getting it used to the level of touch and trust.

- They can be used as an assessment tool.

Tom Bowen had rather idiosyncratic terms to explain which areas of the body he was addressing. For example, 'crowbar' muscles were particularly tight areas such as the latissimus dorsi or the gluteus medius; the gullet muscles might refer to the diaphragm or the sternocleidomastoid muscles. Certainly his anatomical knowledge was largely self-taught and the result of his extraordinarily good observation and palpation skills rather than a conventional approach to functional anatomy that we have today. He certainly would not have been exposed to the kind of research now available on fascia, which helps to explain and refine in detail what Bowen felt and did largely intuitively.

One of the most helpful papers to come out of the Fascia Research Group, which is part of the Division of Neurophysiology at the University of Ulm in Germany, was the paper by Robert Schleip entitled 'Fascial mechanoreceptors and their potential role in deep tissue manipulation' from 2003 (Schleip 2003). Although this paper was largely looking at the effect of therapies such as Rolfing, it has huge importance for the understanding of Bowen work in terms of why we might vary pressure, location and speed of touch depending on what the therapist is trying to achieve. Since the publication of that paper, further research has focused on the function of the numerous mechanoreceptors in the retinacula and subcutaneous tissue, which has further refined our understanding of how the body responds to Bowen moves (Schleip 2014).

Our understanding of fascia has improved vastly over the last 20 years, mostly as a result of the impressive work done in Germany at Ulm, but the general public's understanding of connective tissue in general and fascia specifically is rudimentary, to say the least. If you mention at a party that you work with fascia, most people will assume you work with guttering, soffits and all things related to just beneath the roof. Actually, the use of the word fascia in this context shares the same Latin origin of its use in reference to the body – in other words, a 'band, bandage, ribbon or swathe', which is basically what it does in the body. Fascia wraps organs, blood vessels, nerves, muscles and muscle fibres. It forms 'ribbons' in the body, some of which are very tough, that help support the frame. However, it is also the most richly innervated tissue in the body, with a very high density of sensory nerves, in particular nerves called proprioceptors that help our nervous systems orient to our surroundings. You could say that our fascia is like our antennae, constantly responding to what is going on in our environment and where we are in space.

Dr A.T. Still, the founder of osteopathy, had additional views on the functions of fascia: 'This connecting substance must be free at all parts to receive and discharge all fluids, and use them in sustaining animal life, and eject all impurities, that health may not be impaired by dead and poisonous fluids' (Still 1902, p.61). Thomas Myers, in his book *Anatomy Trains,* has done a great job at identifying some of the key structural bands of fascia in the body, which have such an important and inter-related effect on posture. His identification of what he calls the 'superficial back line' which extends from the plantar fascia of the feet all the way through to the attachment of the paraspinal muscles to the back of the head (and extending to the forehead close to where the dural attachments are at the crista galli of the ethmoid) is a fascial relationship that is addressed a lot in Bowen work. What is interesting is that because there is a clear functional, and therefore anatomical, difference between the superficial back line and the front line, Bowen practitioners work these areas separately, starting with the client lying on their front so the therapist can access the back fascia before turning them over at some point in the treatment and working the front fascia. Actually, much of the front fascia in the human has a very similar construction to that of our four-legged friends. Its function is primarily to support all the organs that hang off the spine such as the heart, stomach, liver and other organs of digestion. In us bipeds, these organs still hang off the spine, supported by the front fascia which has its origins in the attachment sites at the base of the cranium. It's just that because we now stand upright some of those organs tend to hang down a little more (and, unfortunately, more in some of us than others!).

Fascia also creates the ability of the various structures in the body, such as muscles and blood vessels, to move freely one against another. In the neck for example, the sheets of fascia that envelop these structures appear like tubes, whereas in the back they form great sheets which come together to tether at the sacrum and iliac crests. These sheets form what are called 'aponeuroses' (Figure 1.1), so called because early anatomists thought they were nerves (and they were not far off the mark). Because these sheets contain and enfold many large muscles, damage such as can be caused by accidents or operations, which involve cutting through several layers of fascia, can cause tethering, which can have effects far beyond the site of the original injury through the reciprocal relationships of what is termed biotensegrity. Serge Gracovetsky, in his wonderful but slightly impenetrable book *The Spinal Engine*, points out the potentially damaging consequences of operations that affect the lumbar fascia, particularly when the ilium is used as a 'bone bank', thereby affecting the attachment sites of the lumbodorsal fascia (Gracovetsky 2008, p.222). A more accessible explanation of Serge Gracovetsky's concept of the evolution of the spine as an 'engine' vital to movement is found in Eric Dalton's invaluable book *Dynamic Body* (Dalton 2012, p.308).

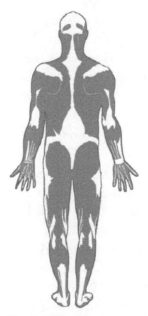

Figure 1.1 The body has numerous aponeuroses
Source: Martin Gordon

Tensegrity and Biotensegrity

When looking at possible mechanisms for how the Bowen Technique works, it is important to differentiate how touch and manipulation affect muscle contraction (or even a lack of tonus in the muscles) as opposed to connective tissue contracture. Many practitioners do not appreciate the difference between muscle contraction, which is described as a high-energy shortening of tissues, and contracture of connective tissue, a 'slow, (semi) permanent, low-energy, shortening process, which involves matrix-dispersed cells and is dominated by extracellular events such as matrix remodeling' (Tomasek *et al.* 2002, p.357).

For efficient functioning of the human system, connective tissues need to hold certain contractive patterns to maintain stability. In dissection you can see clearly that all connective tissues are under stress – for example, dissected nerves and blood vessels have a length of around 25–30 per cent less than their in situ length (Tomasek *et al.* 2002).

Myofibroblasts play a crucial role in maintaining constructive tension within the connective tissue, being a type of fibroblast – the 'building block' cells of fascia – which have the characteristics of smooth muscle, and their structure and function are affected in many kinds of connective tissue disorders. On the one hand, fibrotic contracture, in conditions such as Dupuytrens, reveal an imbalance in myofibroblast density and function (Naylor 2012). It would also appear that there is some mechanism involved where fibroblasts are encouraged in certain areas of the body to transform excessively into myofibroblasts (Hinz and Phan 2007). This also happens in conditions where 'frozen' type tissue occurs – the lumbar aponeurosis in low back pain and in frozen shoulder, for example.

This complex constructive tension within the connective tissue (which is largely maintained by the action of myofibroblasts) is an essential element of what is sometimes called the body's tensegrity system (Levin and Martin 2012). Tensegrity is a term coined by the sculptor Kenneth Snelson and the celebrated American architect Buckminster Fuller in the 1960s. Tensegrity (the word comes from the two words tensional and integrity) is based on the concept of reciprocal tension or compression between rigid members (bones in the body) and cables (connective tissue). Many elegant structures have been built using these principles, the largest being the Kurilpa Bridge in Brisbane which opened in 2009. In applying the ideas of tensegrity to the human body, various authors use the term 'biotensegrity' to explain the relationship between rigid structures such as bones and the reciprocal tension in the connective tissue (Levin and Martin 2012). Biotensegrity can be used to explain the complex interaction that maintains structural homeostasis in gross anatomical structures such as the spine and joints, and more subtle inter-relationships in the myofascial system (Guimberteau 2010; Guimberteau and Bakhach 2007) and even in the cytoskeleton of the cell (Oschmann 2003). Biotensegrity offers an elegant explanation as to how space is held in the joints of the body and how, when the delicate balance of reciprocal forces that are held by the connective tissue begin to break down, all kinds of musculoskeletal symptoms can begin to emerge (Turvey 2007). This concept is explored in more detail later in this book. Beautiful artistic representations of this are found in Snelson's magnificent sculptures, where none of the rigid structures (the struts of the sculptures; in the case of the human body, the bones) touch each other and often appear to hang in space as though unsupported. The anatomist Tom Flemons (www.intensiondesigns.com) has also made elegant models demonstrating the principles of tensegrity when applied to the human body (see www.biotensegrity.com). Soft-tissue techniques such as the Bowen Technique rely on effecting structural change by directly influencing this tensegrity aspect of the connective tissue, something that is often difficult to explain to clients and involves a different approach to that of chiropractic and other forms of bony manipulation.

The Bungee Effect

As mentioned, in walking and running, all the aponeuroses (particularly the lumbar aponeurosis) display this tensegrity feature to great advantage as they act as a kind of 'bungee' and greatly reduce the amount of effort that is needed to exert via the muscular system. This is demonstrated in the movement of animals such as kangaroos, lemurs and gazelles as well as humans (Kram and Dawson 1998). Where this recoil property is compromised through a lack of hydration and reciprocal tension in the fascia, certain movements such as running and walking require more exertion through the muscular system. All the aponeuroses in the healthy body (Figure 1.1) aid movement in this way and even some muscles.

The gastrocnemius muscles and Achilles tendons use this springy quality to propel us forward by acting with all the characteristics of a catapult (Fukunaga *et al.* 2002). It is quite easy to observe this flexibility (or lack of it) in clients. The elderly (or particularly the chronically inactive) will show little flexibility and 'recoil' in their aponeuroses. It can be enlightening for a practitioner to mimic the posture and particularly the gait of a client as it gives a remarkable insight into how restrictions in one area of the body create discomfort or problems in another.

Take the piriformis muscle, for example. This is a deep muscle in the buttock, which goes from the greater trochanter of the femur to the sacrum. It is a key rotator of the leg, so if there is a problem here (tightness or laxity) it will have a big effect on the knee and ankle. It also depends on a complex but intricate relationship with some other muscles such as the gracilis, sartorius and semitendinosus. Likewise, problems with the gracilis (the long muscle that attaches to the pubis and goes on to insert just below the inside of the knee at the pes anserinus) will often be felt as pain in the knee, and mistakenly attributed to a problem with the knee.

An important question to ask is 'How do our clients engage in being in the world?' Emotional aspects have a big impact on the way we hold ourselves and how we move – it is surprisingly easy to 'body read' someone's emotional state just by observing their posture and particularly their gait. One of the favourite maxims of Rolfers is 'The way one walks through the room is the way one walks through the world.' Shakespeare famously wrote, 'There's no art to find the mind's construction in the face.' Unfortunately, the work of Stephen Porges wasn't around in 1606 because his work shows clearly that there is a very clever and accurate art to finding the mind's construction in the face. If he had been a Bowen practitioner, Shakespeare could have added 'but there is an art to find the mind's construction in the body'. But then that would have ruined the plot of *Macbeth*!

Bowen and Nerves

The Bowen Technique consists of moves over the following structures:

- muscles
- tendons
- ligaments
- nerves
- joints
- dural membranes
- superficial and deep fascia
- blood vessels.

The common thread with all these structures is that they are all enveloped by fascia, or fascia is integral to their structures. Fascia has many types of sensory nerves with different densities depending on where it is in the body and also depending on any potential pathology involved in particular areas. Bowen moves initially involve moving the skin (we call it taking skin slack) before actually activating the connective tissue. Touch of any kind will activate certain sensory receptors in the skin such as Merkel's discs (which relay information about pressure and texture), Meissner's corpuscles (which are sensitive to very light touch) and free nerve endings (which sense mechanical stimuli and pain). Moving the skin also seems to have an effect on the Langerhan cells which are macrophage-like cells living in the Malpighian layer of the dermis (Tremblay 2010). Interestingly, these cells appear to have the function of preventing excessive immune responses in the skin (Kaplan *et al.* 2005), something that is a problem in autoimmune conditions and allergies, which is possibly why Bowen seems to have a beneficial effect on people with autoimmune conditions, but only if light pressure is used. Strong pressure can over-stimulate the immune response in these individuals which can potentially have undesirable side effects in the short term.

Sensory Receptors

When we look at fascia as a whole, there are key mechanoreceptors not only within the fascia but also the subcutaneous tissue, membranes, tendons and many other structures that are activated during a treatment. These are largely Golgi, Ruffini and interstitial receptors. Occasionally, Bowen moves involve a fast release of pressure, which affects the Pacini receptors (involved in proprioception), but these types of move are rare. Mostly, Bowen moves involve taking skin slack, applying a challenge (or gentle push) for a few seconds, and a slow steady move over the structure being addressed. Bowen moves mostly consist of a type described by Schleip (2009) as slow melting pressure. These types of move strongly affect the numerous Ruffini receptors, which are found in the skin and in many deep tissues of the body including the dural membranes, ligaments and joint capsules. The reason that the Ruffini receptors only respond to slow pressure (in other words, they don't respond if the practitioner works with fast moves) is that they are generally found in higher densities in the body where the tissues are regularly stretched in everyday movements, like the outer layer of joint capsules and the ligaments of peripheral joints. They are also especially responsive to tangential forces and lateral stretch (Kruger 1987), such as is used in Bowen moves. Bowen practitioners will have noted that slow moves generally result in deep relaxation by stimulating an increase in the parasympathetic system (measured by an increase in vagal tone), whereas fast moves seem to have the opposite effect (Eble 1960).

Researchers such as Schleip have concluded that when vagal tone is increased through this sort of touch, not only does this trigger a parasympathetic response in the organs (heart, digestion, etc.) but the anterior lobe of the hypothalamus is activated as well. Seminal research by Ernst Gellhorn (Gellhorn 1967) shows that these sort of changes in the hypothalamus have a lowering effect on all muscle tonus in the body as well as quieting the mind and calming the client's emotional state. As we will see later, the Ruffinis also have an important role in changing local fluid dynamics and aiding tissue metabolism, an important factor in Bowen treatments.

There are many moves in Bowen that stimulate the Ruffinis – in fact, you could say that almost any moves done with slow melting pressure will stimulate them. It is interesting, for example, to really slow down the moves when working the paraspinal muscles (the bottom and top stoppers and moves up the back), giving a much longer challenge and slower roll over the muscle. This will nearly always result in someone falling asleep on the couch within a few minutes. Of course, this is not always desirable if one were treating someone who has got to get up a play a round of golf, in which case the practitioner might want to use a different kind of touch. Tom Bowen used to say enigmatically that when you do the first few moves of a Bowen session 'the body knows that the emergency is over'. This kind of research certainly bears that out.

Interstitial Receptors

Other receptors that induce a decrease in the sympathetic nervous system (SNS), and corresponding increase in vagal tone, are the interstitial receptors, which are found nearly everywhere in the body. Some of these receptors (particularly what are called nociceptors) are high-threshold, and known to be involved in chronic conditions, but interestingly about 50 per cent of interstitial receptors are low-threshold fibres and are sensitive to the kind of very light touch (similar to skin brushing) that is used in some Bowen moves. This mechanism explains the deep relaxing effect of Bowen treatments and the crucial healing effect of increased vagal tone even when light pressure is used (e.g. when treating the chronically sensitive and animals such as horses).

If you look at the composition of nerves generally in the body, most are sensory (take the sciatic nerve, for instance), with a small number being motor nerves and only about 10 per cent type I and II (Ruffini, Pacini and Golgi). The rest (type III and IV interstitial receptors) make up the majority. In fact, they are the most abundant receptor in the body, found almost everywhere, but particularly in the periosteum (the membrane that covers the outer surface of bones). There are only a few Bowen moves that are done that come into contact with the periosteum. Some of these are on the coccyx (which interestingly uses very light pressure) and the back of the head (moves 3 and 4 of the neck work), but any Bowen moves done lightly anywhere in the body will stimulate the interstitials.

About half of these receptors are what are called 'high-threshold' fibres – in other words, they need quite a lot of stimulus to fire them off – whilst the other half are extremely sensitive and are responsive to the kind of touch used when lightly brushing the skin. Robert Schleip has written that the interstitial receptors can function both as mechanoreceptors and as pain receptors, which means that they are very important to address in situations of chronic pain and sensitivity. What seems to happen in situations that involve chronic pain, inflammation and tissue damage is that these receptors become over-sensitized, leading to strong and chronic firing. This means that pain can often exist without specific mechanical irritation of nervous structures (Liptan 2010).

Nociceptors are usually mostly high-threshold fibres that need a fair amount of stimulation for them to respond. What happens as a result of prolonged inflammation and tissue damage is that these nerves become hyper-sensitized, leading to people actually feeling a lot more pain than they should. This situation can, over time, spiral into an activation of the sympathetic nervous system where sufferers will often experience feelings of restlessness, an over-active mind, difficulty in sleeping and even depression (see Chapter 6).

There are many situations where this might occur – basically any condition that ends in '-itis' or '-osis' (inflammation and/or tissue damage) as well as the multitude of different conditions nowadays that are poorly understood but affect the connective tissues (such as fibromyalgia) and result in chronic pain and tiredness.

The best way of working with these receptors therapeutically appears to be working very gently (i.e. not getting a pain response) with the intention of re-sensitizing (or effectively re-calibrating) these receptors, particularly the nociceptors which have become hyper-sensitized and over-active. The key to knowing if you are getting a result is if the client's body displays an autonomic reaction – in other words, goes sleepy, clammy or cold, etc. Interestingly, when they are stimulated, these particular receptors (type III and IV) also have an effect on heart rate, blood pressure and respiration so it is not uncommon to also see changes here during a treatment.

Practitioners often claim that Bowen has an effect on blood pressure (BP) – someone with high blood pressure will experience a lowering of BP after a treatment with the reverse happening with someone with elevated BP. This might appear far-fetched and wishful thinking until you understand that research has shown that stimulation of type IV receptors tends to increase blood pressure (Coote and Pérez-Gonzáles 1970) whereas stimulation of type III receptors can both increase and decrease blood pressure. Several studies have also shown that an increase of static pressure on muscles such as is used in a Bowen move tends to lower arterial blood pressure (Schleip 2003). Schleip points out that it would appear that one of the major functions of the interstitials is to influence the autonomic nervous system to regulate blood supply according to local demands, which might be one reason why clients often notice a change in blood supply to the extremities after a treatment.

Golgi Receptors

On a more structural level, Bowen moves affect the Golgi receptors (found in myotendinous junctions, ligaments and the deep fascia) by using slightly more pressure, longer holding times and working close to origins and insertions. It has been suggested that manipulation of these receptors causes the firing of alpha motor neurons resulting in a softening of related tissues. This process also seems to happen via gentle stretching of the tissues such as in yoga. Although there has been some debate on how much manual therapies can actually activate the Golgi receptors (certain massage techniques that involve stretching the tissues probably don't), it is clear that cross-fibre moves close to the attachment sites (i.e. close to the bone) certainly have the potential to activate them.

Muscles themselves are stimulated by the 'challenge' in a Bowen move, which activates the muscle spindles in response to the stretch on the muscle fibres. Much of this response is mediated at the level of the spinal cord, but some impulses do make their way to various areas of the brain such as the cerebellum, the basal ganglia, the reticular formation and the brain stem, before being coordinated in the thalamus and sent back down the various motor nerve tracts to the muscles or organs (Wilks 2007).

It seems to take around two minutes for muscles to respond in this way, so it is interesting that it is normal practice for Bowen practitioners to leave a two-minute break between the various activations or moves. However, when working the Golgi receptors, practitioners often leave longer (up to ten minutes) as it takes that amount of time for the muscles to respond to the response initiated by the Golgi receptors. This can be seen when working on the heads of the hamstring, the gracilis and the psoas, for example. It would appear that by inputting targeted, but minimal, sensory stimulus during a Bowen session without extraneous interference, it allows the body to re-calibrate. For example, Dietz and others (Dietz 1992) have shown that the central nervous system (CNS) can reset Golgi tendon receptors and related reflex arcs so that they function as delicate antigravity receptors (Schleip 2003). One thing students of the Bowen Technique are taught is always to get clients up at the end of a treatment so that both feet land on the ground at the same time, thereby stimulating a response in the many Golgi receptors in the plantar fascia of the feet.

There are many moves in Bowen that involve a stimulation of the Golgi receptors and working them has a profound effect on posture. Golgi receptors can be found in all dense connective tissue, particularly in the junctions between tendons and muscles, but also in ligaments and joint capsules. Some moves, particularly around the pelvis where there a lot of attachments of various important structural muscles, really do have to be performed close to the bone, otherwise the slack is taken up by the muscle itself and the Golgi receptors are not activated in the same way. These types of move need some explaining from the practitioner as they are inevitably close to areas such as the sitting bones (ischial tuberosities), the pubis (where the adductors attach) and the front of the pelvis (where the longest muscle in the body, the sartorius, attaches). Apart from requiring stronger and longer challenges, these moves also need a longer wait time (sometimes 10 to 15 minutes) as the relaxing effect on the attached muscles can take that long to work.

Pacini Receptors

The Pacini receptors tend to be more stimulated in other therapies such as chiropractic and osteopathy rather than Bowen, but they provide a very important role in terms of proprioceptive feedback that helps coordinate movement. Pacini receptors only respond to stimuli such as sudden pressure release, high velocity adjustments, vibrations and rhythmic movements such as shaking and rocking, most of which are not used in Bowen.

However, there are a number of Bowen moves that involve rapid pressure change – for example, on the patella tendon, or the gracilis, as well as some 'jarring' type moves that affect the shoulder, the ankle, the elbow and the hamstrings. The Pacini receptors are actually slightly closer to the bony attachments sites, so it is even more vital to be very close to the bone if the practitioner wants to influence them. The question is why would a practitioner need to adapt the moves in this way? The answer is simply that certain conditions and certain types of people have problems with a lack of proprioception, which can make people quite unsteady on their feet. Working with the Pacinis has a particularly powerful local effect on proprioception, so for people who have specific areas (particularly joints) that are a problem (e.g. a knee that constantly feels unstable) working them can be very beneficial. Two of the most obvious conditions where people have a more general problem with proprioception are Parkinson's disease and multiple sclerosis (MS) (see Chapter 16) but others include spinal cord injuries, hypermobility syndromes (such as Ehlers-Danlos), post-operatively (for example, after cruciate ligament reconstruction) and ageing (particularly if there is osteoarthritis involved). In these types of client it is often inappropriate to use any kind of forceful manipulations, so other approaches such as the Alexander Technique, Feldenkrais and yoga can be very useful in improving proprioceptive sense and stability.

There are also some excellent remedial exercises called the Cawthorne-Cooksey exercises which can help improve not only proprioception but also balance, dizziness, Ménière's disease and vertigo. These are simple exercises which need to be done at least three times a day, starting with the person performing them lying down to eventually standing and moving around.

What is significant from the research into how these receptors respond to different levels of pressure, touch and speed is that the practitioner can constantly vary his or her approach (and location) depending on what is needed. For example, if a client is having problems with proprioception, the practitioner can do moves that affect the receptors that increase proprioception. If the problem is chronic pain or inflammation, a different approach will be needed.

If one were to summarize the effects of Bowen moves on the body according to Schleip, one would say that Bowen moves:

> involve a stimulation of intrafascial mechanoreceptors. Their stimulation leads to an altered proprioceptive input to the central nervous system, which then results in a changed tonus regulation of motor units associated with this tissue. In the case of a slow deep pressure, the related mechanoreceptors are most likely the slowly adapting Ruffini endings and some of the interstitial receptors; yet other receptors might be involved too, (e.g. spindle receptors in affected muscle fibers nearby and possibly some intrafascial Golgi receptors). (Schleip 2003, p.6)

There is also a clear differentiation between 'Bowen type' moves and other forms of deep tissue work (and even some other forms of Bowen – derived body work) as strong, sudden, deep touch will induce muscle contraction rather than relaxation (Eble 1960) and certainly won't encourage an increase in vagal tone, something vital if repair and healing are to take place.

Certain factors are important for a successful Bowen treatment, critically that there is not excessive stimulation of the central nervous system (particularly the reticular activating system) by an unnecessary number of moves or by distracting the client. Even playing music in the treatment room can stimulate areas of the nervous system unnecessarily. A lack of extraneous stimulation is particularly important when there is a general sensitization of nerve pathways and tissues, as is the case in chronic pain, which is why a favourite Bowen maxim is 'less is more'.

Fascial Fitness

As well as its effect on the mechanoreceptors, Bowen affects the fascia directly through encouraging hydration, as this process is assisted by gentle stretching, repetitive squeezing and release with pauses (i.e. pressure applied and then waiting) – all elements of a Bowen treatment. The waiting time would appear to be essential as there is a significant increase in hydration after half an hour (Schleip and Klingler 2007).

Addressing the key issue of fascial fitness (Muller and Schleip 2012) in terms of tissue hydration, balance and composition of collagen fibres is an essential adjunct to Bowen treatments, which is partly why it is so important to enlist the active participation of the client in recovery. Fascial health is influenced by a number of factors including diet (pH and inflammatory markers), hydration, exercise (including stretching; see Myers and Frederick 2012), gentle therapeutic approaches (such as the Bowen Technique) and managing stress levels. Prolonged inflammation has been shown to have a deleterious effect on many structures and mechanisms in the body and may derive from a variety of causes – for example, old injuries, operations, inflammatory conditions such as endometriosis and so on. It is well known that inflammation in the gums (gingivitis) or in the jaw after root canal fillings can affect organs such as the heart and cause joint and muscle pain. Frequently the original site of the inflammation is asymptomatic but will have effects elsewhere in the body. Diet also has a profound effect on inflammatory markers, which can be increased by eating pro-inflammatory foods (such as grain-fed animals and fish) and reduced by adopting a low-inflammatory diet (Hankinson and Hankinson 2012, p.147; Reinagel 2007). This is discussed in Appendix 2. Long-term inflammation and tissue damage can also have an activating effect on the sympathetic nervous system, leading to symptoms such as panic attacks, anxiety, lowering of vagal tone and a racing mind.

The Structure of Fascia: Fibroblasts and Myofibroblasts

Another important mechanism to understand in seeing how Bowen affects the body physiologically is the function and relationship between those ubiquitous fascial cells, fibroblasts and myofibroblasts. Myofibroblasts (which are fibroblasts that have some of the characteristics of smooth muscle) are affected in many kinds of connective tissue disorders such as frozen shoulder and low back pain. Bowen affects myofibroblasts directly as they contract and expand slowly in response to factors such as pH and stress (Schleip 2009). This occurs over a period of minutes or hours, so expansion or relaxation of myofibroblast activity will certainly occur during the length of a Bowen treatment (normally 30–45 minutes) as the person relaxes. Soft-tissue techniques such as Bowen rely on effecting structural change by directly influencing the biotensegrity aspect of the connective tissue via their action on myofibroblasts, which is partly why Bowen has such a powerful and measurable effect on posture. When it comes to the way that myofibroblasts operate to maintain structural integrity, it is important to understand the difference between muscle function and connective tissue function:

> Viewing connective-tissue contracture simply as a result of muscle-like contraction of myofibroblasts is an oversimplification, and leads to the misconception that myofibroblast function is simple and muscle-like. From our present understanding, it is reasonable to conclude that myofibroblasts are predominantly responsible for contracture, whereas smooth (and skeletal) muscle cells act by contraction. Although some mechanical contraction is an inevitable part of the process of contracture, the reverse is not necessarily true. (Tomasek *et al.* 2002, p.357)

In the fascia, Transforming Growth Factor (TGF β1) is released from the extracellular matrix (ECM) in response to contraction in myofibroblasts (Wipff *et al.* 2007). This is significant therapeutically, as changes in myofibroblasts (i.e. contracture or otherwise) are initiated by a variety of different factors, including bodywork (such as the Bowen Technique), exercise, diet, stress and inflammatory conditions. TGF β1 is a protein that is secreted by many kinds of cell and plays a crucial role in many cellular functions including cell division and proliferation. In fact TGF β1 has a key role in the creation of the extracellular matrix that is critical in determining tissue characteristics in general. The level of expression and effective dispersion of TGF β1 would appear to be critical in fascial health, particularly as its expression can be influenced in a variety of ways. TGF β1 has been used experimentally in wound healing and is key in the formation of scar tissue and, in excess, fibrosis (Li *et al.* 2004).

There are mechanisms for the way TGF β1 is dispersed in the fascia. These have ramifications for therapies such as the Bowen Technique, as well as the choice of exercise regimes, specifically in what would potentially help or hinder recovery. This is partly to do with what is called myofascial force transmission, which is the complex interaction of stress on the various components of fascia, muscles and tendons, which could potentially influence the expression of TGF β1. Wipff and colleagues (2007) show that contraction of myofibroblasts encourages expression of TGF β1 into the extracellular matrix. Conversely, mechanical loading that might occur with some types of exercise or deep manual therapy may interact with cytokines such as TGF β1, thereby activating an inflammatory response resulting from tissue microinjury (Masi 2011). This could be why too much stimulation of the myofascia (by excessive pressure, too much work in a treatment or, in the case of exercise, too strong a regime) tends to have an adverse effect on some sensitive patients.

Tissue laxity and fragility is determined by the action and composition of collagen fibres (particularly the ratio of type I to type III) and factors such as TGF β1 production. It is known, for example, that TGF β1 promotes changes in myofibroblast function and morphology as well as the formation of stress fibres. This has been shown to correlate with an increased generation of contractile force within myofibroblasts, which undoubtedly has implications in terms of treatment approaches for individuals suffering from an imbalance in this area (particularly the hyper- or hypo-mobile clients) and also more generally with people who have any kind of local tissue stiffness.

Interestingly, one very gentle approach used in craniosacral therapy (CST) relates directly to the rhythmic oscillations that myofibroblasts exhibit (Follonier *et al.* 2010). This rhythm has a period length of 99 seconds, which correlates to the 'long tide' oscillations that Dr Sutherland described. Because myofibroblasts are in close proximity in the body, they tend to express this rhythm universally, so it is possible to palpate this tide-like rhythm with sensitive hands anywhere in the body (although it takes a bit of practice!).

Fascia as a Communication Network

There is considerable interest amongst therapists in the concept of fascia as a communication medium in the body (Oschmann 2012). It has been known for many years that piezoelectric effects initiated by stressing collagen fibres have a strong healing effect on tissues (Becker 1985). There is no doubt that something of this kind is occurring during a Bowen treatment because the impulses created by stressing collagen fibres in the challenge and roll of a Bowen move can be felt clearly with sensitive palpation. Although there other mechanisms involved in encouraging hydration into local tissue (mostly through the action of the mechanoreceptors), these impulses seem to have the effect on the tissues of freeing areas of fascia that are 'stuck', a process Deane Juhan (2002) refers to as thixotrophy. Mae Wan Ho has studied these effects in reference to acupuncture meridians (Ho and Knight 1998). In relation to Bowen, the findings might be summarized as follows:

1. Impulses are created in the collagen fibres by very light pressure. The type of stretching that is used in Bowen creates a stronger piezoelectric current than just pressing on it (such as might be used in Rolfing) or going along the length of it (as might be used in massage). The fact that impulses can be generated

by heat may give a clue as to why clients are asked to avoid exposing the area treated to extremes of hot or cold after a session. The conductivity of collagen is strongly dependent on how hydrated it is. This means that the impulses created during a treatment will travel much more effectively if the fascia is hydrated. This is probably why some people respond better to treatment than others – babies, animals and those who practise yoga all tend to have a much more hydrated and fluid system. Hydration of the fascia generally decreases with age and under-use (but not necessarily).

2. Impulses created in the fascia are amplified via the action of proteins in liquid crystals. Mae Wan Ho describes fascia as essentially liquid crystalline in nature – in other words, highly responsive to electrical charge and able to carry electrical impulses very fast. There also seem to be other mechanisms as to how impulses travel through the body which are more based on fluid dynamics. Some commentators have likened this to a soliton wave which can travel over long distances without losing its speed, power or merging with other waves.

3. Fascia responds as a single coherent system, rather like the liquid crystal display that is used in computer monitors. In other words, the fascia will respond as a whole to stimulation, not just locally, and it will respond in large part directionally, determined by how the impulses travel through it. This in turn is determined by the orientation of the collagen fibres, which in turn is determined by use.

In terms of how Bowen affects the fascia, my own clinical experience of using Bowen on scar tissue has been enlightening. Scar tissue that is raised and red responds to Bowen moves by becoming visibly less fibrotic and less inflamed quite quickly. This means that there is some physiological change in the tissues, specifically in the ratio of type I and type III collagen. This is significant as this ratio is a crucial element in the make-up of fascia in terms of laxity. Because scar tissue can also cause restrictions through the tissue field and affect areas at some distance from the scar (not only structurally but also in terms of communication) it can be very useful to work directly on it (Wilks 2007).

The exquisite images in the various fascia DVDs produced by Dr J.-C. Guimberteau (to date he has produced five DVDs with the most recent looking at the formation of scar tissue) show clearly why techniques such as Bowen, which encourage more fluidity in the fascia, would have a profound effect on vascular and nerve supply by freeing up the connective tissues that surround capillaries, veins, arteries and nerves (specifically arterial supply to nerves). Local vascular supply is an issue for many clients and it would be interesting to find out if slightly longer rest times between Bowen moves would assist in the process of revascularization.

The Esoteric

Bowen's interesting explanation of the stoppers helping to contain an uprising force in the spine has correlations with many ancient healing traditions. The idea of an inherent healing intelligence in the body has been central to all healing traditions throughout the ages, including being the basis of osteopathy. This is sometimes perceived as a powerful uprising force originating at the base of the sacrum (or the muladhara chakra in Sanskrit). In Western healing this uprising healing force is represented (some would say mistakenly) by the caduceus, the symbol of the British Medical Association, which is a graphic depiction of the nadis or subtle nerve channels depicted in many ancient Sanskrit texts, whilst in Christian traditions it is mentioned in the writings of many mystics, including St Thérèse of Lisieux and Hildegard of Bingen.

The way the caduceus is represented shows two snakes intertwined around the central channel or sushumna. These represent the Ida and Pingala or the 'moon' and the 'sun'. They are also sometimes referred to as 'Ha' and 'Tha', from which we get the term Hatha Yoga.

The practice of yoga was originally perceived to have a balancing effect on these two subtle nerve channels. Again, superficial parallels are not always useful, but there are some similarities here with the sympathetic nervous system and its plexuses. Some writers have also written on the parallels between the chakras and the endocrine system, although the subtleties of the different systems can get lost with comparisons such as this.

In his treatise 'Devatma Shakti', Vishnu Tirtha describes this force as 'liquid light' (Jee 2011), which is also a term used by Dr Sutherland to describe the 'Breath of Life' or the 'highest known element' – in other words, consciousness itself. Some writers have also used the words 'liquid light' to describe the liquid crystalline nature of fascia.

Talking to many practitioners from different traditions, it is clear that these powerful healing properties have close parallels in the expression of embryonic forces throughout life and a longing in the human being to get back to a primal state of health, wellbeing and connection with our true nature. Many clients report exactly this after a Bowen treatment – feelings of being at peace, a lifting of anxiety and connection to self.

What We Do

The effectiveness of the Bowen Technique in its treatment of a wide range of conditions is borne out by clinical experience and, although more research needs to be conducted, it is clear that there are well-researched mechanisms by which the Bowen Technique can assist in terms of fascial fitness, reducing stress levels, increasing vascular supply and improving mobility and posture (Wilks 2004).

To summarize the research in this area:

- Bowen helps hydration of the myofascia.

- Bowen stimulates efficient nerve and blood supply by creating more fluidity in the surrounding connective tissue.

- Bowen aids relaxation by lowering the stress response and increasing vagal tone.

- Bowen allows proprioceptive pathways to change, resulting in long-term changes in posture.

The following chapters will look more specifically at how Bowen helps in different conditions and different situations. The key to being a successful therapist is not being complacent but trying to get to the real root of the client's problem, whether that is physical, emotional or even spiritual. We do an injustice to our clients when we apply 'recipes' to them. Assessment (particularly in relation to fascial lines) will be looked at later in this book, but it has been, and always will be, an essential and highly individual starting point for determining how to apply the Bowen Technique with each client. For every client presenting with lower back pain there may be a thousand different reasons for those symptoms. A Bowen treatment will therefore never be the same from client to client even though they may present with identical symptoms. There are many variations in touch (speed, depth of pressure, etc.) that are possible even when working in similar areas of the body.

A medical colleague rather shockingly said to me recently, 'I love evidence-based medicine (EBM) – it means I don't have to think.' The Chinese writer Lin Yutang (1937) summed it up beautifully: 'A doctor who prescribes an identical treatment in two individuals and expects an identical development, may be properly classified as a social menace.'

The abiding principles of all complementary therapists should ideally be: 'How can I listen more with my hands? How can I be more responsive to what I am feeling? What is really going on with this client that is causing their disease? How deep can I listen with all my senses? How can I hold a safe and nurturing space for them to heal?

References

Becker, R. (1985) *The Body Electric*. New York: Harper.

Coote, J. and Pérez-Gonzáles, J. (1970) The response of some sympathetic neurons to volleys in various afferent nerves. *Journal of Physiology* 208 (2), 261–278.

Dalton, E. (2012) *Dynamic Body*. Oklahoma City: Freedom from Pain Institute.

Dietz, V. (1992) Regulation of bipedal stance. *Experimental Brain Research* 89 (1), 229–231.

Eble, J. (1960) Patterns of response of the paravertebral musculature to visceral stimuli. *American Journal of Physiology* 198, 429–433.

Follonier, C. *et al.* (2010) A new lock step mechanism of matrix remodeling. *Journal of Cell Science* 123, 1751–1760.

Fukunaga, T., Kawakami, Y., Kubo, K. and Kanehisa, H. (2002) Muscle and tendon interaction during human movements. *Exercise and Sport Science Review* 30, 106–110.

Gellhorn, E. (1967) *Principles of Autonomic-Somatic Integrations.* Minneapolis: University of Minnesota Press.

Gracovetsky, S. (2008) *The Spinal Engine.* St Lambert, Canada: Serge Gracovetsky.

Guimberteau, J.-C. (2010) *Muscle Attitudes.* DVD, EndoVivo Productions.

Guimberteau, J.-C. and Bakhach, J. (2007) A fresh look at vascularized flexor tendon transfers. *Journal of Plastic, Reconstructive and Aesthetic Surgery* 60 (7), 793.

Hankinson, M. and Hankinson, T. (2012) Nutrition model to reduce inflammation in musculoskeletal and joint diseases. In R. Schleip, T.W. Findley, L.Chaitow and P. Huijing (eds) *Fascia: The Tensional Network of the Human Body: The Science and Clinical Applicatoins in Manual and Movement Therapy* (1st edition). Edinburgh, New York: Churchill Livingstone.

Hinz, B. and Phan, S.H. (2007) The myofibroblast – one function, multiple origins. *American Journal of Pathology* 170, 1807–1816.

Ho, M.-W. and Knight, D. (1998) The acupuncture system and the liquid crystalline collagen fibres of the connective tissues. *American Journal of Chinese Medicine* 26 (3–4), 251–253.

Jee, S.V.T. (2011) *Devatma Shakti.* Nabu Press.

Juhan, D. (2002) *Job's Body – a Handbook for Bodywork.* New York: Station Hill Press.

Kaplan, D. *et al.* (2005) Epidermal Langerhans cell-deficient mice develop enhanced contact hypersensitivity. *Immunity* 23 (6), 611–620.

Kram, R. and Dawson, T.J. (1998) Energetics and biomechanics of locomotion of red kangaroos. *Comparative Biochemistry and Physiology*, Part B 120, 41–49.

Kruger, L. (1987) Cutaneous sensory system. In G. Adelman (ed.) *Encyclopedia of Neuroscience* 1: 293. Boston: Birkhäuser.

Levin, S. and Martin, D.-C. (2012) Biotensegrity: the mechanics of fascia. In R. Schleip *et al.* (eds) *The Tensional Network of the Human Body.* London: Churchill Livingstone, Elsevier.

Li, Y. *et al.* (2004) Transforming Growth Factor-β1 induces the differentiation of myogenic cells into fibrotic cells in injured skeletal muscle. *American Journal of Pathology* 164 (3), 1007–1019.

Liptan, G. (2010) Fascia: a missing link in our understanding of the pathology of fibromyalgia. *Journal of Bodywork and Movement Therapies* 14 (1), 3–12.

Masi, A. *et al.* (2011) Integrative structural biomechanical concepts of ankylosing spondylitis. *Arthritis* 2011. Available at www.hindawi.com/journals/arthritis/2011/205904, accessed on 8 May 2014.

Muller, D. and Schleip, R. (2012) Suggestions for a fascia-oriented training approach in sports and movement therapies. In R. Schleip *et al.* (eds) *The Tensional Network of the Human Body.* London: Churchill Livingstone, Elsevier.

Myers, T.W. (2013) *Anatomy Trains: Myofascial Meridians for Manual and Movement Therapists* (3rd edition). Edinburgh: Churchill Livingstone.

Myers, T. and Frederick, C. (2012) Stretching and Fascia. In R. Schleip, T.W. Findley, L. Chaitow and P. Huijing (eds) *Fascia: The Tensional Network of the Human Body: The Science and Clinical Applications in Manual and Movement Therapy* (1st edition). Edinburgh, New York: Churchill Livingstone.

Naylor, I. (2012) Dupuytren's disease and other fibrocontractive disorders. In R. Schleip, T.W. Findley, L. Chaitow and P. Huijing (eds) *Fascia: The Tensional Network of the Human Body: The Science and Clinical Applications in Manual and Movement Therapy* (1st edition). Edinburgh, New York: Churchill Livingstone.

Oschmann, J. (2003) *Energy Medicine in Therapeutics and Human Performance.* Oxford: Butterworth-Heinemann.

Oschmann, J. (2012) Fascia as a body-wide communication system. In R. Schleip, T.W. Findley, L. Chaitow and P. Huijing (eds) *Fascia: The Tensional Network of the Human Body: The Science and Clinical Applications in Manual and Movement Therapy* (1st edition). Edinburgh, New York: Churchill Livingstone.

Reinagel, M. (2007) *The Inflammation-Free Diet Plan.* New York: McGraw-Hill.

Schleip, R. (2003) Excerpt from: Fascial plasticity – a new neurobiological explanation. *Journal of Bodywork and Movement Therapies* 7 (1), 11–9 and 7 (2), 104–116.

Schleip, R. (2009) Fascia as a sensory organ. World Massage Conference (online), November.

Schleip, R. (2014) Fascia as a sensory organ. Presentation at the British Fascia Symposium, 11 May, Windsor, UK.

Schleip, R. and Klinger, W. (2007) Chronic back pain may originate from sub-failure injuries in lumbar fasciae. *Proceedings of the Biological Science* 268, 229–233.

Still, A.T. (1899) *Philosophy of Osteopathy.* Kirksville, MO: Academy of Osteopathy.

Still, A. (1902) *The Philosophy and Mechanical Principles of Osteopathy.* Kansas City: Hudson-Kimberly.

Tomasek, J. *et al.* (2002) Myofibroblasts and mechano-regulation of connective tissue remodelling. *Nature Reviews* 3 (May), 349–363.

Tremblay, L. (2010) Powerpoint presentation, International Bowen Conference, Sydney, Australia, 16 October.

Turvey, M.T. (2007) Action and perception at the level of synergies. *Human Movement Science* 26 (4), 657–697.

Wilks, J. (2004) *Understanding the Bowen Technique.* Lakewood, CO: First Stone Publishing.

Wilks, J. (2007) *The Bowen Technique, the Inside Story.* Sherborne: CYMA.

Wipff, P.-J. *et al.* (2007) *Myofibroblast contraction activates latent TGF-β1 from the extracellular matrix.* Laboratory of Cell Biophysics, Ecole Polytechnique Fédérale de Lausanne, CH-1015 Lausanne, Switzerland.

Yutang, L. (1937) *The Importance of Living.* New York: Important Books.

2

Fascia, Tensegrity and Assessment

Kelly Clancy

Fascia is the organ of structure. It is the overall fabric that makes up our body. It includes the dense planar tissue sheets such as septa, joint capsules, aponeuroses, organ capsules and retinacula. It also encompasses local classifications of the network in the form of ligaments and tendons. It includes the softer collagenous connective tissues as well as the dura mater, the periosteum surrounding bones, the perineurium, surrounding nerves, the fibrous capsular layer of the vertebral discs, the organ capsules, the mesentery of the abdomen and the bronchial connective tissue. It is the fibrous connective tissue enveloping, separating and binding together our muscles, organs and all of the structures within the body. Fascia has normally been thought of as a passive structure that transmits mechanical tension generated by muscular activities or external forces throughout the body.

Recent research by Robert Schleip, director of the fascial research group at Ulm University, suggests that fasciae might be able to contract independently and thus actively influence muscle dynamics (Schleip, Klingler and Horn 2005). Dysfunctions within this organ may exist higher or lower in the structural chain than the location of emanating pain complaints. Often there cannot be long-lasting resolution of symptoms in many cases until the whole pattern of dysfunction in the fascial system is identified, evaluated and treated accordingly. Meanwhile, no one is looking at the fascial system, a structure of connective tissue that surrounds muscles, groups of muscles, blood vessels and nerves, binding some structures together while permitting others to slide smoothly over each other.

Dr Ida Rolf was one of the first scientists to emphasize the importance of the fascial network within the anatomical system. She called it 'the organ of structure'. Rolf was a research biochemist whose concepts are taught through the Rolf Institute of Structural Integration. She observed that when the body organized itself around a vertical line it was better able to respond to all of life's demands and to accommodate the ceaseless influence of gravity. She saw that structure and function are interdependent and that change at the structural level of organization will inevitably evoke changes at all other levels, including the functional, emotional, psychological and perhaps even spiritual. In *Rolfing: The Integration of Human Structures*, Rolf wrote:

> In the myofascial system as a whole, each muscle, each visceral organ, is encased in its own fascial wrapping. These wrappings in turn form part of a ubiquitous web that supports as well as enwraps, connects as well as separates all functional units of the body. Finally, these elastic, sturdy sheets also form a superficial wrapping, serving as container and restraining support for the whole body. This is the so-called superficial fascia, lying just under the skin. (Rolf 1977, p.38)

Fascial researchers and clinicians are beginning to further understand and recognize the crucial role played by the fascial network in creating efficient movement patterns and optimal functional abilities.

Fascia has existed all along, but we could not see the relationship of its connections clearly until now. It has been impossible to see the role of active fascia directly in preserved dissection and so we have ignored it in our primary evaluations, when we should have been treating it, possibly, as our primary intervention. Now, with endoscopic visualization in live tissue, we can see the complex connective tissue matrix in the whole system and its organization or disorganization in the entire body.

The work of Jean Claude Guimberteau, a French hand surgeon, demonstrates the existence of this complex extracelluar matrix throughout the whole organism. Guimberteau documented his in vivo endoscopic exploration of fascia while studying flexor tendon excursion in his film *Strolling under the Skin: Images of Living Matter Architectures* (2005) and has since gone on to study in vivo tissue endoscopically as it covers other connective tissues such as muscles, skin and scars. Guimberteau and others have shown that fascia exists as a superficial layer below skin, then dives into and encapsulates compartments of muscle, then individual muscles and then myofibrils themselves. Fascia also exists on a cellular level; it provides structure in a three-dimensional way both macroscopically and microscopically throughout the body's systems.

Tensegrity

Connective tissue determines our shape through its actions, restrictions, inhibitions and performance. We are tension-based structures: fascia imparts a continuous tension to our system. Donald Ingber, a pioneering scientist who works with the biological application of tensegrity, describes it as 'a system that stabilizes itself mechanically because of the way in which tensional and compressive forces are distributed and balanced within the structure' (1998, p.48). Fascia holds together all tissue – muscular, skeletal, neural, visceral, lymphatic and vascular. It also provides communicating links, both mechanical and chemical, between the body's parts through the extracellular matrix. Connective tissue transmits these tensegrity forces.

An understanding of biotensegrity is especially relevant to the Bowen practitioner who treats a client with issues in their upper extremity because our upper extremities are responsible for executing such a vast majority of our body's everyday tasks. When clients present with pain or dysfunction in the upper extremity, fascial imbalances – and imbalances in the biotensegrity of their fascia throughout their whole body – are often an underlying root cause of their pain.

Viewed as a model for the skeletal system of any vertebrate species, the tensegrity model of the icosahedron, with the bones acting as the compressive elements and the soft tissue as the tension elements, will allow the whole organism to be stable in any position. Therefore, shortening one soft-tissue element will have a rippling effect throughout the whole structure. We see this in nature: when a tree stands up to the forces of wind in a continuous manner, that tree will then modify its growing pattern and distort into a structure that is altered in its vertical alignment by laying down more bark and trunk growth in a different plane of motion to withstand the forces. The human body will do the same and transform into the positioning that is required to perform a task repeatedly. The body will lay down additional tissue in a particular region to create stability; such is the case with a dowagers' hump to support the weight of the head in an individual with forward head posture. Our biology becomes our biography as we perform repetitive activities over time and our tensegrital alignment of compression forces and tensioned forces will modify themselves to meet the demands of the environment.

One of the first clinicians to start applying tensegrity concepts to complex biological organisms was Dr Stephen Levin, an orthopaedic surgeon. He developed the term 'biotensegrity' to describe the application of tensegrity principles to biological systems, including our bodies. Biotensegrity represents a significant conceptual shift from the simpler view that our bones are the load-bearing structures in our bodies, like the framing of a house. Levin makes the compelling point that if our bones operated as a system of continuous compression members, like the beams and rafters of a house, then the force of regular, daily loads on our bodies would result in the shearing and crushing of our bones. It is only by modelling the transmission of forces in the tensional members of our bodies – the muscles and connective tissue – that we can account for our ability to perform everyday tasks.

In addition to Ingber and Levin, other scientists have taken this further by training in clinical practice that integrates the effects of fascia. One such scientist is Louis Schultz, a former biology professor and an advanced certified Rolfer. Schultz states in *The Endless Web: Fascial Anatomy and Physical Reality* (1996, p.32) that:

> The old paradigm of looking at the body was one of the skeleton as being the organizing force of the body which was surrounded by connective tissue. The new paradigm which explains and confirms mobility and agility is the concept of connective tissue as the actual supportive aspect of the structure. Bones are spacers, serving to position and relate different areas of the connective tissue.

Bones are not the supporting structures of the body; the connective tissue serves this function. Muscles provide the source of directional movement and execute motility. The spinal column is lengthened by a combination of the narrower coiling of the connective tissue and the pressure of the compressed fluid between bones. Support in a moving structure arises from the organization and arrangement of the connective tissues – the reciprocal, balanced planes of connective tissue supporting both muscle and bones by their elastic capability. All joints should lengthen with movement as the connective tissue wraps and supports the joint capsule.

Research during the past 30 years by Ingber, Levin, Schultz and others has taken these concepts of tensegrity and biotensegrity to new heights of understanding of how to apply this knowledge to clinical practice. There has been an exponential increase in the number of scientific presentations and publications which investigate various aspects of these concepts, beginning with the First International Fascia Research Congress held at Harvard University in 2007, where clinicians and researchers from various fields came together to develop novel approaches to understanding and researching fascia. Ingber presented the following at the 2007 Fascia Research Congress:

> Anyone who is skilled in the art of physical therapy knows that the mechanical properties, behavior and movement of our bodies are as important for human health as chemicals and genes. However, only recently have scientists and physicians begun to appreciate the key role which mechanical forces play in biological control at the molecular and cellular levels. … Molecules, cells, tissues, organs, and our entire bodies use 'tensegrity' architecture to mechanically stabilize their shape, and to seamlessly integrate structure and function at all size scales. Through the use of this tension-dependent building system, mechanical forces applied at the macroscale produce changes in biochemistry and gene expression within individual living cells. This structure-based system provides a mechanistic basis to explain how application of physical therapies might influence cell and tissue physiology. (Ingber 2008, p.198)

Clearly, the biotensegrity model of the body's structure, with its support coming from the prestressed, tensioned members of our connective tissue and fascia, provides the most complete explanation for the structural functioning of our bodies. And if fascia truly supplies the majority of the body's structure and function, then the role of fascia in any kind of injury or presentation of pain must become central to our assessment and treatment approach.

As we transpose these tensional and compressive elements to the biotensegrity model of the body, we can see that the disruption to one part of the body's fascia necessitates tugging and pulling on the body's connective tissues. The balance of compression and distraction forces within the overall system determines how much overall give the structure has to weather such disruptions. Once the fascia is severely disrupted, physical interventions in the form of bodywork or movement therapies are necessary to return the body's structure to its original state of optimum support for the entire body.

Within the fascial system lie the musculoskeletal, vascular, nervous and lymphatic systems. Any adverse presentation of those isolated or combined systems would be directly influenced by the health and positioning of the connective tissue matrix. By treating the fascial system directly, all these systems will potentially be self-regulating and restored by returning the body's fascia to its original length, strength and function.

Fascial Lines, Postural Assessment and Myofascial Length Testing

Thomas Myers, a structural integrator and founder of the Kinesis school of Structural Integration, describes common pathways of functional force transmission through a term he coined, 'anatomy trains'. In his book, *Anatomy Trains: Myofascial Meridians for Manual and Movement Therapists* (2009), he describes in detail the concepts of tensegrity and myofascial meridians. He follows the grain of the myofascial fabric from structure to structure and labels common force patterns that not only make up our structure but allow for stability, reciprocal movement patterns and alignment of the joints and surrounding structures. These anatomy trains, or myofascial meridians, are common, continuous networks of fascial fabric throughout the body.

In vivo human surgical dissections using light microscopy (magnification × 25), undertaken and video-recorded by Guimberteau (2005) have confirmed the complexity of fascia and its multidirectional influence on the musculoskeletal system. In his film we see that a tug in the fascial web is communicated across the entire fascial 'fabric' like a snag in a sweater or a pull in the corner of an empty woven hammock. One disruption to the tensional network can have far-reaching effects in other parts of the system, but multiple 'snags' in the structure can have a devastating impact on the stability and mobility of the whole body system. Though Myers describes nine common lines that intersect throughout the system, connecting the upper body to the lower body, many other fascial lines exist within the body.

Fascial Lines

Each of these fascial lines warrants discussion in further detail as they relate to pathology that we may see in our clinic settings as Bowen workers. Tissue treatment and assessment is performed from a superficial to deep manner, making sure that the superficial structures are restored to their ideal balance of mobility and tensegrity before the deeper layers are addressed.

These diagnoses listed in each later section are not mutually exclusive to each of these lines because a change in one line will directly affect the tensegrity balance of the other lines. This is why treatments such as Bowen work can be so effective in so many conditions because it is based on the premise of balancing out the body three-dimensionally.

BACK AND FRONT FUNCTIONAL LINES

The first and most superficial of these lines are the back and front functional lines. These lines act like an overcoat on the body. These continuous fascial networks consist of the vastus lateralis, gluteus maximus and the opposite latissimus dorsi posteriorly, and the adductor longus, rectus abdominus and the opposite pectoralis major. The functional front and back lines are important for reciprocal movements involving power of the shoulder and hip. These lines become important to assess and treat with injuries to the back, hip and shoulder, and they need to be considered first in treatment sessions because of their superficial nature. Just as mobility can be altered if one is wearing too small an overgarment, the functional line's overall mobility and length is important to obtain full range of motion between the relationship of the hips and the shoulders.

SUPERFICIAL FRONT AND BACK LINES

The next two lines, which also need to be balanced in their length and strength, include the superficial front and back lines. The superficial back line includes the plantar fascia at the bottom of the feet, the gastrocnemius and soleus, the hamstrings and the sacrotuberous ligament into the paraspinals, ending at the scalp fascia. This line is balanced by the superficial front line, which begins at the dorsum of the foot and includes the muscles within the anterior crural compartment of the lower leg, the quadriceps, the rectus abdominus and into the sternalis and sternocleidomastoid (SCM). These lines can be altered through many causes, such as engaging in habitual repetitive activities, having poor core stabilization strength, or undergoing abdominal or back surgeries, to name a few. A single alteration within one of these lines will affect the tensegrity balance of the corresponding muscles of the other line, which together create a 'force couple' to promote stability within the joints and overall structure.

LATERAL LINE

The next line, which provides a base of support for the shoulder and hip, is the lateral line. The lateral line begins at the fibularis and extends through the iliotibial (IT) band and tensor fasciae latae (TFL) into the internal and external obliques and through the axillary fascia into the SCM and splenius capitus. Injuries or changes to the balance of this line will lead to disruptions to the base of support of the hip, shoulder and/or head positioning.

Spiral Line

The spiral line is a bit more complex in description. It begins on one side of the head at the splenius capitus. It then crosses over to the opposite rhomboid and into the serratus anterior and from the internal oblique to external oblique. It then goes down to the TFL and IT band, the fibularis and the base of the first metatarsal, where it connects to the anterior tibialis, to the lateral hamstring of the biceps femoris, to the sacrotuberous ligament, into the paraspinals, and then back to the base of the skull. As you may notice, many of these fascial lines have intersecting muscles that can be found in other lines, but it is their fibre direction and the forces placed on them which determine their functional pattern. Spiral line issues present at foot and ankle rotations and pelvic and thoracic rotations.

Arm Lines

The arm lines are two superficial and two deep lines within each arm. The superficial back and front arm lines balance the rotational aspects of external rotation and supination. The deep arm lines promote internal rotation and pronation.

Superficial Back Arm Line

The superficial back arm line (SBAL) begins on the wide origin of the trapezius muscle, the nuchal line of the occipital bone, nuchal ligament (nuchal line to C7) and spinous processes of C7–T12. All of the fibres of the trapezius muscle converge on the spine of the scapula and then continue into the deltoid muscle. The middle and lower trapezius fibres continue into the posterior deltoid, the cervical trapezius fibres are continuous with the middle deltoid and the occipital trapezius fibres continue into the anterior deltoid. The three heads of the deltoid converge on the deltoid tubercle on the humerus. The SBAL then continues along the lateral intramuscular septum to the lateral epicondyle of the humerus. From here, the line melds into the common extensor origin and follows the wrist and hand extensor muscles under the dorsal retinaculum and then on to insert on the carpals and phalanges. Common diagnoses seen within this line include shoulder pain, lateral epicondylitis and dorsal wrist tendonitis. It is balanced by the superficial front arm line.

Superficial Front Arm Line

The superficial front arm line (SFAL) begins on the sternum, clavicle and ribs at the origin of the pectoralis major muscle. Although the latissimus dorsi comes from the back of the body, it is a part of the SFAL due to its anatomical and functional relationship to the pectoralis major. The latissimus dorsi inserts on the medial bicipital groove and, along with the pectoralis major, connect here to the medial intramuscular septum along the humerus. The intramuscular septum is then continuous with the common flexor tendons that originate at the medial epicondyle of the ulna. Finally, the SFAL passes through the carpal tunnel and ends in the insertion into the palmar surface of the fingers. The common diagnoses seen in this line include medial epicondylitis, forearm and wrist tendonitis, as well as carpal tunnel syndrome.

DEEP BACK ARM LINE

The deep back arm line has two origins. One begins at the origin of the rhomboids (C7–T5 spinous processes) and follows the rhomboids over to their insertion on the medial border of the scapula. From here, the line continues on the fibres of the infraspinatus and teres minor muscles (two of the rotator cuff muscles). The second origin of the deep back arm line begins on the lateral occiput at the origin of the rectus capitus lateralis and continues to the transverse processes of the cervical vertebrae. From here the line continues down the fibres of the levator scapula to the superior angle of the scapula and melds into the supraspinatus muscle in the supraspinous fossa of the scapula. The supraspinatus is another rotator cuff muscle, and it is here that the two origins converge on the head of the humerus. The rotator cuff muscles keep the ball of the humerus in the socket of the glenoid fossa of the scapula. From here, the deep back arm line connects into the triceps brachii muscle and proceeds down to the olecranon process of the ulna. The line continues along the periosteum of the ulna to the hypothenar eminence. Diagnoses commonly seen here include thoracic outlet syndrome (TOS), ulnar nerve compressions and ulnar sided wrist disorders.

DEEP FRONT ARM LINE

The deep front arm line begins on the third, fourth and fifth ribs at the origin of the pectoralis minor, which inserts on the coracoid process of the scapula. From there, it is continuous with the short head of the biceps brachaii muscle all the way to its insertion on the radius and deep along the periosteum of the radius, across the scaphoid to the thenar eminence of the thumb. The deep front arm line includes the pectoralis minor, biceps, brachialis, into the supinator and radial periosteum to the thenar musculature. Disorders to this line include nerve entrapments to the median and radial nerve in the forearm, thumb tendonitis and carpometacarpal (CMC) arthritis of the thumb.

DEEP FRONT LINE

Last and most core is the deep front line. The functional implications of this are vast. The involvement of the respiratory diaphragm is an integral part of our core stabilization, and therefore our breath. This also alludes to the core stabilizing function of the hyoid muscles, the core implications of our pharyngeal raphe (throat) and scalene muscles, and lastly the importance of the activation of the longus colli and longus capitus in anterior neck stabilization.

The deep front line is not only the most complex, but is perhaps the most important myofascial network in our body. The last important piece is the connection of the pelvic floor to the pubic bone (via the pubococcygeus muscle) and on to the linea alba up to the umbilicus (navel). At the deepest level, this connection wraps around the entire abdomen via the transversus abdominis muscle (the deepest of the abdominal muscles). This line begins at the intrinsics of the foot and extends into the deep compartment of the lower leg, including the posterior tibialis, the adductors of the thigh, into the pelvic floor, the psoas, quadratus lumborum, the diaphragm, the mediastinum, the deep cervical musculature including the scalenes, longus colli and capitus, the jaw muscles, and finally into the tentorium (part of the dural membranes) of the skull. Some of the diagnoses within this line may include bunions, leg asymmetries affecting the knee and hip joints, pelvic floor dysfunction, breathing disorders, TOS, temporomandibular joint disorders (TMJD) and headaches.

Posture

Posture is the position of the body with respect to its surrounding space. It is determined and maintained by coordination of the various muscles that move the limbs, by proprioception and by our sense of balance. It is also an attitude of the body that is usually considered to be the natural and comfortable bearing of the body. It can also be described as the body mass distribution in relation to the force of gravity.

When the integrity of postural muscles is compromised, the whole skeletal system is affected and misalignments lead to abnormal wear and tear on joints. Additionally, misalignments will cause musculoskeletal breakdown, injury and pain, affecting the optimal functioning of internal systems. Compensated and dysfunctional posture can result in the body's joints bearing weight abnormally. The muscles can become imbalanced and may not function to their optimal levels. The nervous system can become tractioned, compressed, or often both.

A typical client that we might see in our clinic would be one with tight upper cervicals and weak neck flexors which would result in a forward head posture, a kyphotic thoracic spine with tight upper chest and pectorals that would put the scapula into protraction and the glenohumeral joints into internal rotation, weak abdominal and tight erectors which could lead to low back discomfort and tight ankles which would create a poor base of support to the whole body. A client presenting in this pattern may have a diagnosis or site of pain anywhere within their body's structure, but each of these previously listed factors of postural asymmetry will have a directly adverse effect on the client's structure. Treatment, however, cannot have long-term success without addressing the whole system and the tensegrital balance of all of these structures in relation to each other.

This is the reason why postural assessment is so important. Assessment tells the practitioner what is happening, where to find the origin of the problem, how to organize the application of the Bowen moves and why one would choose those procedures.

How to Perform a Standing Postural Assessment

There are five aspects of performing a standing postural assessment:

1. Look globally at the client, obtaining a general silhouette of their overall structural condition, observing the big picture of their organization.

2. Examine the organizational relationship of the body parts through joints in gravity.

3. Examine the kinaesthetic experience of 'taking on the client's posture,' thus allowing the practitioner to feel the kinaesthetic and emotional general being of the client.

4. Assess the movement available within the client's structure by trying to place the body manually into alignment.

5. Perform myofascial length testing (MFLT) both in and out of gravity to determine the specific limitations in fascial mobility, at specific areas, which will affect the overall structural balance of the system. For more information on MFLT, see later section in this chapter.

The practitioner must also understand what normal alignment looks like:

- The head should be neutral over the yoke of the shoulders.

- The cervical spine should have a normal curve, with a slight concavity anteriorly.

- The scapula should lie flat against the thorax, with the medial borders being perpendicular with the spine.

- The thoracic spine should have a normal primary curve, slightly convex posteriorly.

- The lumbar spine should also have a normal curve, slightly concave anteriorly.

- The pelvis should be in a neutral position, anterior superior spines in the same vertical plane as the symphysis pubis. There is some debate among different schools of thought and between the sexes, what these exact angles should be, but, in general, we are looking at a level pelvis.

- The hip joints should be in a neutral position, neither flexed nor extended.

- The knee joints should also be in a neutral position, neither flexed nor hyperextended, and the ankle joints in neutral.

Common Postural Patterns

There are four common postural patterns that are typically seen in the human body.

1. The first pattern is normal alignment, as outlined above.

2. The second is the kyphosis-lordosis posture, which is an excessive exaggeration of the primary and secondary curves of the spine. The primary curve of the thoracic spine becomes excessively convex posteriorly, which will drive the secondary curve of the lumbar spine excessively concave. This will lead to changes throughout the structure, including scapular protraction and a forward head posture.

3. The next common postural pattern is the sway back posture. This is usually driven by an anteriorly tilted pelvis with excessive lordosis, followed by a posteriorly displaced thorax. This will also lead to a forward head posture and often hyperextension at the knees.

4. Last is the flat back posture, which is a loss of the normal primary and secondary curvatures of the spine, leading to an appearance of a 'flat back.' This will also lead to scapular and glenohumeral dysfunctions, secondary to the loss of a proper base of support of the scapula, and may limit the excursion of spinal mobility overall.

During the movement assessment portion of the evaluation, assuming the client's habitual standing patterns in your own structure can create a kinaesthetic experience within the practitioner's own body, allowing one to experience the 'stress points' or areas of tension which are required to maintain a particular posture in gravity. The practitioner can then attempt to reorganize the client's standing posture through palpation with the intention of establishing the best alignment to gravity as possible. This can help identify what parts of the structure can and cannot move and the compensation that may be necessary to obtain vertical alignment.

Myofascial Length Testing

Up until this point, we have had no way to measure the influence of fascia during evaluation or as a means of tracking client progress and outcomes. Practitioners have been limited to relying on a client's report of pain and function as well as a clinical evaluation of the isolated location of pain. However, a diagnostic procedure has been developed, called myofascial length testing (MFLT), which objectively measures the function of the muscles and fascia in an individual's whole body.

MFLT, an objective measure and evaluative technique, provides quantifiable physical measurements, pre- and post-treatment, to determine the direct effects of the therapeutic intervention on the connective tissue system. When used in addition to the client's objective reports, standing postural assessment, provocative testing measures and functional outcomes, MFLT can lead to a comprehensive picture of the client's overall state of physical health. Combining these sources of data collection and tracking provides detailed, comprehensive information that can provide accurate assessment of a client's state and rate of progress over time, leading to greater whole body outcomes. By further understanding the importance of global and specific evaluative measure, therapeutic interventions and treatments directed at balancing the whole system, we are then able to restore not only the muscular and fascial system back to its tensegrity balance but also potentially all systems to a more self-regulating level of homeostasis.

Donna Bajelis, PT, CHP, SMS, the founder and owner of the Institute for Structural Medicine, developed myofascial length testing as a way to test objectively the fascial restrictions within the body (Bajelis and Duben 2012). She combined principles of muscle testing taken from physical therapy with proprioceptive neuromuscular facilitation (PNF) patterning and the fascial lines, to determine where primary restrictions may be located, as well as the compensatory patterns that have developed which may be contributing to pain symptoms. By utilizing a formal objective assessment technique for both pre- and post-treatment testing, the practitioner is able to determine exactly where the restrictions are located within the structure and thus can target the treatment to these areas, making treatment more efficient and cost-effective. This also gives the practitioner tools of objective testing that can be used in documentation, allowing greater communication between the practitioner and the referral source, insurance companies, or other providers involved in the client's overall care.

Following a standing postural assessment, specific passive MFLT is performed. For the upper extremity, the scapula is addressed first, assessing the ability of the scapula to organize itself toward depression, allowing the shoulder to passively flex and adduct. This biomechanical pattern is paramount in normal functioning of the shoulder which creates the normal scapula/glenohumeral rhythm in shoulder mobility. The scapular mobility is 100 per cent dependent upon the thoracic alignment because of its floating position on the rib cage.

Once the scapula's ability to 'seat' is evaluated, meaning its ability to depress, then the testing procedures for the superficial front and back arm line can be performed. This testing will include passive shoulder flexion, external rotation and adduction, while maintaining the forearm in full supination and wrist in a neutral position.

- For the superficial back arm line (Figure 2.1), while the scapula is placed in its end range depression position, the arm is passively flexed and horizontally adducted while maintaining end-range external rotation and forearm supination. This tests the total end-range capacity of the fascial fibres of the superficial line.

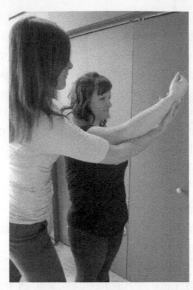

Figure 2.1 Superficial back arm line (SBAL) testing

- Likewise, the superficial front arm line (Figure 2.2) is tested with the scapula seated, while maintaining the external rotation and supination components of the 'wind up.' The arm is then passively moved into shoulder extension at approximately 30 degrees of abduction. The practitioner must ensure that the client is not positioning the elbow in valgus to achieve this orientation.

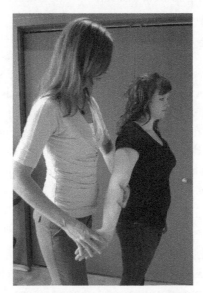

Figure 2.2 Superficial front arm line (SFAL) testing

The deep front and back arm lines are tested in the same fashion, except the shoulder is positioned this time in full internal rotation and with the forearm in pronation.

By approaching the client in this systematic manner, taking into consideration the whole body's fascial alignment both in and out of gravity, the practitioner is able to effectively and efficiently determine which procedures are appropriate to effect whole body change and to honour Tom Bowen's theory of providing 'less is more' within the treatment session.

References

Bajelis, D.F. and Duben, I. (2012) *Myofascial Length Testing: Practical Assessment Tools for the Myofascial Therapist*. Twisp, WA: Institute of Structural Medicine.

Guimberteau, J.-C. (2005) *Strolling under the Skin: Images of Living Matter Architectures*. Film directed by J.-C. Guimberteau.

Ingber, D.E. (1998) The architecture of life. *Scientific American* 278, 48–57.

Myers, T.W. (2009) *Anatomy Trains: Myofascial Meridians for Manual and Movement Therapists* (2nd edition). Edinburgh: Elsevier.

Rolf, I. (1977) *Rolfing: The Integration of Human Structures*. Santa Monica, CA: Dennis-Brown.

Schleip, R., Klingler, F. and Horn, F. (2005) Active fascial contractility: fascia may be able to contract in a smooth muscle-like manner and thereby influence musculoskeletal dynamics. *Medical Hypotheses* 65 (2), 273–277.

Schultz, R.L. (1996) *The Endless Web: Fascial Anatomy and Physical Reality*. Berkeley, CA: North Atlantic Books.

3

Fluid Flow, Nature and Embryological Development

Our Fluid Bodies

Bodily Fluids

Now we get on to some of the more hypothetical explanations for how Bowen works and the various effects it has on the body. Practitioners have for many years pondered why is it that doing medial moves in the opposite direction (i.e. laterally) or doing anterior moves in a posterior direction seem to have very different effects on the body. The various discussion forums on the web are full of debates of this sort, but most are inconclusive. The main thing on which there is consensus is that there is a difference in clinical outcome dependent on the direction of a move. Because most Bowen moves are performed cross-fibre, on a physiological level (i.e. how the move might affect the various receptors in the connective tissue) it is not clear why it would make a difference whether the move was done medially or laterally. Tom Bowen himself (rather unhelpfully!) used to advise his 'boys' that if a medial move doesn't do the trick, then try a lateral move. Some Bowen instructors have opposing views about the different effect of the direction of Bowen moves, including Julian Baker (Baker 2013, p.37), but most agree that direction is important, even if they cannot explain why.

If we look at how water moves in nature and how the all the various fluids move in the body, we can get some clues as to why direction of moves matter and why they might have different effects in terms of strengthening or releasing muscles and other forms of connective tissue.

There are many types of fluid in the body:

- blood (the plasma), flowing through veins, arteries, capillaries and other vessels such as the venous sinuses in the cranium

- cerebrospinal fluid, produced in the brain (in the choroid plexuses of the ventricles) but which flows mostly within the enclosed space created by the dural membranes

- interstitial fluid (the fluids between the cells)

- intercellular fluids (water within the cells)

- lymph

- fluids within the urinary and digestive tracts such as stomach and intestinal contents (urine, etc.)

- other fluids such as synovial fluid, serous fluid and mucus, etc.

Most of the fluid in our body is held within the cells themselves. In fact around two-thirds of our body water is held here. This is why although it might appear that people who are overweight have more fluid in relation to their body weight, they actually have less. For example, an 80 kilogram male will be carrying a total of 48 litres of body water around with him all day. Of that 48 litres, intracellular fluid will be 32 litres and extracellular fluid will be 16 litres, of which 12 litres will be interstitial fluid. For some reason, if you are a female, then your total body fluid will be less than a man's at 40 litres and your total interstitial fluid volume will be 10 litres.

As we shall see, the various fluids in the body have a tendency to move in particular ways, ways that are remarkably similar to the way water flows naturally in our environment and in nature. In fact, the anthropologist and author Loren Eiseley observed: 'Not for nothing has the composition of mammalian blood led to our description as "walking sacks of seawater"' (Eiseley 1946).

Fluid Flow in Nature

Early scientists were fascinated by organizational patterns in nature. Two of those of particular interest to us are Lawrence J. Henderson and Viktor Schauberger. Henderson (1878–1942) was something of a polymath, being a biochemist but with a deep interest in philosophy and sociology. In his book from 1913, *The Fitness of the Environment*, he discusses at great length the particular and unusual properties of water that are essential for supporting life. His writings and vision formed the basis of the concepts of dynamic equilibrium and the Gaia hypothesis.

In a thought-provoking article on water in the journal *The Scientific Monthly*, Henderson wrote:

> There is a good deal of resemblance between the salts dissolved in our blood and the salts dissolved in sea water. It has been suggested by Professor MacCallum that our blood is, so to speak, descended from sea water, that in the course of evolution somehow or other the fluids of the body originated as sea water. Of course single-celled organisms have no blood. When multi-cellular beings came into existence, where did the fluid which bathes the cells come from, provided multi-cellular beings did develop from the unicellular? It is not a wild

assumption to suppose that sea water furnished the inter-cellular liquid, that it was the material that first surrounded the several cells making up the complex organism. If you look into the whole story of comparative physiology that idea, while it must not be pushed too far, seems not an extravagant one and, if so, it is interesting to reflect that in that original simple fluid, simple compared with our blood in most respects, there were nevertheless a vast number of substances that had been leached out of the earth's crust in the course of millions of years.

This peculiarity of sea water depends on the fact that water is, among all the liquids that we know, on the whole the best solvent, the one that can dissolve the greatest number and the greatest variety of substances of all kinds.

Later he writes:

One of the factors that greatly influence the circulation of water on the earth is the way in which it clings in the soil. Indeed water clings better, on the whole, than any other substance. This is due to the phenomenon which everybody has heard of as capillarity, and which is well illustrated by the action of a sponge in soaking up water. If you study this process you will find that it is easy to represent the sticking power of a liquid in the soil or in any finely divided matter by the height to which it can rise in a small capillary tube, in a very fine tube. Water rises to a very great height relatively to other substances in such a tube, and for the same reason it sticks very tight in the soil and water rises to a great height in the soil. That is one reason why great portions of the earth are habitable, or at least can grow crops. If water did not stick as well as it does, a large portion of the fertile earth would be sterile.

But here again we have come upon a property of water which is just as important in the body as it is in the meteorological cycle. The living cell may be compared to a microscopic swamp, to a swamp of inconceivably fine dimensions. There is water running through it, and it consists of a very intricate meshwork of only partly known nature. In this swamp – this microscopic swamp, if I may call it that – these same forces, these same capillary forces, are of decisive importance. And here again it is the particularly great capillary activity of water that is one of the factors that determine the nature of physiological processes. (Henderson 1922, pp.409–413)

Whilst Henderson was interested in studying blood and other bodily fluids (the term 'Henderson equation' which explains how the body manages to maintain equilibrium in pH is named after him), Viktor Schauberger (1885–1958) studied how water behaved in nature. He was an Austrian forester and inventor, whose designs for water flow, storage and turbines created the basis for efficient designs that are still in use today.

From his observations of fluid flow in nature, Schauberger described two forms of motion in nature (which are sometimes described as centripetal and centrifugal forces) – an outward, expanding flow that is used to break down and an inward-spiralling force which nature uses to build up and energize. One of the things that greatly dismayed Schauberger was how mankind uses the former to create energy, which he viewed as being inefficient and destructive to the environment as it creates a lot of heat and waste as byproducts. Frequently critical of conventional science and of his less imaginative colleagues, he once famously uttered, 'It would have been better if Newton had spent more time thinking about how the apple got up there in the first place'!

Many people wonder why water appears to spiral one way in the northern hemisphere and the opposite direction in southern hemisphere. This, unfortunately, appears to be one of those urban myths which deserves to have an airing on the panel game *QI*, because although a force called the Coriolis deflection causes large things such as cyclones and our oceans to rotate clockwise in the northern hemisphere and anticlockwise in the southern hemisphere, the force is too miniscule to have an effect on the water in your sink or bath. In the same way, the gravitational pull of the moon is too weak to create the tide-like movements of cerebrospinal fluid in our bodies.

Schauberger's notion that natural forces that create spirals towards a centre in some sense give vitality to water was not new. In his book *Hidden Nature, the Startling Insights of Viktor Schauberger* (2003), Alick Bartholomew points to the fact that nature primarily uses centripetal type forces moving slowly from the outside towards a centre with increasing power and velocity. This can be seen everywhere from cyclones, tornadoes, water flows in streams, to the way gases and liquids move and even galaxies form.

The crucial thing to understand about Schauberger's work was his discovery that inward-spiralling movements and lateral forces (i.e. from a point or midline outwards) have very different effects in nature. His grandson, Dr Tilman Schauberger, described the outside – in forces (which might relate to medial moves in Bowen) as structured, concentrated, intensifying, condensing, dynamic and self-organizing. Certainly my experience of medial moves, particularly the bottom stoppers, is that they have also have a very strong intensifying effect, which is possibly why some people feel they have so much energy after a Bowen session. It is interesting to experiment with the effect of moves in different directions. If you perform a series of moves up the back which are all in a lateral direction, for example, many clients will feel this as energetically draining. We normally refer to medial moves as relaxing and calming, which is interesting as Schauberger used to point out that in the centre of the spiral there is calm – 'everything that is natural is silent, simple and cheap,' he used to say.

The opposite (which might be related to lateral moves in Bowen) were described by Schauberger as releasing, inefficient and producing heat. This principle is seen in the way we produce energy nowadays – in the internal combustion engine or, in an extreme example, nuclear energy, where the bound energy of something small (petrol or the atom) is released outwards from the core to produce large amounts of heat, friction and waste products.

If we apply the same principles to the body, then lateral moves appear to do the same thing (i.e. release areas that are solid or stuck), something that has been explored by teachers such as Alastair McLoughlin. One of the common misconceptions about these areas of the body (whether it is tight muscles, 'frozen' connective tissue or areas of the body that express a lack of movement) is that they are somehow low-energy places, which need to be given more energy to release and flow. In fact, the opposite is true. Most of these places are areas where a huge amount of energy is bound and unable to express itself in the tissues. John Upledger, an osteopath and developer of craniosacral therapy, described these sites as 'force vectors', which are areas of the connective tissue (particularly the fascia) that contract to contain forces (such as falls and blows) that enter the body. They do this as a protective mechanism and so these 'force vectors' have to maintain high levels of energy to maintain their protective effect. Some practitioners are particularly adept at feeling these, whether through palpation off the body (heat, cold energetic flows), on the body (lack of response in the fingers when performing a move, or sensation of energetic release) or observation (noticing areas of the body which don't move – this is particularly obvious when observing people walking). Palpation of the superficial and deep fascia by very light palpation can also give clues as to where these stuck areas are. The easiest way is to allow the hands to rest on the body as though resting on the surface of the water and sensing an elastic type pull into areas of the fascia which are holding such patterns. In his book *Foundations in Craniosacral Biodynamics*, Franklyn Sills uses the term 'fulcrum' to describe how these sites effectively form a non-moving centre around which the body has to compensate.

So lateral moves appear to have the effect of liberating areas of the body that are stuck and high energy (Tom Bowen described this as unfreezing the tissues, which is essentially true if we look at Mae Wan Ho's research; Ho and Knight 1998). It is also true that medial moves can have the same releasing effect, and one of the byproducts of releasing stuck tissue is heat and a release of energy which clients often feel in their bodies after these types of move.

Fluid Spirals in the Body

Spiral flow is found everywhere in the body. Even the air we breathe is spiralled in opposite directions in each nostril to create positive and negative ionization, a process that changes from left to right every few hours during the course of the day. Much is unknown about this 'nasal cycle'. In fact, most people only breathe out of one nostril at a time, something that was noticed by a German nose specialist back in 1895 and is still not yet explained (Flanagan and Eccles 1997). Even stranger is that a study from 1988 shows that breathing through your right nostril significantly increases blood glucose levels while breathing through your left nostril has the opposite effect (Backon and Kullok 1998). Also, for some strange reason, if you breathe through your left nostril, the right hemisphere of your brain (the creative or imaginative side) will be more active, something that novelists suffering from writer's block might like to consider (Schiff and Rump 1995)! If you breathe through your right nostril, you use more oxygen, apparently.

Energetically, many writers have speculated on spiral energy flows in the body, and some artists such as Alex Grey have produced wonderful paintings and drawings showing these energy patterns. In his book *Energy Medicine*, James Oschman describes our bodies as reflecting the shape of the torus, a shape that is that found everywhere in nature – in atoms, cells, seeds, flowers, animals, planets, galaxies and even the cosmos.

The fundamental structure of the torus is what Buckminster Fuller called the vector equilibrium, which is the only geometric form in which all forces are equal and balanced. These forces then express themselves on a larger scale through patterns that are called the Phi spiral – this can again be seen everywhere from ferns to galaxies, and even in the proportions of the human body. These principles of ratio and form also apply fractally, something that Dr Guimberteau has discovered more recently in his investigation of fascia.

So, in the body we find spirals in:

- DNA
- collagen fibres
- amino acids and protein molecules
- cerebrospinal fluid flow
- blood flow and within the heart
- umbilical flow
- lymph fluid flow
- kidneys
- the small intestine
- air flow as it enters the body.

Spirals seem to be the most efficient way of creating the building block of our bodies. Professor Jayanth Banavar and his colleagues at Penn State University have experimented with every possible shape when trying to create artificial proteins and concluded that the spiral is by far the most efficient shape. 'We have discovered a simple explanation, based solely on principles of geometry, for the protein's preference for the helix as a major component of its overall structure', he said – an idea that was expanded in the 20 July 2000 issue of the journal *Nature* (Maritan *et al.* 2000).

Language often reflects the notion of spirals in our bodies. The Greeks call the belly button *bembix*, which means whirlpool. The Germans have referred to the spine as *Wirbelsäule* (spiral). Even Leonardo da Vinci noticed that blood flows in spirals through the body. In his early drawings of the heart he portrays how the heart creates a 'spin' in the blood to create a vortex spiral. Today a company in Scotland makes artificial replacement blood vessels using a process called 'Spiral Laminar Flow™'. The reason for this is that surgeons have found less need to replace them if the blood is encouraged to spiral through veins and arteries. Spiral flow also seems to allow fluid to travel through vessels such as veins more efficiently with less drag, perhaps one explanation why it would appear that blood flow is not just dependent on the action of the heart as a mere 'pump'. According to practitioners of manual lymph drainage, lymph also flows in spirals. Food passes through the small intestine in a spiral movement. Cerebrospinal fluid does the same as it passes through the ventricles of the brain.

Cerebrospinal Fluid

Cerebrospinal fluid (CSF) is interesting stuff. Clear and colourless, studied for years by craniosacral therapists and given almost mystical qualities by the originators of cranial osteopathy, it appears to have a subtle but palpable flow which can be tracked at around 10–12 cycles a minute. Other tide-like movements can also be felt – a slower 'potency' tide at around two and a half cycles a minute and a very slow tide of around 90 seconds, which may well be created by the slow pulse-like action of myofibroblasts in the fascia. As adults we produce around half a litre of CSF a day but only have around 150 ml in our system at any one time, which means that the turnover of the entire volume of CSF happens three or four times a day. CSF is produced in the choroid plexuses of the lateral and third ventricles and absorbed by the arachnoidal villi at the top of the head at the sagittal sinus. It also seeps out and mixes with extracellular fluid as the various nerve roots exit the spine (there are also absorption mechanisms around the spinal nerve roots themselves). This is perhaps why Dr Sutherland, creator of craniosacral therapy, used to say that CSF expressed itself throughout the body. He also used to say that CSF filled the room as 'liquid light', but that is another story!

There is a lot more to be discovered about the relationship between CSF and other fluid mechanisms in the body. For example, there is a clear relationship between the venous system, the lymphatic system and CSF absorption which is effectively unidirectional. Because this absorption happens mostly via the cervical lymph nodes as well as at the cribriform plate of the ethmoid (i.e. just behind the top of the nose), injuries to these areas (e.g. whiplash or blows to the bridge of the nose) can have serious consequences, as the lymphatic system has an important role in maintaining a normal intracranial homeostasis (Pollay 2010). This was discovered by restricting the CSF outflow at the cribriform plate of some poor unsuspecting sheep.

Fascia as Fluid

As stated earlier, fascia itself has been described by biologists as being essentially liquid in form or as 'liquid crystal' (Ho and Knight 1998). Fascia needs to be highly hydrated to enable the sliding of one structure against another. For this reason there are various ways that water molecules are in contact with the collagen fibres of the fascia.

1. Water is bound within the triple helix of the collagen molecules.

2. Water molecules are bound on the surface of the triple helix.

3. Free water lies within the space between the fibrils.

Collagen molecules are rods of about 300 nm long which form into a triple helix. These spontaneously self-assemble end to end into long fibrils which in turn form fibres and then larger bundles or sheets (Ho 2006). Mae Wan Ho, in collaboration with Franco Musumeci at the University of Catania, has identified that the water associated with collagen is highly structured and that at critical points of hydration (or lack of hydration) an abrupt transition occurs analogous to ice structures. This is no doubt why, in our work, hydration of the tissues is so important, why Tom Bowen often referred to tissue as 'frozen' and why this concept is so laboured in this book! Hydration, hydration, hydration should be the mantra of all therapists.

Bowen practitioners will have noticed that many Bowen moves are done in a spiral direction in relation to the body. Moves down the arm and up the spine are all spiral in direction. Could it be that there is also some as yet undiscovered reason why spirals are so prevalent in nature and in our bodies? Certainly, Viktor Schauberger's ideas lend credence to the idea of life-giving forces being created or channelled through these types of flow. It is an idea that has even been explored at the Max Planck Institute:

> Could life in deep space be made from mere inorganic particles of dust? According to a computer simulation, electrically charged dust can organize itself into spiral structures that behave in many ways like living organisms; reproducing and passing on information to one another.
>
> 'It has a lot of the hallmarks for how we define life,' says Gregor Morfill of the Max Planck Institute for Extraterrestrial Physics in Garching, Germany. Morfill and colleagues simulated what happens to dust immersed in an ionized gas. The team found that the dust sometimes forms double helices, the same shape as DNA and, like DNA, they can store information. (Tsytovich *et al.* 2007, p.263)

The Body's Midline

Spiral-type movements, which have as their reference the midline of the body, are many and varied. It all starts at around 14 days after conception when a highly significant event occurs. A primal midline is established in the form of a furrow in the developing embryo. This primal midline is called the 'primitive streak' and it starts its uprising journey towards our embryonic heart at around the level that is later to become the coccyx and sacrum in the adult.

Why is this important? First, the midline would appear to arise from something outside of natural cell division. What exactly initiates it is something of a mystery, but it forms the basis around which the whole body organizes itself. One embryologist even referred to the emergence of the primitive streak as the 'finger of God'. If one sees a movie of this, the nearest thing it looks like is someone drawing a line or furrow in the sand with a finger. The eminent embryologist Dr Blechschmidt explained that because of its position and particularly its quality of stillness 'the developing body orients all of its growth to it' (Shea 2007, p.180).

For a start it establishes a reference line for front/back, left/right and top/bottom. The primitive streak is referred to as an 'embryonic organizer' as it establishes a basic 'body plan'. Different levels of the primitive streak determine the development of different areas of the body. For example, the 'head centre' goes on to form the heart, brain and eyes, the middle centre the gut and trunk, and the tail centre the pelvic organs and the neural tube. In terms of left and right, it determines the fact that the liver is on the right and the stomach on the left and the fact that the apex of the heart points to the left.

The primitive streak is something of a mystery to embryologists – it has been discovered that grafting of the primitive streak can cause an entire secondary axis to form around which cells will organize.

What is interesting for us as Bowen practitioners is the importance of the primitive streak in terms of developing bones, muscles, organs and connective tissue. What happens is that, as it emerges, it generates three definitive germ layers from the epiblast – endoderm, mesoderm and ectoderm. The mesoderm goes on to form somites at around day 20 when they first appear either side of the midline. These somites then go on to form the vertebrae and the limb buds of the arms and the legs.

The fact that so many clients experience an uprising force is interesting as their sensations correspond exactly to embryonic development as if those embryological forces were still present within the adult body. In craniosacral therapy it is quite possible to palpate this uprising force by tuning into the notochord whose remnants still exist in the centre of the inter-vertebral discs and the apical ligament which connects the axis with the occiput.

In embryological terms, what happens is that, after the emergence of the primitive streak, the midline it creates enfolds in on itself (literally bowing to the heart) to form the neural tube which then goes on to form the brain, spinal cord, the autonomic nervous systems (sympathetic and parasympathetic) and the neural crest.

Neural crest cells are very interesting as they migrate to various areas of the body during the development of the embryo. For example, they help form the inner membranes surrounding the brain and spinal cord (particularly the pia and arachnoid membranes as well as myelin sheaths of nerves). In the coccyx procedure we move directly over the dura, arachnoid and pia membranes as they attach to the coccyx in the form of the filament terminalis. Both L4 (where we do the bottom stoppers) and C7 are also both highly significant in terms of the legs and arms in that these levels of the spine are where the buds which form the legs and arms grow out of. These levels are sometimes referred to as axial midlines.

When we talk about accessing a tissue memory of deep embryological organizing forces, we are talking about cellular memory, particularly in the fluids and the liquid crystalline connective tissue of collagen fibres. The embryological development of collagen fibres is fascinating as it starts in the mesoderm (the middle layer between the ectoderm and endoderm) as fibrils, differentiates out to form different kinds of connective tissue in the body and then infuses all the layers of ectoderm and mesoderm. In other words, it becomes the basis of tissue throughout the body. It is well researched by Mae Wan Ho and others that collagen holds memory and that it is highly adaptable at registering new experience.

Embryological development of tissue is very important in terms of referred pain. 'Head' zones are well-known phenomena where, for example, someone might experience pain in their right shoulder as a result of a problem with their gallbladder. This is as a direct result of the embryology of the development of mesoderm, endoderm and ectoderm.

Another consequence of embryological development is the fact that blood supply and nerve supply to tissue are inextricably linked because of their derivation from the same embryological tissue. Some commentators have even claimed that, because individual muscles form and come into action at different times in our early development, certain emotional and psychological qualities can be ascribed to different muscle groups.

Is it possible that by stimulating the fascia we are in some way allowing the body to access and re-orient to these deep ordering forces held in the collagen at a cellular level in the body? From clinical observation, something of this kind certainly seems to be happening.

References

Backon, J. and Kullok, S. (1988) Changes in blood glucose levels induced by differential forced unilateral nostril breathing, a technique which affects both brain hemisphericity and autonomic activity. *Medical Science Research* 16, 1197–1199.

Baker, J. (2013) *Bowen Unravelled.* Chichester: Lotus Publishing.

Bartholomew, A. (2003) *Hidden Nature. The Startling Insights of Viktor Schauberger*. Edinburgh: Floris Books

Eiseley, L. (1946) *The Immense Journey.* New York: Vintage Books.

Flanagan, P. and Eccles, R. (1997) Spontaneous changes of unilateral nasal airflow in man: a re-examination of the 'nasal cycle'. *Acta Oto-Laryngologica* 117 (4), 590–595.

Henderson, L.J. (1992) Water. *The Scientific Monthly*. New York: The Science Press.

Ho, M.W. (2006) Collagen water structure revealed. *Isis Report* (23 October).

Ho, M.W. and Knight, D. (1998) The acupuncture system and the liquid crystalline fibres of the connective tissues. *American Journal of Chinese Medicine* 26 (3–4), 251–263.

Maritan, A. Micheletti, C. Trovato, A. and Banavar, J.R. (2000) Oprimal shapes of compact strings. *Nature* 406 (6793), 287–290.

Oschman, J.L. (2000) *Energy Medicine: The Scientific Basis* (8th edition). Edinburgh, New York: Churchill Livingstone.

Pollay, M. (2010) The function and structure of the cerebrospinal fluid outflow system. *US National Library of Medicine* (June).

Schiff, B. and Rump, S. (1995) Asymmetrical hemispheric activation and emotion – the effects of unilateral forced nostril breathing. *Brain and Cognition* 29 (3), 217–231.

Shea, M. (2007) *Biodynamic Craniosacral Therapy Vol. I* (1st edition). Berkeley, CA: North Atlantic Books.

Sills, F. (2011) *Foundations in Craniosacral Biodynamics: Breath of Life and Fundamental Skills.* Berkeley, CA: North Atlantic Books.

Tsytovich, V. *et al.* (2007) From plasma crystals and helical structures towards inorganic living matter. *New Journal of Physics* 9, 263.

4

Bowen and the Acupuncture Connection

The fact that Tom Bowen had a deep interest in acupuncture and shiatsu is well documented. However, in the spirit of 'a little knowledge is a dangerous thing', it can be easy, and sometimes confusing, to draw too many superficial parallels between specific organs that might be affected by Bowen moves over acupuncture meridians (acupoints). Acupuncturists spend many years studying the philosophy and understanding of acupuncture before they are ready to apply these principles to treating people.

There have been many attempts to equate the fascial network as being the basis for the acupoints and meridians in the body (Bai *et al.* 2011) and there are certainly some very interesting parallels. Some studies have looked at the relation between Tom Myers's anatomy trains model and specific acupuncture meridians (Finando and Finando 2011). For a good overview of the subject, Dominik Irnich and Johannes Fleckenstein's chapter in the *Tensional Network of the Human Body* (Schleip *et al.* 2012, pp.349–357) is a very useful start.

Acupuncture
↶ Titus Foster

Acupuncture is just one aspect of Chinese medicine and has been gradually evolving to its present form. Significant acupuncture texts such as the Nei Jing date from well over 2000 years ago. Over the centuries acupuncture has travelled and simultaneously evolved in countries such as Japan, Korea and Vietnam and is now practised in countries all over the world.

Acupuncture's unique gift is that it measures health in terms of chi or vital energy. This can regulated by means of stimulating acupuncture points which are located all over the body and correspond to the 12 organs. Each organ can be accessed by specific acupuncture points, which are usually distant from the area to be treated. For example, we can treat the lungs by using 11 points on the radial aspect of both arms. Each point has a different action: 'Lung 10' has a specific effect on the throat whereas 'Lung 5' treats a cough with phlegm.

Furthermore, in regulating the chi by using a variety of points, the skilful acupuncturist not only treats symptoms but also regulates the body's complex web of interconnected metabolic function and thus brings it to a state of balance and homoeostasis. In Chinese medicine terminology this is known as the balance of Yin and Yang. Acupuncture therefore seeks to harmonize the opposites; interior/ exterior, hot/cold, excess/deficiency. Diagnosis is achieved by examining the tongue and feeling the pulses, as well as observation, listening, palpation and taking a case history, making special note of traumas and emotions which may have a profound bearing on the patient's diagnosis and prognosis. It is worth mentioning that, within Japanese acupuncture, protocols have evolved which reflect the recent advances and catagorizations of Western medicine. Examples are specific points and protocols for immune system, adrenal exhaustion, thyroid and pituitary imbalances, and even detoxification protocols for substances including pharmaceuticals. However, many acupuncturists regard skilful acupuncture as not only resolving symptoms but, more importantly, connecting the patient with 'the spirit'. Indeed, there are even specific protocols for patients who have, for one reason or another, lost this connection to spirit or the heart.

The Chinese have an interesting perspective on the body, which they see as a kingdom. The heart is the emperor or prime minister and the different organs are seen as ministers. When the emperor rules the kingdom fairly, in harmonious balance with his ministers, there is peace within the kingdom of the body. Each organ not only has its own particular acupuncture points but is seen as having unique properties such as a particular emotion and element. For example, the lung's element is metal and its emotion is grief. The lungs rule skin and it is often found that people develop skin conditions after a profound grief in their life. Not only do the organs support each other but they also exercise a dynamic communication with each other. This means that individual organs are less likely to get out of sync and unbalance the harmonious running of the kingdom. We can see this clearly in a situation where there is a benevolent leader in a particular country whom the ministers and the general population respect and look up to. Indeed, this leader does not even have to be a political one in order to exercise a balancing and regulating effect on the country as a whole. Of course, this same principle applies with the internal dynamics of organizations and even families.

The heart is seen not only as the physiological centre of the human organism but also as its spiritual centre. Hence the importance of spiritual practice, ethics and morals. All these are seen by the Chinese to cultivate and nourish the different aspects of the human organism and yoke them to the supremacy of the heart as our true centre. Interestingly, although Western culture has finally embraced the importance of food and its profound effect on the body, sadly it appears much less aware of the importance of feeding and nourishing the mind. The subtlety and delicacy of the mind and heart is habitually assaulted by a torrent of information and images from various media sources that muddies our ability to perceive clearly and profoundly. Chinese philosophy understands the value of good actions and thoughts as these expand and clarify the mind and give joy to the heart.

As Bowen practitioners, it is true to say that virtually every single Bowen move is either on an acupuncture point or meridian. 'Hitting the Lat' is often accompanied by a gurgle from the stomach because of its location on the stomach meridian. All of the organs of the body can be accessed on the back by acupuncture points at the level of the erector spinae which are worked on extensively in Bowen sessions in the mid-back work. For example, the lungs and the heart are represented at the level of T3 and T5 respectively. Similarly, T11 and T12 correspond to digestive function, whereas the area between L2 and L3 corresponds to the kidneys. In Chinese medicine the kidneys rule the low back and the Bowen 'bottom stoppers' are vital preparatory moves for any back problem. Moves 12 to 15 as performed in the kidney procedure logically have a profound effect in regulating the organs energetically and are neurologically linked to that area. Similarly, the carpal tunnel procedure is performed over the heart and pericardium meridians which not only affect the functioning of the heart but also treat psychological states such as anxiety and hyperactivity of the mind. This is a perfect example of how treating one area on the body can profoundly influence the functioning of another.

A further example is the spleen meridian. Starting at the big toe, it travels up the medial aspect of the leg and comprises a total of 21 points, many of which are stimulated by Bowen moves. Examples of the astonishing variety of symptoms treated are as follows. 'Spleen 6' is *the* great women's point, treating everything from infertility to period and menopausal problems, whereas 'Spleen 10' treats skin problems and 'Spleen 1' has the ability of stopping bleeding.

Here are some more interesting correlations between Bowen moves and acupuncture points:

- Top stoppers relate to Bladder 17 which opens the diaphragm.

- Temporomandibular Joint procedure involves points on the Stomach, Triple Heater, Small Intestine and Large Intestine meridians.

One of the principles of acupuncture is to treat points both local and distal to the problem area. The meridian system helps us to realize that moves such as 3, 4, 5 and 6 on the occiput affect the Bladder meridian which extends down the entire length of the back, continues through the gluteals, hamstrings, gastrocnemius muscles and finishes in the little toe. We should never underestimate the power of a single Bowen move nor its ability to affect apparently unrelated imbalances.

To sum up, Bowen and acupuncture practitioners provide a therapeutic culture where the patient has time to speak and be heard. Our therapeutic interventions, far from being repressive and invasive, are respectful and non-invasive, as befits the astonishing complexity and subtlety of the human organism. Bowen is also empowering, as it works by a subtle stimulation of the patient's own healing mechanism. Certainly, for the Bowen practitioner, a little knowledge of the principles of Chinese medicine can be of great value.

&

References

Bai, Y., Wang, J., Wu, J., Dai, J. *et al.* (2011) Review of evidence suggesting that the fascia network could be the anatomical basis for acupoints and meridians in the human body. *Evidence-Based Complementary and Alternative Medicine.*

Finando, S. and Finando, D. (2011). Fascia and the mechanism of acupuncture. *Journal of Bodywork and Movement Therapies* 15 (2), 168–176.

Schleip, R., Findley, T.W. Chaitow, L. and Huijing, P. (eds) (2012) *Fascia: The Tensional Network of the Human Body: The Science and Clinical Applications in Manual and Movement Therapy.* Edinburgh, New York: Churchill Livingstone.

5

Back Pain

Back Pain: A History

Back pain is a costly business. A recent National Institute for Health and Care Excellence (NICE) report from the UK (NICE 2009a) estimated that treating back pain costs the NHS £1 billion per year with lost production costs of at least £3.5 billion. In the USA total costs (i.e. treatment and lost production) related to low back pain (LBP) exceed an astonishing $100 billion annually, according to another study, done by osteopaths (Crow and Willis 2009).

Strangely, there has been little advance in our understanding of the pathology of low back pain in the last 25 years, with the term chronic (i.e. more than 12 weeks) non-specific low back pain (CNSLBP) being used to describe something that is difficult to classify and even more difficult to treat effectively using conventional means.

Recent NICE guidelines for treating LBP in the UK suggest an exercise programme supported by some kind of manual therapy such as physiotherapy, osteopathy or acupuncture. Other investigations such as X-ray or MRI scans are only recommended if there is a potential need for surgery, such as spinal fusion (NICE 2009b). However, when it comes to the whys and wherefores of back pain, it is interesting that certain markers such as disc prolapse and disc degeneration have failed to be accurate markers of the extent and degree someone will experience pain.

Other seriously detailed studies have also evaded a diagnostic consensus and certainly lack agreement on successful treatment (Adams *et al.* 2002). These include ligament pain, muscle pain, muscle spasm, trigger points, iliac crest syndrome, segmental dysfunction and dural pain. As the authors conclude:

> Although many lesions have been implicated as the cause of low back pain, few are supported by objective evidence. Tumours, infections and fractures are rare. Ligament sprains and muscle sprains are attractive explanations for acute low back pain, but there are no clinical features by which these conditions might be reliably and validly diagnosed. (Adams *et al.* 2002, p.78)

The authors do, however, agree that according to data the following are probably the leading sources of chronic lower back pain (but not acute back pain):

- the sacro-iliac joints – 20 per cent of patients
- the zygapophysial joints (sometimes referred to as Z-joints or facet joints) – 10–15 per cent
- the inter-vertebral discs (discogenic pain and disc prolapse) – 40 per cent.

It is common for clients presenting with back pain to say that X-rays have shown that they have disc degeneration, and they automatically conclude that this is the cause of their pain, which usually it is not. An understanding of the spine as a tensegrity system as outlined in this book will explain why therapies such as Bowen that encourage more hydration and space in the inter-vertebral joints can help, even where there is severe degeneration in joints. Those more interested in the role of connective tissue and fascia in LBP point the finger at the sensory nerves (mechanoreceptors) in the dense connective tissue – particularly around the sacrum and the thick areas known as aponeuroses, which can get hypersensitive. What is clear is that there is a highly complex interaction of tissues of different density in the pelvis and spine that depends on a sophisticated interaction of different kinds of forces exerted on it as we move, walk or run. These forces vary from stretching to compression, from recoil to force transmission, which is possibly why a clear and consistent approach to understanding and treating back pain has so far been elusive. The work of Serge Gracovetsky (2008), Emilie Conrad (Gintis 2006), Andry Vleeming (Vleeming *et al.* 2007) and others describes in detail how free movement combined with joint stability (integrity) and the right combination of elasticity and tension in the tissues is essential for a healthy back – and the requirements needed for that complex interaction vary considerably depending on where in the body we are talking about. This is where Bowen really comes into its own because it is precisely targeted at allowing hydration and free movement between muscle groups and other structures in the body.

Bowen and Back Pain

Perhaps two of the main factors that affect the sacroiliac joints, the inter-vertebral discs and the facet (zygapophysial) joints are poor posture and ergonomics – in other words, what people have inherited and habituated, and what they are doing at work or at home to aggravate their symptoms.

Acute back pain is usually fairly straightforward to treat with Bowen (see case study below) and the sooner someone is able to have treatment after injuring themselves the better because it stops the body going into a protective or compensation pattern. More often than not, someone's back pain has been caused by lifting something awkwardly, particularly in situations where they have lifted and twisted at the same time. This is a disaster for the lower back as the lumbar vertebrae are not designed to twist in relation to each other (unlike the neck vertebrae). Looking after one's spine is not something that is generally taught in schools, so most people have no idea what kind of activities they should be careful with. For example, just bending forwards puts a huge amount of extra pressure on the inter-vertebral discs in the lumbar spine. In fact, when lifting a 50-pound weight, the compressive force on the 5th lumbar increases to 855 pounds (Strait *et al.* 1947, cited in Oschman 2000, p.152). This will increase dramatically if the activity is done quickly. It is not surprising then that the sacro-tuberous ligament itself can withstand around 7000 kilos of tensional strain.

Awareness

Doing activities fast (such as digging or even lifting things out of a car) puts much more strain on the tissues than doing something slowly. It's always a good idea to encourage people to slow their movements down. For a start, doing things more slowly and more mindfully is a lot more enjoyable; it calms our sympathetic nervous system and brings us more 'into the moment', as well as giving us better body awareness where we are much less likely to strain ourselves. In fact, most injuries seem to happen through a lack of awareness and when people push themselves beyond what their body is telling them is safe or appropriate. You see this a lot at airports where people are stressed and tired, trying to yank their cases off the carousels. I think it would be safe to say that if we brought mindfulness into an awareness of our everyday activities, we would probably cut our injury rate by at least half. Unfortunately many gyms nowadays actually discourage an awareness of body sensation by having TV screens and loud distracting music. This is unfortunate, as it is known from the work of Peter Levine and others (Levine 1997) that a sure-fire way of calming people down and getting rid of their stress is to bring their attention into present-time body sensation. This is also a tenet of the mindfulness meditation developed by Jon Kabat-Zinn and used in his stress reduction programme in many businesses across the world. A lot of gym work (and even some forms of yoga) actually encourage an activation of our sympathetic nervous system, which is regrettable. This is a far cry from practices such as Continuum, the Alexander Technique, T'ai Chi and some forms of yoga that demand slowing down and getting in touch with sensation. These practices are also known as 'somatic' practices and are discussed later in the book.

Posture

Bowen practitioners put a lot of emphasis on treating imbalances in posture, and the changes can be dramatic after even a few Bowen sessions. Certain types of posture tend to put excessive strain on the lower back, particularly the kind normally referred to as 'head forward posture'. This is endemic in our culture and effectively means that many people are leaning forward all the time. Although this puts massive strain on the lower back, the key to successful treatment requires that the reasons behind it are addressed, which are sometimes not so obvious. We have inherited certain instinctual tendencies from our furry ancestors, one of which involves an activation of our adult 'startle' reflex (babies have a simpler startle reflex which activates different muscle groups to the adult). Unfortunately, because our way of life is so different from our ancestors, when our autonomic nervous system evolved, we tend to go into instinctive patterns unconsciously whenever we are stressed. Many neurologists point out that actually our 'fight-or-flight' system is activated most of the time because of our exposure to constant auditory and visual stimulus, particularly when we don't have the means to release the high charge created in our sympathetic nervous systems through movement. Unfortunately, most of us are highly sedentary creatures these days, which doesn't help. Sometimes there are other reasons for 'head forward posture'. Sitting at a desk is one of them, particularly if one's eyesight is not as good as it once was. Most people also now tend to use mobile phones, laptops or tablets which involve the head looking down for long periods of time. This is storing up a whole host of problems for future generations. This is discussed in Chapter 7.

Head forward posture involves the maintained activation of a cascade of related muscle groups (remember that this reflex was only ever designed to be a short-term measure to get us out of danger when we were being chased by a bear or sabre-toothed tiger). The general idea can be seen clearly in Figure 5.1, which I am sure you will recognize in many clients and colleagues, if not yourself.

This posture involves the following cascade of compensation patterns:

1. The head coming forward in relation to the trunk to orient to any potential threat or danger. This involves a tightening of key muscles in the front of the neck.

2. A tightening of the superficial muscles in the upper back, such as the trapezius, to counteract the effect on gravity (the trapezius attaches to the back of the head and goes over the shoulders which is why many people with lower back pain also have tight neck and shoulders).

3. A pulling down in the muscles around the top of the chest, restricting breathing and therefore the movement of the diaphragm. Seeing that the action of breathing is vital not only for the intake of oxygen into the system but also elimination, and that the action of the diaphragm is vital for the movement of the lymphatic system and health of the digestive tract, it is not surprising that bad posture has such ramifications for the poor client.

4. The pelvis coming forward in relation to the knees and feet.

5. Weakness in the abdominals.

6. A strong tightening of the muscles in the lower back to counteract the effect of the change in the centre of gravity. This is easy to feel on yourself – in a standing position, place your fingers on the erector spinae muscles just either side of the lumbar spine. Now raise your arm in front of you and see how the muscles respond by tightening. Now try bringing your head forward as though you were peering to see something, and notice what happens with those muscles. The effect is extreme and in the case of chronic head forward posture it is long-term and tiring.

7. Tightening in the front of the legs down towards the knee.

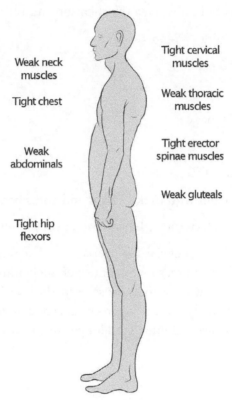

Figure 5.1 Head forward posture
Source: Martin Gordon

This whole cascade of tight and weak muscle groups expends a huge amount of energy (actually about 75 per cent of all our energy goes into our muscles), so it is not surprising that when someone's posture improves after a Bowen treatment, their energy levels increase massively as a result. This is seen again and again, along with the very common comment that they feel 'as though a weight has been lifted off their shoulders'.

Back Pain and the Workplace

For treatment to be successful it is vital to address what habitual movements or postures people are maintaining in their workplace, often unconsciously. For example, most people don't think that spending six hours a day typing would have an effect on the back. Consider the fact that each arm weighs around 4 kilos and most people don't use a wrist rest when they type: that is a lot of weight to hold for most of the day, and nearly all of that will be held in the muscles of the upper back and shoulder.

Bringing more awareness into everyday activities is vital. For example, most people don't realize how much the following activities increase the pressure on the inter-vertebral discs in the lumbar area (Nachemson and Elfstom 1970):

- coughing or straining – 5–35 per cent

- laughing – 40–50 per cent

- walking – 15 per cent

- side bending – 25 per cent

- small jumps – 45 per cent

- bending forward – 150 per cent

- lifting a 20 kg weight with back straight and knees bent – 73 per cent

- lifting a 20 kg weight with back bent and knees straight – 169 per cent.

This is why walking is so beneficial for people with back pain as it puts so little pressure on the lower back, but also why some seemingly innocuous activities, such as bending forward to pick up a toothbrush, can (believe it or not) be seriously dangerous. This is particularly the case when certain areas of the body that have been exposed to years of excessive tension are no longer able to maintain their stabilizing function.

Assessment

An intriguing question to ask oneself when observing someone's posture is 'Where is it originating from?' Many years ago I was flicking through a dental journal and came across two X-rays of a 16-year-old boy, before and after treatment for a minor malocclusion. It was easy to observe how the bite (and particularly the function of the temporomandibular joint (TMJ)) had such a massive effect on posture, something that has been observed by a number of dentists (Levinkind 2008). In fact, in this case the imbalance in the bite was quite small (around 2 mm), but it was easy to see the impact a minor adjustment to his bite had on his whole body.

Chronic lower back pain that started in the teens can also, quite commonly, be related to a problem with bite. It is therefore essential that this is addressed in order to bring about a successful resolution to these clients' back pain. There are reasons why small imbalances in the cranium have such a big effect on posture and we will explore this in Chapter 8. One reason is that most of the connective tissue and fascia is attached to the base of the cranium and so imbalances at the top end tend to get magnified down below in the spine and pelvis. Specific Bowen work at the TMJ has a powerful effect on helping to realign the jaw and this will have ramifications throughout the body.

The Pelvis and the Psoas

There are many muscles and different types of connective tissue that help maintain our healthy relationship to gravity. Many of these attach to the pelvis and help keep it in perfect relationship to the trunk and legs with the least strain.

One of the key muscle groups that help maintain good posture is the ilio-psoas. These are a complex group of muscles that attach on to the inner rim of the pelvis (the ilia), the top of the inside thigh (the inner side of the femur), the pubis and all the vertebrae of the lumbar spine (including the inter-vertebral discs) and the back of the diaphragm. Tightness in these muscles tends to create a posture reminiscent of Neanderthal man and can be seen in many of our clients today – in other words, classic head forward posture. It is also interesting to observe young people mimicking the posture of their idols, many of them with appalling posture.

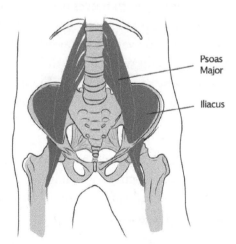

Figure 5.2 The psoas major and iliacus
Source: Martin Gordon

There are usually two types of scenario that have an effect of either shortening or tightening the psoas group (Figure 5.2). Primarily, the psoas muscles have an instinctual reflex to contract and curl in response to danger. You can see this in all animals if they suddenly perceive something that is a threat to their existence – they will contract through their abdominals, arch their back and their head will come forward to orient to any perceived threat. This is activated when someone is subjected to any situation where the body perceives it might be in danger. These sort of situations might be anything from car accidents, psychological or physical abuse, bullying, falls (e.g. off horses or ladders) and even a difficult or traumatic birth. What tends to happen is that the body will hold on to these patterns, which can then be reactivated by any subsequent trauma or even by incidents that might appear fairly innocuous (Koch 1997). For example, I remember treating a man whose back had gone into severe spasm after what appeared to be a minor car accident. It turned out that, as a child, he had had been bullied at school and on one occasion beaten up in the playground. What had happened in this case was that his psoas muscles had gone into a strong intractable protective pattern because the body perceived it was under threat, only this time from the car accident. This sort of situation can lead to chronic back pain and needs a gentle and safe environment to allow these muscles to release and for the trauma to be safely released from the body.

The other common scenario is a chronic dehydration of the psoas group through under-use (or occasionally over-use). Typically, this is as a result of too much sitting (office workers and taxi drivers are some of the worst affected). What happens then is that because the psoas is one of the juiciest and most fluid muscles in the body (not for nothing is the 'fillet mignon' prized for its succulent taste and texture), a lack of use causes dehydration and therefore shortening of the muscles. Bowen work addresses the psoas group in several powerful ways. There are procedures which work the psoas both directly and indirectly with moves over the tough insertion at the top of the femur as well as the diaphragm and close to where it attaches on to the spine. The iliacus can also be addressed in Bowen with a move on the inner rim of the ilium and this can be particularly important where there are rotational issues affecting not just the pelvis but the whole spine and shoulders. The main thing, however, is to adopt a softly, softly approach to the psoas because otherwise it can have a tendency to go into its protective pattern, which then may increase the symptoms temporarily. Liz Koch describes the psoas as a 'messenger muscle' and, as she says, 'You don't shoot the messenger!' Resting postures such as the 'constructive rest position', as described by Pete Egoscue and Liz Koch, can be immensely helpful in lengthening the psoas or allowing it to release and soften. Correct posture when sitting is also vital (with the knees a few inches lower than the hips).

How Bowen Can Help

There are specific 'procedures' in Bowen that help back pain. Many of these involve addressing some of the key fascial bands that help create a good balance in the pelvis in relation to gravitational forces, as well as restoring integrity to the tissues and lowering sensitivity in the nerve pathways. One of the key ways our body responds to the forces of gravity (and we are fairly unique in this regard because of our upright posture – most other mammals don't have to do nearly so much work as we do in terms of maintaining a highly delicate relationship with gravity) is through our sense of proprioception.

Proprioception is to do with how we perceive our body in relation to the space around us – that is, where we are in our surroundings (our environment) and where we are in relation to gravity. Interestingly, in certain conditions, our proprioceptive sense becomes diminished and this can have a big effect on posture and our ability to move easily through the space around us. As we age, our sense of proprioception can become significantly impaired, leading us to become unstable on our feet (Stelmach and Sirica 1986). However, such a decline is certainly not inevitable, as many practitioners of yoga and other forms of exercise such as dance have shown. Some people retain high levels of proprioception and exquisite balance through continued use and stimulation of these receptors. In the case of Emilie Conrad, the founder of the system of fluid movement known as Continuum, despite her venerable age she managed to deport herself with the body of a 30-year-old. As she never tired of saying, 'Movement is what we *are*, not something we *do*.'

One of the key elements that allows for efficient locomotion is the elasticity of the lower spine facilitated by the thick areas of fascia known as aponeuroses, which are large flat tendon-like sheets of fascia that extent from the sacrum over the back of the pelvis and up the lower back. This is something that Bowen addresses very directly, with most Bowen treatments starting in this area. Aponeuroses were so called because originally when early anatomists dissected them they thought they were nerves – not far off the mark actually, as they are one of the most highly innervated areas of the body with sensory nerves. Elasticity is dependent on the fascia being hydrated and this is where Bowen is really effective, something that will be greatly aided by work such as gentle stretching which the client can do at home between sessions.

Bowen has a specific effect on proprioception because we work on the Golgi receptors, which are to be found in the junction between tendons and muscles as well as ligaments around joints. These kind of receptors have been found to act as highly sensitive and responsive anti-gravity receptors, constantly responding to the shifts in centers of gravity as we move. It is also possible to 're-calibrate' these receptors by putting a fairly strong challenge on them as we do in certain Bowen moves. Most of these types of Bowen moves are done close to the bone and performed cross-fibre. It seems from research that actually this might be the only way to activate them as simply the stretching-type moves along the orientation of the fibres, such as is done in forms of massage, are unlikely to make them respond (Schleip 2012, p.143). Other very important proprioceptive feedback mechanisms that are worked in Bowen arise from various sensory nerves in the inner ear and within muscles such as the muscle spindles (stretch receptors).

Another important factor in low back pain that is addressed in Bowen is the increased sensitivity of the nerves in the thoracolumbar aponeurosis. It seems as if (Schleip *et al.* 2010) various changes occur in the lumbar fascia, particularly in people with LBP – for example, a thickening of the posterior layer of the lumbar fascia, a higher density of myofibroblasts (cells with similar properties to smooth muscles) and/or increased inflammation with corresponding alterations in neural adaptions (i.e. hypersensitivity). Bowen seems to help address this by gentle stimulation of the mechanoreceptors in the lumbar fascia, allowing a re-calibration of the neural feedback loops. There are also mechanisms where it would also appear to have a role in decreasing the inflammatory response in the tissues.

The Sacroiliac Joints

When you mention the sacroiliac joints (SIJs) to many people, a puzzled look comes over their faces as they try to imagine where they are and what they do (Figure 5.3).

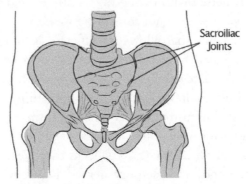

Figure 5.3 The pelvis and sacroiliac joints
Source: Martin Gordon

Strangely, it is often not considered important as to whether the SIJs move freely or not. After all, the monkey has no movement at all in its SIJs and still manages to get around, albeit with a distinctive and slightly unattractive gait. The monkey also has a lack of lordosis (natural curve) in the lumbar spine, which probably adds to its comical walk (something that, although funny to watch, is unnervingly common in the general population, particularly amongst the elderly).

Among even highly experienced manual therapists there is a huge debate about how much movement is actually possible at the SIJs. Even their real function is unclear. Some commentators consider that their chief role is as shock absorbers; others say it's all to do with force transmission between the legs and the spine. However, to the Bowen practitioner several qualities are important:

1. a degree of movement between the ilia and the sacrum (some researchers have put this at as little as 2 mm of 'glide' with about 2 degrees of rotation but in clinical observation it looks far more)

2. hydration of the tissues and SIJs themselves

3. a lack of sensitivity in the tissues around the SIJs (a big problem in low back pain)

4. a lack of repeated stress on the joints (which might be caused by poor pelvic alignment, the sacrum having to compensate for a leg length discrepancy or repeated types of movement or activity, such as standing on one leg as many shop assistants do).

Free movement of the sacrum between the two ilia is one of the cornerstones in craniosacral therapy and cranial osteopathy. Part of the reason for this is the strong attachment sites of the dural membranes that surround the spinal cord and the brain. These strong membranous attachments at the coccyx, sacrum, lower lumbars, top of the neck and within the cranium mean that restrictions at the sacrum (where the dural membranes attach at S2) will inevitably result in, among other things, a restricted neck movement. One of the fascinating things to witness during the back pain course I have run for many years, when the therapist works on the sacrum (having first checked on any restrictions in the client's neck movement), is their amazement at how neck restrictions frequently improve dramatically and immediately after freeing the SIJs by doing the Bowen sacral procedure.

Our four-legged friends appear to be much less prone to what is termed sacroiliac joint dysfunction (SIJD) (i.e. too little or too much movement) although they are still prone to arthritis in the SIJs, which can limit movement and cause pain (inflammation in these joints is a common and painful problem). Other mammals have a very different weight distribution to ours – they take about two-thirds of their weight through their front legs and a third through the back, putting much less pressure on the sacrum (unless of course they are a horse or a camel with a rider on their back).

At some point in our evolution, it was advantageous for us to become bipeds (and there are a lot of intriguing theories as to why that happened). Upright posture puts an inordinate amount of strain on the SIJs from where, effectively, all the weight of the upper part of our body is suspended (from the waist up) by a whole series of very dense ligaments.

It is not surprising that certain activities will create a locking in the SIJs. These include the obvious lifting and twisting, but it also can be caused by a lack of movement – too much sitting, for example (the old abuse/under-use scenarios that are the causes of so many types of joint dysfunction). Because the nerves that exit the sacrum (particularly the sciatic nerve) have to negotiate their way through some very strong muscles and ligaments, restrictions here will tend to be felt often as sciatica and also as stiffness in the lower back, or what used to be called lumbago.

A large number of clients also present with what is effectively hypermobility in the SIJs. This can arise during pregnancy as the ligaments relax because of hormonal changes due to an increase of the hormone relaxin. Relaxin is also a factor in the menstrual cycle, which is why traditionally women are much more prone to SIJD and used to be advised not to do heavy manual work at the time of their periods. Tom Bowen devised a clever procedure for treating women during pregnancy if they were suffering from sciatica. This involves a strong move over the sacro-tuberous ligament followed by a locking in over the ligaments that suspend the sacrum between the wings of the ilia. Excessive yoga can also create a similar scenario, as can too much chiropractic or osteopathic manipulation.

It is not difficult to observe when a client has an SIJ dysfunction. They will often have difficulty getting in and out of a chair, putting on shoes and socks, etc. Also, their gait may be distinctly 'monkey-like' if it is restricted – in other words, as they step forward their hip will rise and swing forward, although there might be other factors involved in this kind of gait. As the heel strikes the ground there will be a noticeable jar through the ilium as well. This might also be because the SIJs are failing in their job as shock absorbers.

The other major structure that affects the SIJs is the piriformis muscle, which goes from the greater trochanter of the femur (the bone that people often call their hip) to the sacrum. The sciatic nerve travels beneath, but adjacent to, this muscle, so tightness (which could either be spasm or excessive stretching) will result in inflammation and pain. This is often caused by something as simple as a wallet being carried in the back pocket, putting unnecessary pressure directly on the piriformis. Because the piriformis is a rotator muscle for the femur, tightness here will also have a big effect on the knees. An observant therapist will notice this and treat accordingly.

The tail-like segments of the sacrum don't really fuse until the late teens/early twenties. This means that the sacrum of a child with a pelvic imbalance will adapt as the child grows – something that is easily seen in many dissection labs where the sacrum has adopted some weird and wonderful compensation patterns at an early age.

Because there are so many possible permutations of torsions, shears, slips, compression and tension between the various articulations of the pelvis and sacrum, it is sometimes difficult to accurately assess what is going on. One of the apparent anomalies that puzzled me for many years was the fact that quite a number of clients, when doing a standing assessment, present with a higher iliac crest but a lower ischial tuberosity on the same side, with a narrowing of the two on the opposite side – an apparent impossibility. This puzzled me for ages until a colleague from the USA came up with a possible analysis: namely, where there is a torsion and/or rotation between the two ilia it will appear that there is a lengthening on one side. Actually, what is happening is, because of the torsion pattern, the iliac crest is either anterior or posterior whilst the ischial tuberosity may be posterior or anterior in a similar manner. This may need some thinking about, but thanks to Claire Darling for enlightening me!

Bowen and the Pelvis

Balance is the key to successfully addressing back pain, not only in terms of our posture and relationship to gravity but also in terms of the exquisite balance of tension and integrity (tensegrity) required in the tissues. There are a number of specific 'procedures' taught in Bowen courses and each of them has specific effects on different structures. When I was first studying Bowen, I used to hear it said many times that 'Bowen moves would go to where they are needed in the body'. This always seemed to me to be something of a cop-out, as though it didn't really matter where you worked in the body because the impulses would go to the right spot anyway, a bit like a genie on a magic carpet. I thought this whole idea absurd until I read the work of Mae Wan Ho and realized that actually what is happening is that impulses created by Bowen moves travel freely in the body if the tissues are hydrated but where they meet resistance (i.e. a lack of hydration or 'frozen' areas of the body) then the impulses start to have the effect of 'unfreezing' them and the person will often feel this as sensation (tingling, heat, pulsations, etc.). Having said that, it is much better if the Bowen practitioner can target areas of the body intelligently. In relation to back pain, the specific procedures that help are:

- moves that address the 'diaphragms' of the pelvic floor and the respiratory diaphragm, partly because both help support the back, but also because they tend to reflect horizontal compensation patterns

- moves that specifically address movement in the SIJs

- moves that address the complex tensional relationships in the pelvis – for example, between the hamstrings and the psoas or the piriformis and the adductors

- moves that create more hydration and integrity in the aponeuroses of the lumbar, thoracic spine as well as the IT band and Achilles

- moves that address the core itself, such as the coccyx

- moves that help lower the firing of sensitive neurons in the tissues around the spine and sacrum.

The Sciatic Nerve

As we have said, back pain can often be caused by something as simple as having a wallet or keys in a back pocket. This will put unnecessary pressure right on the nerve pathway of the sciatic nerve itself as well as tipping the pelvis at an angle. This then means that the lower lumbar vertebrae have to compensate. It is not surprising that this results in sciatica, and it is extraordinary that so many highly intelligent people continue to have something in their back pocket without a second thought to the structures underneath. When most people imagine a trapped nerve, they have in their mind an image of a poor old nerve caught somehow between two vertebrae as it exits the spinal column. However, unless there really is a true bony entrapment such as a stenosis, or narrowing of the foramina, or an exostosis which might involve a build up of bony deposits around a foramen, none of that is necessarily going on.

Nerves are sensitive creatures that hate being compressed, stretched or rubbed. If they are, they tend to get inflamed and then they swell up, making the symptoms worse. There are several areas where the sciatic nerve can get entrapped, for example, where it exits the spine it is surrounded by a sleeve of dural membrane which then becomes fascia. In fact, the distinction between fascia and membrane is somewhat academic as the dura is sometimes referred to as meningeal fascia anyway.

If there is a restriction locally in the spine (a so-called subluxation), then this will tend to create a tethering of the movement of the dural tube. This can result in certain movements such as twisting or bending, aggravating the sciatic nerve as it exits the spine. In this case the straight leg raise test or the slump test can be useful for diagnosing this, although it will only show up an issue if there is inflammation involved (in the same way that it will normally only pick up a prolapsed disc if there is inflammation).

The spinal cord is designed to move fairly freely in the vertebral canal as it is only tethered at the coccyx, sacrum, lumbar and top of the cervical spine (unless you have a condition such as spina bifida occulta, which is surprisingly common and often undiagnosed). Small subluxations can cause unnecessary tethering that can result in irritation and pain from specific twisting and bending movements.

As the sciatic nerve exits the spine, one of its branches passes underneath the iliolumbar ligament which runs from L4/L5 to the ilium close to the posterior superior iliac spine (PSIS). The categorization of this is somewhat academic as in children it's actually a muscle. This can be a common area of entrapment but it is actually quite easy to diagnose. If you press just medially and slightly superior to the PSIS, then the client is likely to get a radiating pain on that side which may well go down their leg. One effective way of working this area with Bowen (apart from addressing any underlying rotational issues) is to perform the kidney work a little lower (in other words, closer to the PSIS). This then becomes a cross-fibre move over the ligament itself, allowing it to relax and create more space for the passage of the sciatic nerve.

The Piriformis Muscles

The piriformis can be tricky to treat as it has a tendency to go into a protective stabilizing mode if there is instability in the sacroiliac joints. The key to successful treatment is to bring back integrity and strength to the joint. The piriformis works in conjunction with the adductors so it can be important to work these as well (another reason why it is often helpful to work the pelvis and the sacrum together).

Piriformis issues are relatively easy to spot because they will affect the rotation of the leg. There are basically two possibilities, which might both result in similar symptoms. The piriformis can either be tight (or even in spasm) or it can be stretched under excessive tension. Either situation may result in an impingement of the sciatic trunk, resulting in specific and deep pain in the buttock or even further down the leg. It may also result in tenderness at the greater trochanter of the femur and, over time, may end up creating a bursitis there. There is an optimal angle of rotation of the leg, termed the Fick angle, and, interestingly, many people from hunter-gatherer societies will have a tendency to have more external rotation than those in the West.

Internal or external rotations of the leg can have interesting effects on the ankle, knees, hips and back. Turning your toes to point more towards the front tends to stress the knees and make people walk more upright but with a rigidity in the spine (perhaps one reason that models and girls at finishing schools used to be taught to walk that way). Conversely, excessive external rotation will affect the knees adversely.

Disc Problems

For most people suffering from a herniated disc with nerve impingement, their condition was an accident waiting to happen. There are actually several things that can happen to a disc and none of them involves 'slipping'. One of the culprits can often be the psoas major, partly because it has attachments on to the discs themselves but also because any contraction or shortening through one side will tend to pull inferiorly and anteriorly on the vertebrae in the lumbar spine, creating more space on the opposite side for a possible herniation or prolapse of the disc. This is made more likely because of the psoas's attachments on to the transverse processes which, because they are more lateral to the midline of the body, will tend to create more of a lever. I see this a lot with people who have had car accidents where the seat belt has inhibited the action of the psoas to curl them into a protective pattern but where the impetus to contract is still there. This is why, even though there may be a disc pain on one side, the originating problem (and tighter psoas) will often be on the opposite side.

Compensation Patterns

There are many techniques to assess the origins of back pain but it is important to understand that observations made whilst the client is standing will change when they lie down and the effect of gravity is removed. There are some interesting (and sometimes heated) debates about which is the most useful way of assessing clients. There is no doubt that it is quite difficult to get an accurate assessment when observing someone standing because instinctively they will try and straighten themselves up. Karel Aerssens, a Bowen instructor in Holland, has a clever way of getting people to relax. Having first observed them standing, he then thanks them and tells them he has seen what he needs. Immediately they will relax and revert to their habitual posture.

One of the outstanding features of Bowen is its ability to change the relationship of horizontal or transverse relationships in the body and practitioners see these changes on a daily basis. One of the most intriguing cases recently was a client who presented with chronic low back pain and had a fairly extreme pelvic imbalance where his leg was around 2 cm longer on one side. This meant that his whole pelvis was tilted, his lower back was compensating, which resulted in a very painful nerve entrapment around L4. The imbalance was so bad that he had been referred by his doctor to a biomechanical podiatrist who was currently making a shoe with an inch lift on his left heel.

On the first treatment he had to lie on his side as he was in so much pain and I did minimal work on him. When he returned the following week he seemed to be moving more easily and he reported less pain. What was really interesting was the fact that his pelvis had completely changed in relation to the legs, so that it was now dead level in relation to the floor. During the following two treatments I did some more work on him and the pelvis subsequently remained level, up to when I saw him six months later for a check-up. Interestingly, when the aforementioned orthotic appliance arrived, wearing it made the symptoms return so it is now firmly kept in his wardrobe, where doubtless it will remain!

Looking at the compensation patterns in someone's body is a bit like a domino effect – if one of these horizontal relationships is affected, all of them will be in one degree or another, so it is the job of the therapist to discover which one is the originating cause. This can be more complicated than it seems because posture can be influenced by ascending factors – poor footwear, old ankle injuries, knee, hip or pelvic imbalances, or descending factors such as jaw and neck issues.

The main ascending influences are:

1. the plantar aspects of the feet (i.e. where the feet contact the ground)

2. the ankles (particularly the lateral aspects)

3. the knees

4. the hip joints

5. the pelvic floor

6. the sacroiliac joints.

Conversely, the main descending influences (at least in terms of Bowen work) are usually:

1. the temporomandibular joints (the TMJ)

2. the junction between the occiput and the atlas – sometimes called the 'rocker' (hence the expression 'off your rocker') or occipito-atlanteal joint (O/A junction)

3. the shoulders and thoracic inlet

4. the diaphragm.

Descending influences on posture tend to start early in life unless the client has had a whiplash injury or extensive dental work. It can be useful to ask the simple question, 'Do you remember as a teenager having a bad or "weak" back?'. They will generally remember this more clearly as a teenager rather than as a child as the body goes through a series of growth spurts. If so, one of these descending influences may need to be addressed.

Another way is to look carefully at facial structures. The possible reasons for facial asymmetry are numerous and may arise from birth patterns (see Chapter 13) or feeding patterns or later dental or orthodontic work. Even though some of these patterns may have been established a long time ago, it is still possible to work on them effectively. Compensation patterns, for however long they have been going on, are still held in the present time as highly energetic contained vortices, even if the need for that holding pattern is no longer relevant. However, because these patterns usually originated earlier in life, it might be necessary to work on them over a longer period and not expect miracles overnight.

Osteopaths have remarked for many years on the similarity in construction between the TMJs and the hips, and also the pubis and the mandible, and how they will tend to reflect each other in terms of compensation patterns.

Many clients have suffered a minor or major car accident (though of course there are many other ways to sustain such an injury, for example horse riding). Whiplash injuries tend to put a lot of strain on the upper cervical region, in particular the junction between the atlas and the occiput. The muscles at the base of the occiput tend to be quite short and are therefore prone to damage, inflammation and atrophy after whiplash.

One pair of muscles, the rectus capitis posterior minor, is particularly vulnerable. It attaches on to the very base of the occiput beneath the trapezius and the semispinalis and runs down on to the posterior arch of the atlas. It also has attachments to the dural membrane that surrounds the spinal cord and it would appear that one function of this little muscle is to stop the dura becoming enfolded when the head and neck is extended (Hack *et al.* 1995); any atrophy of this muscle will inhibit this function, with possible resultant irritation of the dura causing pain and possibly headaches.

Bowen moves address this area very directly and it is a place that can be very sensitive if there is an imbalance or tension here. As well as going over the occipital lymph nodes, these particular moves (3 and 4 of the neck procedure) are very effective when used to address the whole relationship between the head and neck, and you often get strong responses and major postural changes from working here. You can feel these little muscles on yourself by placing your middle fingers just below your occipital crest and a finger's width below. If you maintain gentle pressure here whilst just moving your eyes left and right, you will notice a subtle movement of this muscle under your fingers. This instinctual movement is the remnant of a primitive head-orienting response that develops in the womb and during the first years of life that is mediated by nuclei in the brain stem.

The Diaphragm and Emotional Links to Back Pain

This dome-shaped muscle and tendon is a major stabilizer for the back. It is hard to see and even harder to palpate, but it is an important horizontal structure in its own right and will tend to influence and be influenced by everything above and below it. A lot of us hold all kinds of emotional and deep-seated angst in and around it. First, of course, there is the vulnerability of the solar plexus. Having the umbilical cord cut too early (i.e. before it has stopped pulsating) can be a severe shock for the new-born baby – a shock that can be held long into life and which is referred to by perinatal psychologists as umbilical affect (see Chapter 12).

A remnant of our umbilical vein forms our falciform ligament which goes right the way through our liver, and it is common for umbilical shock to be fed right into that area, partly because some very rapid changes have to happen in the liver right after birth. The diaphragm also has deep connections with the psoas major and can hold deep and primal feelings to do with survival and fear. The area of the back where the posterior attachments of the diaphragm are found (around T12) is incredibly important posturally, being a kind of fulcrum for the body in the relationship between the trapezius and the psoas. Research has shown (Kolar *et al.* 2012) that in people with chronic low back pain both the position and the height of the diaphragm are affected, something that is examined in detail in the chapter by Aline Newton in Eric Dalton's book *Dynamic Body* (Dalton 2012, pp.248–273). This is why working the diaphragm can be an important ingredient in treating low back pain and why Bowen moves (which go over the attachment sites of the diaphragm just below the ribs and the sternum) have such an effect on creating more movement in the diaphragm, thereby aiding breathing and stimulating the lymphatic system.

The Neck

Tom Bowen had a particular interest in the neck and remarked in his 1973 interview with the Osteopathic, Chiropractic and Naturopathic Committee that he found the majority of his patients had trouble in the cervical region. Many other therapists have observed the same thing – it is also the cornerstone of certain branches of chiropractic, for example – because imbalances in the neck can be a major descending influence on the spine and pelvis in addition to creating local restrictions. Bowen had specific ways of addressing the neck, which we will look at in the next chapter.

CASE STUDY

| *Joanna Austen, Bodmin and Liskeard, Cornwall,*
| *England (www.bowenincornwall.co.uk)*

A young woman in her 30s, with children, who used to hold down an office job, run, ride horses and muck out, presented with severe low back and right leg pain. She was unable to carry out any normal tasks and had lost her job due to the condition. Sleep was difficult and she had nightmares. She had suffered for six months and had received a referral from her GP to the pain clinic. An MRI showed disc bulge at L5/S1. She was taking Naproxen, Amitriptyline, Co-Dydramol and sleeping tablets daily.

She received physio treatment and sports massage. She was then offered surgery to perform a discectomy at L5/S1 and was on the waiting list when she came in to try Bowen after a recommendation from a friend. Her pain score on the day was 10/10 and she was unable to stand straight, bending forward from the waist. This was now her posture.

She received a Bowen treatment which incorporated some release on the psoas and illiacus, and also a pelvic procedure. One week later when she returned she reported that the leg pain had gone the day after treatment, the back pain had dissipated to a dull ache, she had only taken one dose of the prescribed anti-inflammatories and was able to more feel refreshed on waking. However, she still could not sleep on her right side and sleep was still being disturbed.

A second Bowen treatment was carried out which followed a similar format to the first, but incorporated TMJ work. The following week on her return she reported no dreams, better sleep, no tablets and she had been able to join a march which included some running and dancing. She had undertaken household tasks and dog walking, with some discomfort afterwards, but this had improved with rest.

Two further treatments were carried out, one after three weeks, the other after four weeks at which time she was fully recovered. She had got a new job, was back running and riding. Needless to say, no surgery needed.

Rebecca writes: 'Since the day after my very first treatment, the pain reduced around 90 per cent. I cannot believe that I was in agony for six months taking all sorts of tablets and feeling so miserable when one treatment took away 90 per cent of my pain. I can smile again. It's amazing and I would recommend Bowen therapy to anyone!'

CASE STUDY

| *Rosemary MacAllister, Symington, Kilmarnock, Scotland*

Jim, male, 51 years of age, worked as a civil servant three days a week and as a photographer, which involves carrying heavy equipment and working in awkward positions.

Sudden onset occurred when client was preparing to get ready for work. Whilst pulling on trousers back suddenly 'went'. Difficulty moving or sitting. Went to work but was sent home after a few hours. On arrival at clinic, client was obviously in excruciating pain, shuffled in, could hardly move and had great difficulty placing his glasses on a low table or getting prepared for the treatment. His wife had to drive him in as he was in no fit state to drive. Client was unable to bend in any direction. Great difficulty with mobility, only able to 'shuffle' along. Client eventually managed to get on to treatment couch but was extremely tender over lumbar region.

Treatment consisted of basic relaxation moves (with long breaks): kidney, respiratory supine, pelvic and psoas. He still appeared to be in a lot of pain when he got up, though pain score was now about 6 out of 10 and he did appear to be moving a little easier. Because the pain had been so severe I strongly recommended him to attend GP or A&E.

On leaving he informed me he had a friend's wedding to attend two days later to do the photography! It was to my amazement that a few days later I received the lovely testimonial enclosed. He had managed the photo shoot and was almost pain free!

I am a 51-year-old male who works as a part-time civil servant (sedentary – in front of a PC for most of my three days per week). I also practise photography and can be on my feet for long periods; sometimes carrying heavy equipment (lighting rigs, backdrops, etc.).

On Monday, 4 November 2013, I was getting dressed for work when I suddenly experienced a sharp pain in my lower back, right of the base, which radiated through my right buttock into the back of my right leg, causing me to fall on the bed. I had been bending whilst pulling up a pair of trousers. I tried to stand up but the pain in my back and leg was so severe that I could not get out of a seated position. Eventually, after figuring out the least painful way of standing up, I managed to move across the bedroom by holding on to furniture and by leaning against a wall. The excruciating pain continued (a score of 8 or 9). I was in tears. However, I needed to get to work, so after a very time-consuming journey downstairs, I managed to haul myself into the passenger side of my car. My wife drove me to work. On arrival, it took 15 minutes for me to find the least painful way of getting out of the car. I did so eventually by gripping the doorframe and pulling myself up using arm strength. I was in agony, but made it to my desk after some considerable shuffling and holding on to anything and anyone that was nearby.

I took the lift to the second floor of the office, made it to my usual seat and felt slightly more comfortable when sitting in my chair, which has an air-filled lumbar support (pain now 6–7). I worked for about 30 minutes on a PC but when I attempted to stand up I could only do so by pushing my hands on the desktop to lift my whole body weight up from the seat. My assumption was that I had a trapped sciatic nerve.

I found that if I attempted to walk as normally and as fast as possible, I could tolerate the pain a bit more easily (when consciously trying to walk normally, the pain was about 5 at this point). I only stayed a few hours as I was sent home as it was obvious I could not work properly being in so much pain. On the assumption that this was a temporary situation, I did not take any medication at that point. My over-riding thought was that I needed to be better asap (although pretty much out of my control) as I was booked for a friend's wedding photography shoot on the Friday of the same week.

I contacted Rosemary MacAllister, a Bowen practitioner who I had attended several years ago regarding a trapped nerve in my neck/shoulder. This was a success after only one session, so I had always kept her number handy, in case anything like it should occur again. First available appointment was Wednesday 6 November at 09:30. I did not get a decent sleep at all through Monday into Tuesday and called my office to say I would not be at work that day and that I would see how things went following my Bowen treatment. On Tuesday 7th, things got worse (possibly due to inactivity) so I contacted NHS 24 for advice (who agreed that sciatica was the most likely cause of pain) and thought that I may have to present myself at A&E in the hope of a 'quick fix' cortisone injection or some other intervention – I was really concerned about the rising pain level (back up to 8–9). I was also anxious about the prospect of being unable to carry out the pre-planned photography shoot at the end of the week. That day, it took me 45 minutes just to shower and get dried. On Rosemary's telephone advice, I lay on the floor with legs raised on to a seat, but that had no real effect or improvement (in fact I could not get up from the floor on to the seat without help). I did not attend hospital or see a GP as I thought it best to wait to see how the Bowen treatment would help, plus I did not relish the prospect of actually having to make the painful effort of leaving my house.

Another sleepless night (but this time having taken ibuprofen and paracetamol on the advice of NHS 24) and on Wednesday morning my wife drove me to see Rosemary at Whitehill Community Centre in Hamilton for my session. I could hardly walk and not even bend to place or pick up my glasses from a low table. I was in agony. However, after a one-hour session with Rosemary carrying out the Bowen Technique, I felt marginally better and was able to withstand the pain (now around 6–7). I managed to walk out of the Centre unaided and to the car where my wife was waiting to drive home. She was very pleasantly surprised to see the instant improvement on how I was able to walk to and get into the car quicker than any time since the original pain started.

Rather than go home, I asked to be taken to work, where, despite some pain, I managed to do a full day. I regularly got up from my seat and walked around the office and noticed as each hour passed by, the pain was becoming more and more tolerable (eventually, by the time I went to bed on the Wednesday, the pain was around 4). I was really improving as the day went on.

On Thursday 7 November, I got dressed normally (albeit a bit slower and more hesitant than normal) and actually drove my wife to work. The pain was now 2–3 and I felt well enough to carry out my normal every day routine (I was now on my non-civil service working days of Thu/Fri of that week, but needed to prepare equipment for the following day's wedding shoot). No real issues on that day and on the Friday (along with another photographer and an assistant) I managed to carry out the photography duties as planned. I was on my feet from 13:00 to 23:00 that day, as the agreement was to cover the entire event. The next morning (Sat. 9th) I felt a bit stiff (as is normal after a heavy day's shooting) but the original problem of the back and leg pain had almost disappeared!

Two weeks further on and I have had no return of pain, no sick leave, no detrimental impact on my life due to back or leg problems. I am delighted that my recovery was so rapid and can only put this down to the fact I sought help quickly by attending a Bowen session when I did.

CASE STUDY

Alastair McLoughlin, Skipton, North Yorkshire, England (www.MobileTherapyService.com)

Before coming to see me the client had mentioned to her doctor that she was thinking of having Bowen treatment for her back pain. This doctor had expressed the view that she ought not 'waste her time and money' on something that is 'unproven'.

Female aged 68 years. For more than 10 years Mrs G. was troubled with low back pain. She had many sessions of chiropractic treatment during this time. Late in 2008 the pain became much worse and, on occasion, she lost bladder and bowel control. Her doctor referred her for an MRI scan which revealed an 8 mm forward slip of L4 vertebra on L5 (a spondylolisthesis). This can be clearly seen on the MRI image that was taken on 16 December 2008 (Figure 5.4).

This type of back problem resulted in inability to walk very far, constant pain in the hip, groin, thigh and lower leg. She had had cortisone injections prior to starting Bowen treatment. They helped for a while but the pain returned.

After six treatments Mrs G reported she had very little or no pain and that she had just completed a three-mile walk! Additionally, bowel and bladder function had returned to normal. She is very happy with the results we have obtained.

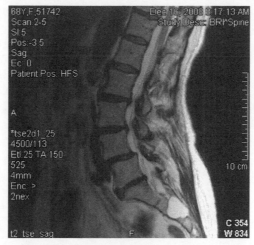

Figure 5.4 Mrs G MRI image, taken December 2008

References

Adams, M., Bogduk, N., Burton, K. and Dolan, P. (2002) *The Biomechanics of Back Pain*. Edinburgh: Churchill Livingstone.

Crow, W. and Willis, D. (2009) Estimating cost of care for patients with acute low back pain: a retrospective review of patient records. *Journal of American Osteopathic Association* 109 (4), 229–233.

Dalton, E. (2012) *Dynamic Body: Exploring Form Expanding Function*. Oklahoma City: Freedom from Pain Institute.

Gintis, B. (2006) *Engaging the Movement of Life*. Berkeley, CA: North Atlantic Books.

Gracovetsky, S. (2008) *The Spinal Engine*. St Lambert, Canada: Serge Gracovetsky.

Hack, G.D., Koritzer, R.T., Robinson, W.L., Hallgren, R.C. (1995) Anatomic relation between the rectus capitis posterior minor muscle and the dura mater. *Spine (Phila PA 1976)* 20 (23), 2484–2486.

Koch, L. (1997) *The Psoas Book* (2nd edition) Felton, CA: Guinea Pig Publications.

Kolar, P., Sulc, J., Kyncl, M., Sanda, J. *et al.* (2012) Postural function of the diaphragm in persons with and without chronic low back pain. *Journal of Orthopaedic and Sports Physical Therapy* 42 (4), 352–362.

Levine, P. (1997) *Waking the Tiger: Healing Trauma – The Innate Capacity to Transform Overwhelming Experiences*. Berkeley, CA: North Atlantic Books.

Levinkind, M. (2008) Consideration of whole body posture in relation to dental development. *Oral Health Report, British Dental Journal Supplement* 1, 1–7.

Nachemson, A. and Elfstom, G. (1970) *Intravital Dynamic Pressure Measurements in Lumbar Discs: A Study of Common Movements, Maneuvers and Exercises*. Stockholm: Almqvist and Wiksell.

NICE (May 2009a) *National Costing Report: Low Back Pain*. London: NHS and National Institute for Health and Care Excellence. Available at www.nice.org.uk/nicemedia/pdf/CG88CostReport.pdf, accessed on 18 June 2014.

NICE (May 2009b) *Low Back Pain – Early Management of Persistent Non-Specific Low Back Pain*. London: NHS and National Institute for Health and Care Excellence. Available at www.nice.org.uk/cg88, accessed on 12 May 2014.

Oschman, J. (2000) *Energy Medicine*. Edinburgh: Churchill Livingstone.

Schleip, R. (2012) Fascia as a sensory organ. In E. Dalton (ed.) *Dynamic Body: Exploring Form Expanding Function*. Oklahoma City: Freedom from Pain Institute.

Schleip, R. *et al.* (2010) The fascial network: an exploration of its load bearing capacity and its potential role as a pain generator. In A. Vleeming *et al.* (eds) *Proceedings of the 7th Interdisciplinary World Congress on Low Back and Pelvic Pain*. Los Angeles, 2010.

Stelmach, G. and Sirica, A. (1986) Aging and proprioception. *Age* 9 (4), 99–103.

Vleeming, A. *et al.* (2007) *Movement, Stability and Lumbopelvic Pain*. Edinburgh: Churchill Livingstone.

6

Chronic Pain and Fibromyalgia

Chronic conditions such as fibromyalgia, chronic fatigue, irritable bowel syndrome (IBS) and chronic complex syndromes such as myofascial pain syndrome present a challenge to the medical profession because there are no simple cures. Sufferers are often complicated patients who frequent their GP with a variety of seemingly unrelated symptoms. This can be a source of frustration to both the patient and the medical professional. The patient may be told that they have a viral condition and will usually undergo a battery of tests which are often inconclusive or give no clear path to recovery. They may suffer increasing pain, requiring stronger and stronger medication, and frequently depression, owing to the chronicity of their condition. This can be exacerbated by the frustration at the inability to discover the underlying cause of their condition. Although doctors do have some useful tools for people suffering from chronic pain, such as cognitive behavioural therapy (CBT), beyond pharmaceutical interventions it is usually only possible to support the patient to manage their condition, with little hope of a sudden cure (Knight 2011, 2013).

In this chapter we will look at these differing conditions and how and why Bowen might help. Readers should refer to Chapter 1, about how Bowen works, and to Chapter 2, about fascia and connective tissues, in order to obtain a full understanding.

Chronic Pain

What is the cost of chronic pain? In purely economic terms, it is estimated to be around £5 billion annually in the UK. Nearly 10 million Britons suffer pain daily, which not only has a major impact on their ability to do normal everyday activities such as going to work, but has a very major effect on their whole quality of life. In the USA, pain affects more people than diabetes, heart disease and cancer combined. According to a recent report published by the Institute of Medicine of the National Academies, the number of sufferers of chronic pain in America is estimated to be as high as 100 million people (IMNA 2011).

Chronic pain may be defined as pain that has lasted persistently for more than three months' duration and often much longer than that (Grahame 2009; Nicholas *et al.* 2005). The pain might start without very obvious incident or resultant trauma; however, *nociceptive pain* is pain whereby tissue damage persists and leads to pain. Examples of this might include cancer, post-operative pain and arthritis (Nicholas *et al.* 2005). *Neuropathic pain*, which may be described as shooting pain or hot pain, occurs due to damage or injury to the nerves. Shingles is a good example of neuropathic pain (Nicholas *et al.* 2005). Neuropathic pain results in changes to the central nervous system (CNS), where the memory of the pain remains and the body continues to respond to pain signals that no longer usefully alert the body to pain. This is how pain becomes chronic, and it can remain unrelenting and often unresponsive to analgesia (Grahame 2009).

Nicholas and colleagues (2005) suggest that 'chronic' pain can share elements of both nociceptive and neuropathic pain, and that there might be an unclear distinction between both types of pain. However, ultimately chronic pain is the result of the body continuing to experience and perceive pain long after an event (e.g. post-surgery) and the pain signals remain active. In the long term this results in changes to the CNS and the nervous system (Nicholas *et al.* 2005). Unfortunately, the reasons for the resultant change in pain response are not fully understood, but ultimately the patient has to endure, cope with and manage them. This is where good pain management is vital (Nicholas *et al.* 2005).

Why Do We Feel Pain?

So, what actually is pain and what are the mechanisms through which we feel it? Is it just a sensation caused by injury and inflammation? Is it the result of nerves becoming hypersensitive? Or is the perception of pain only generated in the mind? Believe it or not, these questions are still a long way from being answered by our current medical understanding. If a common consensus is beginning to emerge, then it is that all these factors (and more) combine to create the phenomenon that can be so debilitating. How much or how little people feel pain seems to be mostly dependent on their emotional state, whether the injury resonates with a previous traumatic event, the level of stimulus through sensitization of nerve fibres and how long factors such as inflammation and tissue damage have been present. One thing that Lorimer Moseley points out is that 'the relationship between pain and the state of the tissues becomes weaker as pain persists' (Moseley 2007a, p.171). This can then have a knock-on effect on movement because the proprioceptive representation of the painful body part changes in the primary somatosensory cortex (Flor *et al.* 1997) leading to further problems. Interestingly, recent research has shown that encouraging proprioception can inhibit the perception of pain as they mutually inhibit each other (Schleip and Müller 2013). Two books by David Butler and Lorimer Moseley called *Explain Pain* (Butler and Moseley 2013) and *The Graded*

Motor Imagery Handbook (Moseley *et al.* 2012) are immensely useful and practical explanations of the pain response and how to modify it, particularly for patients with complex regional pain syndrome (CRPS). For the client, Moseley's *Painful Yarns* (2007b) is a light-hearted, accessible book that uses metaphors and humorous stories to explain this complex subject.

Sensitized Sensation and Pain Amplification

One of the problems in patients with chronic pain is that they very often develop increased sensation and pain amplification in their greatest areas of pain. This is caused by changes to the nociceptive neurons, which are the neurons founds in skin, joint, muscle, fascia and tendon tissues (Shaikh, Hakim and Shenker 2010). Eventually, the nociceptive neurons change in response to trauma or further inflammation and gradually their sensitivity to pain increases over time. This is very difficult to cope with because the increased pain makes the sufferer want to do less in order to protect the area, or they become more anxious that they have reinjured the area or made it worse.

The various theories of pain have their advocates and detractors. Some of these have fancy names such as the Neuromatrix Theory (Melzack and Katz 2013) and Gate Control Theory, but whichever way you look at it there are some strange anomalies when it comes to whether someone will experience pain or not. It is impossible, for example, for even an experienced orthopaedic consultant to accurately assess whether someone will be in pain just by looking at their MRI scan, X-ray, or even a biopsy.

The Link between Inflammation and Chronic Pain

The role of fascia in pain has been studied in relation to fibromyalgia and other conditions, such as Ehlers-Danlos Syndrome (a connective tissue disorder; see Chapter 15) (Schleip 2010) but the principles apply equally to anyone suffering from any condition that involves tissue damage (conditions ending in '-osis') and/ or inflammation (conditions ending in '-itis'). It is postulated that because increased inflammatory markers are found in the fascia in people with fibromyalgia, this creates an increased excitability in the dorsal horn neurons of the spinal cord (Liptan 2010). When these neurons are hyper-excited, this creates a general hypersensitivity to all kinds of stimuli, including stimuli which were previously tolerable (such as going out in the cold, an argument with a spouse, or, importantly, too much or too hard a treatment). There are clear mechanisms by which this happens, often starting with inflammation (which is a natural short-term response of the body to injury) followed by an over-sensitization of the nociceptors, which are normally what are termed 'low-threshold' – in other words, under normal circumstances they need a fair amount of stimulus to activate them. Over time, this can lead to an activation of the spinal cord (often specific segments of it) and eventually an activation of the sympathetic nervous system, leading to symptoms of restlessness, anxiety and a tendency to become irritable, emotional, or even depressed.

In osteopathy this process is referred to as a state of 'facilitation' and has clear markers which are easy for a therapist to track. An over-activation of spinal segments results in:

- a tightness and sensitivity around the erector spinae muscles at that particular level (either bilaterally or unilaterally)

- areas of redness or whiteness emerging after the area has been worked on

- a roughness in the skin around an area of the spine (and sometimes hairy patches).

These markers are very useful for Bowen practitioners as they can help us trace the origin of inflammation and treat accordingly. If the origin is from an organ, it will feed into the spinal cord over several segments. Because any sensory stimulus will result in a corresponding motor response at the same level, it is common for stimulae from the viscera to affect the muscles (by creating hyper-tonus usually) and vice versa. A therapist has to be something of a Sherlock Holmes to find the original cause of inflammation, as there are so many potential culprits; conditions such as endometriosis, local injuries, scars, inflamed or damaged tissue and even root canal fillings can all be triggers.

To really understand the process, it is a good idea to have a good look at charts of the sympathetic and parasympathetic nervous systems which illustrate what might be affecting what. A list of 'viscero-somatic reflexes' is provided on page 109 to show the areas relate to one another (Beal 1985). For the therapist, a few things are worth bearing in mind:

- Sympathetic nerves arise from spinal cord segments T1 to L2. Therefore, activation in any of these spinal segments is likely to result in somato-visceral or viscero-somatic loops – in other words, inflamed tissue affecting organs or inflamed organs affecting tissue.

- As there is no direct neural connection between cervical nerve roots or lower lumbar nerve roots and the viscera, activation of these segments will not spread to the viscera.

- Parasympathetic nerves to the viscera arise from the cranium (the vagus nerve) and from the sacrum. Therefore, sacral spinal cord segments in the lower part of the spinal cord (around T12 to L1, called the conus medullaris and lumbar enlargement) may be involved in parasympathetic facilitation of pelvic organs.

In relation to fibromyalgia sufferers, in common with some other sufferers of chronic pain, their increased sensitivity is also due to higher than normal levels of the neurotransmitter that mediates pain (substance P) in the cerebrospinal fluid, lower than normal glucocorticoid levels and higher levels of activity in the parts of the brain that mediate the emotional and contextual assessment of pain (Sapolsky 2004, p.200).

Diet and Environmental Factors

These days, our bodies are bombarded with all kinds of environmental and dietary stimuli that can set off exaggerated inflammatory responses. The consumption of GM foods, although highly controversial, is now proven to cause inflammatory responses in animals that eat them (Finamore *et al.* 2008; Kroghsbo *et al.* 2008). Such is the concern about the widespread consumption of these foods that the American Academy of Environmental Medicine issued a statement in May 2009 asking physicians to advise the public not to consume GM foods because of their potential link to multiple health problems (AAEM 2009). As far as I know, there is no research to show that humans who eat animals fed GM meal are likely to suffer inflammation, but there is evidence to show that just the consumption of grain-fed animals and fish has this effect (Reinagel 2007). The fact that most animals in the UK (particularly chickens and pigs) are now fed GM food (Wasley 2014) and that 60 per cent of all processed food in the USA for human consumption contains GM ingredients (www.centerforfoodsafety.com) should be cause for concern.

Working with Sensory Receptors

The mechanisms by which Bowen can lower inflammation and nerve sensitivity as well as creating a calmer emotional state (and a lowering of sympathetic nervous system (SNS) activation) are discussed in Chapter 1, and ways of helping lower inflammation in the body through diet and other lifestyle changes are outlined in Appendix 2. Specifically, using light Bowen moves to stimulate the interstitial receptors can be very effective at allowing the nociceptors to become less sensitive. Interstitial receptors are found everywhere in the body but particularly in the periosteum. There are a number of Bowen moves that stimulate these areas directly, notably work on the coccyx, the back of occiput and front of the tibia. The key element to working with the interstitials appears to be performing moves very gently and, crucially, not invoking a pain response. As explained earlier, stimulation of these receptors will result in an autonomic response, such as the client suddenly feeling cold or clammy, showing that the practitioner has definitely 'hit the mark'. If clients can take a bit more pressure (without it being painful), then the slow melting-type pressure that affects the Ruffini receptors is also effective in calming the SNS. This is absolutely crucial as a first step in treating anyone in chronic pain as it is almost impossible for the body to heal if the autonomic nervous system (ANS) is in a hyper-aroused state. Working these receptors also encourages a sense of wellbeing and better sleep patterns almost overnight. In itself, this will begin to turn people around, giving a sense of hope along with a calmer, more positive psychological outlook, allowing them to manage their pain better.

Strategic Approaches

There is a specific strategy to treating chronic pain, which needs a more long-term approach. After a few initial sessions designed to lower their sympathetic activation, the therapist needs to address local hyperactivity in the spinal cord and finally, the original cause of the tissue damage/inflammation needs to be addressed. This might need the involvement of other practitioners, particularly if the complaint is related to organic, dietary, ergonomic or environmental factors. Treatments do not have to be weekly. In many cases, clients in chronic pain actually seem to respond better with longer gaps between sessions. After an initial series, spacing them monthly apart seems to allow many people to integrate the work better and maintain homeostasis.

Studying recent research related to pain has really turned my practice around. I remember treating one lady in her early 50s a few years ago. She had been in constant severe pain for a number of years after a skiing accident where she had damaged her coccyx. Conventional advice given by pain clinics at the time was aimed at getting patients to accept the reality that the pain was not going to go away and therefore the only way to manage their pain was though psychological approaches such as CBT and drugs such as amitriptyline, which is used extensively in the UK for pain management. The irony was that, although patients attending the clinic were actively discouraged from trying alternative approaches such as Bowen, the consultant who ran it used to see her local Bowen practitioner when she herself was in pain! It did not take long for this person to feel considerably better. After coming for treatments monthly for a year, she went to bi-monthly and now, five years later, comes about once a year when she has overdone things. Her pain levels are now non-existent.

Working extremely gently with people in chronic pain can feel counter-intuitive, but is nevertheless highly effective. The worst thing a practitioner of any discipline can do is stimulate the nerve pathways or increase inflammation through too much pressure. A recent client with chronic lower and upper back pain caused by chronic idiopathic inflammation in the tissues reported recently that she had 'got her life back'. This was someone with two small children who was unable to work and for whom even everyday household tasks such as cooking and shopping had become impossible. After two minimal and light Bowen sessions, her sleep had already improved dramatically, with pain decreasing radically. On her fourth treatment she remarked casually that she was going to start looking for a part-time job, something she had thought an impossible dream six months before.

Complex Regional Pain Syndrome (CRPS)

The key symptom of CRPS is continuous, intense pain, out of proportion to the severity of the injury or tissue damage, that gets worse rather than better over time. It used to be referred to as 'reflex sympathetic dystrophy syndrome' or 'causalgia', a term first used during the American Civil War to describe the intense, hot pain felt by some veterans long after their wounds had healed. It usually affects one of the extremities (arms, legs, hands or feet) and is often accompanied by increased sensitivity, changes in skin texture, swelling in the affected joints and a decreased ability to move the affected body part. Often the pain spreads to include the entire arm or leg, even though the initiating injury might have been only to a finger or toe. Pain can sometimes even travel to the opposite extremity. CRPS is an extreme example of facilitation, which has spread to affect the sympathetic nervous system. My experience of working with clients with CRPS has been enlightening because, as well as resulting in more mobility and less pain, skin texture problems and local sensitivity also decline.

Addressing Chronic Pain
ఴ Kelly Clancy

In our current model of disease and dysfunction, we look primarily only at the site of pain. The patient's site of pain or numbness is treated locally, and the patient's symptoms may or may not feel better. This current treatment model is both reductionist and isolated by reducing the patient's complaint to its simplest form, and it becomes very costly, very quickly, as the patient must approach a separate specialist, occupational or physical therapist, or other physician for each isolated physical problem.

In traditional occupational, physical, massage and orthopaedic care, the localized symptoms of pain, numbness, loss of joint motion and loss of strength are the focus. Diagnostic studies of the specific parts are ordered and examined to determine the correct course of care. In the case of chronic pain, the findings often will be minimal or non-existent and the patient will frequently be led from one healthcare provider to another trying to find answers. A common treatment regime will focus on localized treatment to those painful sites, which may include pharmacologic interventions, injections, ultrasound, massage, stretching and strengthening. These treatments may lead to temporary relief of symptoms but may not address the root cause of these often migrating symptoms. If conservative management is not satisfactory, often surgical interventions are implemented to the localized painful area. It is not uncommon for a patient to have multiple surgeries, especially in areas such as the upper extremity, in an attempt to address the many locations of pain, or put out the many fires of complex multi-system symptoms.

This reductionist medical model does not follow the patterning of dysfunctions in the fascial network. We may see but do not recognize that pathology in one place leads to pathology in another place, with a cascading effect through the body's systems. This cascading effect occurs because of the alteration of the fascial network. Without enough give in the system, the fascial connective tissue reorganizes to meet the need of the injured part of the body. Multiple injuries are then created because of the uneven tugging of fascia within the entire structure of the body. We currently are blaming the victim – the place of pain or numbness – for the criminal's activity and the origin of the pattern, which may be proximal or distal tightness in one or more lines of fascia. The lines of fascia, methods of assessing posture and fascial length, and how to use Bowen to address fascial imbalances will be discussed in other chapters.

For complex clients, such as those with chronic pain, practitioners may have to go after one of the body systems as a first priority to help regulate the others; for example, a client who has lived with chronic pain for several years may require a preliminary intervention for his or her nervous system, and a modality such as Bowen can be an appropriate precursor to more intensely focused fascial work. Once the nervous system becomes more regulated, the lymphatic, musculoskeletal and vascular systems will also be more likely return to homeostasis.

Over time, as a client continues to deal with the pain and dysfunction of a chronic issue, the fascial system loses its ability to be flexible and aligned, and therefore throws the nervous system into dysregulation. Then the nervous system starts to affect the function of the autonomic nervous system, endocrine system and the hormonal system. The relationship between fascia and the nervous system has to be addressed in chronic pain conditions to get the rest of the body's systems to start regulating again.

We attempt to regulate the nervous system in Western medicine by using drugs such as gabapentin, pregabalin and beta blockers that affect the nervous systems, which can all change the brain chemistry that affects the nervous system. These drugs have steep side effects, and they may change a client's perception of pain, but they inevitably only put a veil over the client's bodily structure being out of alignment.

Additionally, practitioners prescribe at-home exercise programmes for clients with chronic pain, focused mainly on strengthening. Isolated treatments of the musculoskeletal system fail in clients with chronic pain because the muscles are not the problem. The problem is fascia. Strengthening of an isolated muscle does not restore fascia to its original tissue length. However, strengthening other muscles in relation to postural alignment throughout the body may restore integrity to alignment and thus provide more flexible tensioning in the fascia throughout the whole system.

Positive fascial change is possible when three-dimensional, global approaches are used in the case of a client with chronic pain. This is how Bowen helps people with chronic pain – because it is innately a global approach that can be utilized to treat dysfunctions in the fascia. However, simply aligning the body's structure through Bowen is often not enough to unravel the total effects of chronic pain on a client. The client's structure can be organized fascially, but still produce the same painful sensations in the client's body. The effects of chronic pain may persist, even after structurally reorganizing work such as Bowen, because the client's nervous system may have become overly sensitized to painful sensations in the form of central sensitization.

Butler and Matheson's work in *The Sensitive Nervous System* (2000, p.34) discusses the research on central sensitization in great detail, with a particular focus on clients with phantom limb pain as a way to demonstrate the brain's ability to create painful sensations even when there is no longer a painful part attached to the client's body.

> Phantom limb pains are usually regarded as medical odd baskets, although no one could doubt or fail to feel for clients suffering what must be among the most frustrating of all pains… Phantom pains are more likely and often worse if the amputated limb has been painful… As Melzak…comments, the brain generates the experiences, sensory experiences only modulate it. We should also note that stress such as frustration will make many phantom limb pains worse.

After surviving chronic pain for an extended time, the brain will go into central sensitization and change its threshold of pain, described by Butler and Matheson as sensory cortical reorganization:

> People suffering phantom limb pains have had their brains mapped. The findings are likely to have great relevance to manual therapists. The greater the magnitude of phantom limb pain, the greater the amount of sensory cortical reorganisation… It seems likely that chronic pain anywhere may be linked to plastic changes in the nervous system. However, the very notion of plasticity should lift hopes and expectation in dealing with chronic pain. (2000, p.35)

It is the nature of plasticity in the nervous system that paves the way for Bowen to affect real change in the body systems of a client with chronic pain – by affecting change in the client's nervous system and fascia.

In addition to reorganizing the nervous system via the fascia, the chronic pain client's nervous system must also learn that the body can move correctly, without threat. The nervous system can learn this new information when the body is retrained in functional movement. By engaging in purposeful new movements, the nervous system can learn that this new, specific movement, that previously caused pain, is no longer painful, even when done repetitively. Butler and Matheson describe the brain and nervous system as:

the ultimate 'use it or lose it' machine. It seems clear that functional, meaningful and goal directed inputs will be better accepted by the brain processing. Movements that are feared, avoided and context dependent will have to be presented to the brain in different ways, for example in different environments, or the movement 'broken down' or paced... Clearly, the more functional the movement and the more it links to desired activity and achievable goals, the better. (2000, p.37)

After completing a modality such as Bowen that addresses global chronic pain issues, a medical practitioner can take several approaches to retraining a client in functional movement. Some approaches to movement re-education that encourage nervous system re-patterning are:

1. Gyrotonics, with its approach to global repetition, core strengthening and gross body movement, can effectively reduce distal overuse by training the client on the initiation of power from the core.

2. The Feldenkrais Method® requires a state of awareness of one's own structure and teaches alternate choices in movement patterns, ones that give the system more corrective safe choices over time.

3. The Alexander Technique encourages present moment awareness and, similarly variations of movement that may be more healthy for the individual.

Appropriate forms of exercise are discussed in more detail in Appendix 1. As we see a dramatic rise in the reported cases of chronic pain, including repetitive stress injuries of the upper extremities, back and neck, one cannot help but examine the pace and lifestyle that our society currently demands. The combination of chronic stress patterns, our focus on multitasking and productivity and the fears and economic uncertainty of our time inevitably affect our physical structures and our resultant embodiment of pain. Bowen practitioners can expect to see more clients present with symptoms of pain and dysfunction, especially in their upper extremities and, by treating their fascia and with awareness of their nervous systems, Bowen practitioners can bring about real, lasting change for clients with chronic pain.

෴

Chronic Syndromes

A syndrome may be defined as a group of symptoms that are related to a particular condition. For example, heartburn, gastric reflux, bloating, diarrhoea and constipation might be a collection of symptoms which are related to the medical condition irritable bowel syndrome or IBS (Berne 2002; Farmer and Aziz 2010). There are a group of syndromes, which include IBS, chronic fatigue syndrome (CFS) and fibromyalgia (FM), which might be also known as autonomic nervous system conditions, which have a considerable overlap of symptoms (Knight 2013; Rahman and Holman 2010). Indeed, there are probably many more syndromes that have overlap of symptoms which have common themes – for example, chronic pain, fatigue, etc. (Knight 2013; Rahman and Holman 2010). Syndromes might be described as a group of symptoms that form a known 'condition'. They are frequently difficult for the medical profession to treat because there are often many diverse symptoms. Treatment becomes more about the management of symptoms than curing the disease (Arnold *et al.* 2012; Berne 2002; Knight 2013; Rahman and Holman 2010).

ANS conditions result from altered levels of cortisol, growth hormone and thyroid levels (Berne 2002; Lavergne *et al.* 2010) which cause disruption to the ANS, affecting breathing, blood pressure, bladder and bowel function (Berne 2002). In addition, there might be imbalances in cytokines and in the neurotransmitters, further affecting both the sympathetic and parasympathetic parts of the ANS (Shaikh *et al.* 2010).

Chronic Fatigue Syndrome

Chronic fatigue syndrome (CFS) might be defined as 'a complex illness characterized by incapacitating fatigue, neurological problems and often resembles other disorders such as Fibromyalgia (FM)' (Berne 2002, p.8). People with CFS feel an overwhelming exhaustion, which is often similar for those with FM, along with many of the symptoms experienced by those with FM.

Fibromyalgia

Berne describes fibromyalgia as 'a common, debilitating disorder of widespread musculoskeletal pain, sleep disturbance, fatigue and additional somatic experiences (bladder/bowel problems). FM affects muscles, joints, tendons, ligaments and other soft tissues, most frequently causing pain in the neck, shoulders back and hips' (2002, p.26). There are often multiple points of pain or trigger points, which is partly how the condition is diagnosed (Arnold *et al.* 2011, 2012; Berne 2002; Lavergne *et al.* 2010). It is estimated that 2–5 per cent of the American adult population suffer from FM, with women accounting for 80–90 per cent of those diagnosed (Arnold *et al.* 2011). Diagnosis of symptoms includes chronic widespread pain of long duration and sleep disturbance, and then there are other associated symptoms which include tenderness, stiffness and mood disturbances, including depression and anxiety and also cognitive impairment (sometimes also known as 'fibro-fog') where patients experience difficulty with memory and concentration (Arnold *et al.* 2011). In addition to pain, there are other symptoms such as migraine and IBS (Arnold *et al.* 2011; Berne 2002). Diagnosis is made by taking a detailed clinical history, including looking at sites of trigger points and widespread pain which is characteristic of the condition (Arnold *et al.* 2011; Berne 2002).

Patients with FM are frequently perceived as difficult to treat (Arnold *et al.* 2012) and education is a significant part of the management (Arnold *et al.* 2012). Pain management and goal setting are key aspects of managing the condition, with a slow and low-grade approach and 'pacing of activity' (Arnold *et al.* 2012; Knight 2013). In terms of the pharmacological management, some types of anti-depressants such as amitriptyline and duloxetine are examples of medications used to help with both pain management and sleep, and are issued at lower doses than they might be for depression (Arnold *et al.* 2012). A multidisciplinary model of care is required for FM and conditions such as Ehlers-Danlos Syndrome, including pain management and other psychological-based approaches such as CBT; other non-pharmacological approaches including yoga and massage might be recommended (Arnold *et al.* 2012). Some patients do turn to complementary and alternative therapies – for example, acupuncture (Arnold *et al.* 2011, 2012; Berne 2002).

Ehlers-Danlos Syndrome (Hypermobility-Type)

Ehlers-Danlos Syndromes are a group of heritable connective tissue disorders of which type III was, until recently, known as Type III (Hypermobility-Type), and is now known as 'Ehlers-Danlos Syndrome – Hypermobility-Type' (EDS-HT). Approximately 20–40 per cent of the population (Castori *et al.* 2012) might be considered hypermobile and have no symptoms, just joints with a larger than normal range of movement (highly desirable in the performing arts population), whilst only a very small percentage of those will be symptomatic with the 'syndrome' per se (Castori *et al.* 2012). The types of symptoms that those with EDS-HT have significantly overlap with FM, so the management is similar. For much more information about EDS-HT, please read Chapter 15.

Clinical experience suggests Bowen can help considerably with some of the myriad of symptoms that those with EDS, FM and CFS report, such as widespread pain, fatigue and sleep disturbance. Part of the reason for this is Bowen's profound effect on the ANS. Bowen work also has specific ways to lower sensitivity in the fascia through addressing the intrafascial mechanoreceptors. One of the very interesting aspects of working on people with FM is that their sensitivity to touch reduces markedly after only a few Bowen sessions. Because Bowen has such a beneficial effect on sleep, mood and energy levels, it would be advantageous for medical professionals to consider Bowen as a possible healing modality to help reduce some of the symptoms and improve quality of life for those with this debilitating condition.

Conclusions

'Syndrome'-type patients often present quite a challenge to general medical practitioners (Arnold *et al.* 2012; Knight 2013), where they are frequently under-diagnosed, present to the doctors' surgery very regularly and are often dismissed as hypochondriacs or not believed (Arnold *et al.* 2012; Berne 2002; Knight 2013). It might be that Bowen could be considered a very useful treatment adjunct to the conventional approaches to these syndromes, often with co-morbid symptom overlaps (Rahman and Holman 2010). In addition to the evidence-based management of anti-depressant medication, pain medications and psychological (e.g. CBT) interventions (Arnold *et al.* 2012), Bowen is a worthy consideration.

CASE STUDY

| *Isobel Knight*

Merces is a 59-year-old woman who suffers from fibromyalgia and Ehlers-Danlos Syndrome. In my extensive experience of treating autonomic and chronic conditions such as chronic fatigue syndrome, FM and Ehlers-Danlos Syndrome (a genetically heritable connective tissue disorder – see Knight 2011, 2013), 'less is more' is very important in this patient group, owing to them having very low energy levels and 'reserves'. During Merces' first treatment she was given the first few moves of the lower body relaxation work and the first four moves of the upper body relaxation work, which both work on key areas of the nervous system.

Treatment was gradually increased over the coming few sessions until by her last session she could manage the whole body rebalance, namely the lower body, upper body and neck relaxation procedures.

Merces writes, 'I came for Bowen a couple of years ago and did a couple of sessions for about two months and the results were very good. I noticed an improvement in my balance, coordination got better and more importantly my fibromyalgia became more bearable. I strongly recommend the Bowen Technique; you will notice an instant improvement on your health.'

CASE STUDY

| *Keeley Sissons, West Yorkshire, England (www.thepeoplemechanic.co.uk)*

Susan came to me with chronic back pain, which she had suffered from for four years. It began to be troublesome when she was 27 after her eldest son had hit her at the base of her back on a slide. She also has asthma and depression and has been on anti-depressants for 20 years.

When I first treated Susan she said she felt out of alignment and she was! As she lay on my treatment couch she was a like a zigzag, with her feet, hips, shoulders and head all out of alignment. It was so bad that I wondered how I was possibly going to help her. She could barely stand. It took her a full five minutes to turn over from prone to supine and she got out of breath doing it. The pain was etched across her face. She had endometriosis and had fertility treatment to get pregnant. She had bronchiectasis with normal lung bronchi at the top and huge open ones at the bottom. She also has a heart condition where her heart rate can suddenly peak to 180 bpm.

Although there was severe tightness in her upper back and thighs, this eased considerably after three sessions. By her seventh session, ten weeks after her first one, she had managed to reduce her amitriptyline from the original 50 mg to 10 mg daily. Her peak flow readings improved from 350 to 450 and said that she now barely touched her ventolin.

She has had numerous comments from friends about her appearance being much better. She says her coughing fits that usually start at the beginning of October didn't begin until mid November and she also hasn't had any of the chest pain she usually has. She feels amazing and has dubbed herself 'the Bowen evangelist'!

CASE STUDY

| *Keeley Sissons, West Yorkshire, England (www.thepeoplemechanic.co.uk)*
Joanne was seen by me five times during 2013. She suffered from osteoarthritis in her lower back, two herniated discs in her lumbar region, arthritis and degeneration in both hips, and no sensation in her feet except at night when they would feel like they were on fire. She suffered from general anxiety and paranoia and was undergoing a 24-week CBT course.

Joanne writes:

For over 12 months I have suffered from chronic pain in the majority of my body, particularly my hips and back. This, combined with diabetes and its complications, led to what could be described as an uncomfortable life. I got through the day on high doses of pain relief and survived on little or no sleep which as a full-time mum of three was a struggle. I came across Bowen through Facebook and will be the first to admit I was skeptical regarding anything holistic as a result of anxiety issues but after a friendly informal chat with Keeley I 'bit the bullet' and decided to give Bowen a try and booked my first session.

From the first session I experienced positive results, at first in my feet, where after seven years of numbness I acquired some feeling back. As the weeks went on I noticed I was slowly reducing the stronger painkillers I was on and that my blood sugars were the most stable they had been in years and what's more I had the blood test results to prove it. Due to my diabetes I will never be 100 per cent healthy but with the help of Bowen the diabetes is stable, my pain is significantly reduced, and I have feeling in my feet.

Viscero-somatic Reflexes

Parasympathetic reflexes to the organs are relatively easy to trace. Anything from the mid-point of the transverse colon up (and including the liver, kidneys, pancreas, spleen, etc.) is innervated by parasympathetic supply from the vagus, occiput, C1 and C2. Below the mid-point of the transverse colon (including bladder, ovaries, testes, rectum, etc.) is innervated by S2–S4.

- Ovaries and testes: T10–T11 same side as affected organ.
- Adrenals: T8–T10 bi-lateral.
- Kidneys: T9–L1 same side as affected kidney.
- Bladder: T11–L3 bi-lateral.
- Pancreas: T5–T9.
- Liver and gallbladder: T5–T10 right-sided.
- Gastrointestinal tract:
  - oesophagus has right-sided sympathetic reflex from T3–T6
  - stomach – left-sided sympathetic reflex T5–T10
  - small intestine – bi-lateral sympathetic reflex T8–T10
  - ascending colon – right T11–L1 and descending colon and rectum; left L1–L3.
- Lung: T1–T4 (might be bi-lateral if both lungs affected).
- Heart: T1–T5 (more left-sided).
- Eyes, ears, nose and throat: T1–T5 but the trigeminal nerve is also a common pathway for both sympathetic and parasympathetic innervation of the upper respiratory tract.

References

AAEM (2009) *Genetically modified foods*. Available at www.aaemonline.org/gmopost.html, accessed on 12 May 2014.

Arnold, L., Clauw, D., Dunegan, J. and Turk, D. (2012) A framework for fibromyalgia management for primary care providers. *Mayo Clinical Proceedings* 87, 488–496.

Arnold, L., Clauw, D. and McCarberg, H. (2011) Improving the recognition and diagnosis of fibromyalgia. *Mayo Clinical Proceedings* 86 (5), 457–464.

Beal, M. (1985) Viscerosomatic reflexes: a review. *Journal of the American Osteopathic Association* 85 (12), 786–801.

Berne, K. (2002) *Chronic Fatigue Syndrome, Fibromyalgia and Other Invisible Illnesses*. Alameda, CA: Hunter and House.

Butler, D. and Moseley, L. (2013) *Explain Pain* (2nd edition). Adelaide, Australia: Noigroup Publications.

Butler, D. and Matheson, J. (2000) *The Sensitive Nervous System.* Adelaide: NOI Group Publications.

Castori, M., Morlino, S., Celleti, C., Celli, M. *et al.* (2012) Management of pain in the joint hypermobility syndromes (EDS Hypermobility type) principles and a proposal for a multidisciplinary approach. *American Journal of Medical Genetics, Part A* 158a, 2055–2070.

Farmer, A. and Aziz, Q. (2010) Bowel dysfunction in joint hypermobility syndrome and fibromyalgia. In A. Hakim, R. Keer and R. Grahame (eds) *Hypermobility, Fibromyalgia and Chronic Pain.* London: Elsevier.

Finamore, A. *et al.* (2008) Intestinal and peripheral immune response to MON 810 maize ingestion in weaning and old mice. *Journal of Agricultural and Food Chemistry* 56 (23), 11533–11539.

Flor, H., Braun, C., Elbert, T. and Birbaumer, N. (1997) Extensive reorganization of primary somatosensory cortex in chronic back pain patients. *Neuroscience Letters* 224, 5–8.

Grahame, R. (2009) Joint hypermobility syndrome pain. *Current Pain and Headache Reports* 13, 427–433.

Knight, I. (2011) *A Guide to Living with Hypermobility Syndrome: Bending without Breaking.* London: Singing Dragon.

Knight, I. (2013) *A Multidisciplinary Approach to the Management of Ehlers-Danlos Type III Hypermobility Syndrome: Working with the Chronic Complex Patient.* London: Singing Dragon.

Kroghsbo, S. *et al.* (2008) Immunotoxicological studies of genetically modified rice expression PHA-E lectin or Bt toxin in Wistar rats. *Toxicology* 245, 24–34.

Lavergne, R., Cole, D., Kerr, K. and Marshall, L. (2010) Functional impairment in chronic fatigue syndrome, fibromyalgia and multiple chemical sensitivity. *Canadian Family Physician* 56, 57–65.

Liptan, G. (2010) Fascia: a missing link in our understanding of the pathology of fibromyalgia. *Journal of Bodywork and Movement Therapies* 14 (1), 3–12.

IMNA (2011) *Relieving Pain in America: A Blueprint for Transforming Prevention, Care, Education, and Research.* Washington, DC: National Academies Press.

Melzack, R. and Katz, J. (2013) Pain: Wiley interdisciplinary reviews. *Cognitive Science* 4 (1), 1–15.

Moseley, L. (2007a) Reconceptualising pain according to modern pain science. *Physical Therapy Reviews* 12, 169–178.

Moseley, L. (2007b) *Painful Yarns: Metaphors and Stories to Help Understand the Biology of Pain.* Canberra, Australia: Dancing Giraffe Press.

Moseley, L., Butler, D. Beames, T. and Giles, T. (2012) *The Graded Motor Imagery Handbook* (1st edition). Adelaide, Australia: Noigroup Publications.

Nicholas, M., Molloy, A., Tonkin, L. and Beeston, L. (2005) *Manage Your Pain.* Sydney: Souvenir Press.

Rahman, A. and Holman, A. (2010) Fibromyalgia and hypermobility. In A. Hakim, R. Keer and R. Grahame (eds) *Hypermobility, Fibromyalgia and Chronic Pain.* London: Elsevier.

Reinagel, M. (2007) *The Inflammation-Free Diet Plan.* New York: McGraw-Hill.

Sapolsky, R. (2004) *Why Zebras Don't Get Ulcers* (3rd edition). New York: St Martin's Griffin.

Schleip, R. (2010) Biomechanical properties of fascial tissues and their role as pain generators. *Journal of Musculoskeletal Pain* 18 (4), 393–395.

Schleip, R. and Müller, D.G. (2013) Training principles for fascial connective tissues: scientific foundation and suggested practical applications. *Journal of Bodywork and Movement Therapies* 17 (1), 103–115.

Shaikh, M., Hakim, A. and Shenker, N. The physiology of pain. In A. Hakim, R. Keer and R. Grahame (eds) *Hypermobility, Fibromyalgia and Chronic Pain*. London: Elsevier.

Wasley, A. (2014) How GM food is finding its way into your diet. *The Ecologist*, 22 February. Available at www.theecologist.org/News/news_analysis/2288397/how_gm_food_is_finding_its_way_into_your_diet.html, accessed on 19 June 2014.

7

Arms, Shoulders and Upper Back

Kelly Clancy

Our upper extremities (UE) are an extension of our creativity and practicality, designed to provide both an interaction of sense perception of our environment and practical experiences to meet our survival needs. Because of their near-constant functioning, our UE are susceptible to trauma, overuse or dysfunction, especially if the rest of our system is out of balance. In our clients with injuries related to cumulative trauma and repetitive stress, efforts made by the traditional community to treat their conditions have not produced lasting change and permanent healing in our clients' bodies. Revisions to the traditional treatment of such issues in the UE are called for, and, in my clinical experience, I have used Bowenwork as a crucial element to bring about lasting health and healing for these clients with such pain and dysfunction in their UE.

Common orthopaedic therapeutic approaches to treating these conditions of repetitive stress injuries routinely involve concentrating clinical efforts on the localized site of pain, strengthening the involved muscles, or stretching an involved joint. What this traditionalist approach ignores is the role of fascia and the imbalance of tensegrity in the entire UE. If the balance of tensegrity in the upper body is off, then the upper body will never be able to hold its most efficient, most correct shape until its base is in the right place. The metaphor of a house and its foundation is very apt: if the foundation of a house is not level or balanced, then the entire house will be off-kilter, regardless of how strong the walls above the foundation may be. Without its base in the correct alignment, the entire structure of the house will be lopsided, cracking and eventually will lose its integrity and collapse. The foundation must be fixed before the walls of the house are sound.

Tensegrity in the Upper Extremity

Restoring the tensegrity balance in the fascia of the UE, as a way to promote lasting change and healing in clients with these conditions, is a complex, multi-step process.

Before work can be done on either the superficial arm line or deep arm lines, the back and front functional lines of fascia must be addressed and restored to their ideal balance of tensegrity. Utilizing Myers' *Anatomy Trains* (2009) as a roadmap to therapeutic intervention, we can see how the functional lines, superficial front and back lines, and deep front and back arm lines will all play important roles in promoting balance, length, tensile strength and coordination for everyday functional movement patterns.

In treating conditions of the elbow and wrist, the traditional, reductionist approach taken by occupational therapists (OTs), physical therapists (PTs) and certified hand therapists (CHTs) is to stretch the forearm in a linear line. However, this linear model has been proven ineffective because of what we now know about the spiralling effect of fascia in the UE. When either the front or back arm line is restricted, simply addressing the one imbalanced line in isolation will not produce lasting change. Both the front and back superficial lines must be rebalanced, or unwound, in a three-dimensional fashion in order for effective treatment and lasting outcomes to occur. The structural principle of tensegrity shows us that tension in the superficial front arm line (SFAL) changes the tension of the superficial back arm line (SBAL).

The new paradigm of treatment in the upper extremities is to untwist and derotate along the lines of fascia, in a three-dimensional fashion, in order to restore the balanced tensegrity of the whole structure and to produce lasting change in healing in the client's body. Only when this original, optimal rotation or spiral is restored in the tissue will such lasting healing be possible. These spiralling lines of fascia create unique issues in the distal parts of the UE, namely, in the wrist and elbow, because both the tissue above and below the site of pain and dysfunction must be derotated in order to influence the problematic area. In this way the practitioner must treat the whole line of fascia, rather than only treat the location of pain and dysfunction.

Myofascial Length Testing in the Upper Extremity

Myofascial length testing (MFLT) is the last and most important component of the assessment process. It tells the practitioner what and where are the limitations within the client's structure. It reveals that what is seen in gravity may be the client's compensations to stay upright in gravity, but not the true limitations of their structure. It can help delineate between the primary structural holding pattern versus the secondary compensatory holding pattern required to maintain vertical alignment. This allows the practitioner to choose more effective targeted Bowen procedures and subsequently achieve better outcomes by targeting the primary problem. The assessment process allows the practitioner to determine the end feel of the muscle within the myofascial line. It provides an objective measure to document pre- and post-treatment changes, which can be beneficial for patient education, insurance authorization and for the therapist's confirmation that the correct procedures were applied.

MFLT specifically tests isolated muscles within the myofascial meridians and allows specific objective reporting to determine primary restrictions in the structure. It provides a roadmap for specific treatment interventions and determines the effectiveness of those strategies in an objective, progressive way.

Testing becomes paramount when treating UE injuries because it tells the practitioner what capacity exists in the arm lines to rotate in relation to each other, both in internal and external rotation at the shoulder and upper arm, and in supination and pronation at the forearm. This rotational ability lies at the heart of normal functioning in the upper quadrant. When the rotational functioning is altered, the structures within the arm, including the muscles, tendons, ligaments, nerves, vascular and lymphatic systems, will become altered.

By evaluating the rotational ability of the UE, the practitioner is able to determine where within the arm line the deficits lie and can direct their treatment accordingly. Often, the regions most restricted in mobility will translate into hypermobility above or below that segment. It is critical that the practitioner be able to evaluate these areas of rotational restriction because it is at these locations that the client will compensate into another plane of movement or will become hypermobile just proximal or distal to that site. The areas of compensation or hypermobility are often the same sites that the client identifies as painful, as the structures at that site become irritated, inflamed, tractioned or compressed. In traditional orthopaedic treatment, it is at these sites that the physician, PT or OT will direct treatment, but these painful sites may not be where the origin of the problem lies.

Specific Concerns of the Upper Extremity

First, common pathologic conditions of the UE related to repetitive stress injuries will be described: elbow and forearm pathologies, including medial and lateral epicondylitis; wrist pathologies, including carpal tunnel syndrome, carpometacarpal (CMC) arthritis, de Quervain's tenosynovitis and triangular fibrocartilage complex (TFCC) tears; and shoulder pathologies, including rotator cuff tendonitis and thoracic outlet syndrome (TOS). Next, traditional approaches to the treatment of these conditions, and any drawbacks to those treatment modalities, will be summarized. Then alternative treatment approaches to the same condition will be discussed, namely, a combination of Bowenwork and an at-home exercise programme.

One of the reasons that Bowenwork is an effective approach to treating these difficult conditions of the UE is that Bowenwork directly relieves inflammation in the body's soft tissue and the overall influence of inflammation in the body. Inflammation often accompanies these UE conditions and, as Bowen practitioners know firsthand, if the body is reacting in an inflammatory way, a client will never get optimal results of lasting change and healing. A client must optimize their healing through proper nutrition and hydration, and a Bowen practitioner can create an environment where a client's nervous system can reach a state of parasympathetic normalization. Once a client's nervous system is calmer and the influence of inflammation is reduced, the changes that practitioners and clients make together can produce actual, lasting change that will hold in the client's body long-term.

Elbow Pathologies

Abnormalities within the superficial front arm line (SFAL) will produce pain on the medial aspect of the elbow and involve the common flexor tendons. Lateral epicondylitis is a problem of the superficial back arm line (SBAL) and it involves the forearm extensor tendons at their origin site at the elbow, with pain on the outside of the elbow.

Conventional treatment approaches to medial and lateral epicondylitis include the following:

- ultrasound therapy

- moist heat

- friction massage and general localized soft-tissue massage

- passive stretching of forearm flexors and extensors

- electrical stimulation

- iontophoresis

- corticosteroid injections administered by a physician

- circumventional forearm bracing.

Many of these localized treatment approaches may temporarily reduce pain and dysfunction in the elbow, but they rarely produce lasting change and healing. An imbalanced pattern of fascia will almost always produce pain, inflammation and dysfunction. If this imbalanced pattern is not addressed globally, lasting improvement will not occur for our clients. Progress in the localized, conventional treatments produces short-lived gains; however, the pain at the site of the elbow often moves to another location. That client may discontinue treatment with one provider, after experiencing a short-term gain, only for pain to occur later at another site in the UE. The client may then go on to see a second provider with a speciality in that second site of pain.

In addition to only producing temporary gains, some of the treatments listed above can cause additional pain and dysfunction. For example, forearm bracing is designed to relieve tension at the elbow. However, such bracing often compresses the radial and median nerves at the supinator and pronator to a greater degree, adding additional nerve compression to the pre-existing conditions in the elbow.

An alternative treatment plan, utilizing Bowenwork and an at-home exercise programme, can positively impact clients with medial and lateral epicondylitis. And yet some clients with the same issues may not improve when undertaking the same alternative treatment; their injury may continue until additional interventions are implemented.

1. Bowen procedures to affect elbow pain should address not only localized elbow alignment, but also pelvic positioning in relation to the thorax, neck, shoulder and wrist.

2. An at-home exercise programme would include stretches related to the thorax, shoulder, elbow and wrist complexes – not simply the elbow.

3. Stretching must be implemented in all three dimensions and focus on global issues of fascia and imbalances in all of the arm lines. Such stretches would involve lengthening the latissimus dorsi, pectoralis major and minor, biceps, triceps and forearm flexors and extensors.

Wrist Pathologies

Pathologies within the deep front arm line (DFAL) would include diagnoses of bicipital tendonitis, radial nerve impingements at the forearm and thumb-related disorders. These specific conditions can present in isolation or in combined pain complaints in relation to the altered tensegrity of the DFAL itself and its relationship to the other fascial lines within the arm. Because the end-range test positioning of the deep arms involves an internal rotation and pronation pattern, we often see deep structural imbalances within this line affecting the anterior labrum of the shoulder, the deep rotation patterns of the forearm, and subsequently the alignment of the carpals within the wrist and thumb.

Carpal Tunnel Syndrome

Carpal tunnel syndrome directly involves the SFAL. The SFAL begins proximally at the latissimus dorsi and pectoralis major, and then extends into the medial intramuscular septum to the wrist and digital flexors.

The structure of the carpal tunnel forms a passageway for eight flexor tendons, two to each finger, and the median nerve as they pass through to the hand. Whenever there is asymmetry in the carpal bones, or an inflammatory process that involves the tendons or outlying structures, the tunnel pressures will increase in the carpal tunnel, thereby compressing the median nerve. This median nerve compression will result in a client experiencing paresthesias or numbness in the first three digits of the hand. Compression of the median nerve may be at the wrist itself, or the site of compression may be proximal to the wrist, based on the orientation of the fascia and the structures influenced by the SFAL. Traditional diagnostic studies to rule out or rule in the diagnosis of carpal tunnel syndrome include electromyogram (EMG) studies, provocative percussion testing such as Tinel's test, and compression testing such as Phalen's and Durkan's tests. These tests can determine if there is a localized site of compression at the carpal tunnel but will not determine if there are other sources of tractioning or nerve irritation that may be contributing to the distal symptoms.

Current traditional OT/PT treatment approaches to carpal tunnel syndrome include:

- night splinting
- placing the wrist in a neutral to 15 degrees extension positioning to maximize the carpal tunnel opening
- ultrasound
- phonophoresis – the use of ultrasound to deliver corticosteroid medication
- rest
- localized stretches to the forearm and flexor tendons
- active tendon and nerve gliding exercises
- ergonomic interventions.

When traditional, conservative interventions fail, then surgical intervention is applied. The carpal tunnel is enlarged by transecting the transverse carpal ligament, thus creating a larger space for the median nerve and flexor tendons to glide and thereby reducing compression of those structures.

However, Bowenwork is an excellent first line treatment for carpal tunnel syndrome, and an alternative treatment plan focused on a structural model for carpal tunnel syndrome might include the following:

1. Therapeutic interventions for carpal tunnel and nerve compressions in the forearm should address pelvic positioning in addition to the thorax, neck, shoulder and wrist alignment.

2. Like the programme for medial and lateral epicondylitis, an at-home exercise programme would include stretches related to the thorax, shoulder, elbow and wrist complexes – not simply the wrist alone.

3. Stretching must be implemented in all three dimensions and focused on global issues of fascia and imbalances in all of the arm lines. Such stretches would involve lengthening the latissimus dorsi, pectoralis major and minor, biceps, triceps and forearm flexors and extensors.

4. The fascial lengthening programme requires cueing for end-range positioning to ensure that the client is not compensating in another plane of movement if the normal end-range length of the connective tissue is not available. This can be quite problematic in the UE due to the complex spiral nature of the arm. Clients frequently will compensate into a valgus positioning at the elbow, an anterior subluxation at the humerus, or an ulnar deviation pattern at the wrist, as a means to compensate for a loss of mobility anywhere within the fascial lines. It is imperative that the practitioner monitor these movements carefully, as it is these compensations that are often the primary pain complaint.

5. Clients with issues in the carpal tunnel would also benefit from proximal stabilization exercises of the shoulder blades, specifically the scapular stabilization muscles encouraging scapular depression and retraction.

6. Distal strengthening at the wrist and forearm is counter-indicated for this condition initially until the proximal structures can resume their stability function in UE movement patterns.

7. Once the connective tissue has been reorganized in a more aligned and balanced position, nerve glide exercises may be added to the exercise programme. A common mistake is to assign nerve glide exercises too early, before the fascial structure has been reorganized.

CMC Arthritis, de Quervain's Tenosynovitis and TFCC Tears

When the DFAL is restricted, the client will lose the ability to fully extend the elbow due to bicep shortening, and the elbow will be forced into a valgus positioning with abduction of the lower arm. Forearm end-range supination will be lost, and compensatory patterns at the wrist will be reinforced leading to overuse of the CMC joint at the base of the thumb, de Quervain's tenosynovitis affecting the thumb extensor and abductor, and triangular fibrocartilage complex (TFCC) disruptions in the ulnar wrist.

Traditional treatment strategies again would include:

- ultrasound
- phonophoresis
- iontophoresis
- isolated joint splinting of the thumb and wrist
- local cortisone injections.

When conservative management fails, then surgical intervention is undertaken in the following forms:

- bone excisions

- tendon transfers

- extensor compartment releases.

Clinically, it is not uncommon to see clients who have multiple surgeries of the UE in an attempt to alleviate the myriad of symptoms they present.

For clients with such symptoms, fascial interventions that affect the relationship of the deep front line to its corresponding anatomical fascial lines are imperative. A structural, postural approach which addresses the fascial superficial and deep arm lines would be warranted as a first line in therapeutic intervention to restore the tensional balance of these structures, thus taking off the tension patterns that are leading to arthritic changes, tendon irritation and cartilage damage. After first restoring the tensegrity balance throughout the UE, the practitioner's goal should be to ensure that these new postural patterns are further engrained within the client's nervous system patterning. At this point, a treatment plan might include:

1. movement lessons

2. proximal stabilization exercises

3. ergonomic education

4. manual therapy.

Shoulder Pathologies

Pathologies within the deep front and back arm lines include proximal issues related to the rotator cuff musculature and distally in the thumb and carpals. Tensegrital imbalances affecting these lines will affect all of the muscular balancing of the glenohumeral joint, elbow and wrist. The deep back arm line includes the levator, rhomboids, infraspinatus, supraspinatus, subscapularis, teres minor into the triceps, ulnar periosteum to the ulnar wrist, and hypothenar musculature. When these imbalances occur proximally, the deep external rotators will cinch the posterior capsule and shear the anterior humerus forward. Limitations will be present in abduction, flexion, horizontal adduction and external rotation.

Rotator Cuff Tendonitis

The rotator cuff is a complex of four stabilizing muscles and tendons, including the infraspinatus, teres minor, subscapularis and supraspinatus. They naturally hold the humerus in the glenoid fossa, allowing the joint to be stable and mobile for three dimensional movements of the UE. When the tensegrital balance is altered – whether due to scapular dysfunction, postural asymmetries such as a forward head posture or kyphotic thoracic positioning, trauma, or surgical intervention – then dysfunction will be present.

Again, with these disorders, typical treatment interventions involve:

- localized splinting to immobilize these regions

- corticosteroids

- ultrasound

- electrical stimulation

- strengthening exercises.

These treatments can lead to temporary reduction in symptoms but again will not heal the postural dysfunction. Balancing the fascial tensegrity will be the only way that the tension and compression forces can be restored and lead to long-term resolution of symptoms. Often, when localized modalities and treatments are applied, we either see a temporary change in symptoms that is short-lived, or we will see a translation of symptoms proximally or distally within the fascial line into the elbow, shoulder or neck.

An alternative treatment plan might include:

1. Treatments such as Bowenwork, which address the pelvis, thorax, neck, shoulder, elbow, forearm and wrist as part of a balancing session, would naturally affect all of the fascial arm lines and other lines that influence them. This will lead to a normalization of the tensional balance of the lines and subsequently the joint positioning throughout the upper quadrant.

2. Movement lessons, shoulder range-of-motion exercises and postural retraining can be helpful, as well as stabilization strengthening once the alignment has been restored.

3. Ergonomic education regarding work-station positioning, home computer set-up and postural positioning with activities of daily living are also essential in promoting long-term optimal alignment of the tensional patterns of the upper quadrant.

Thoracic Outlet Syndrome

Thoracic outlet syndrome (TOS) is a condition most often seen in populations where UE repetition is involved. Previously, it was seen in clients who were performing overhead activities in a sustained fashion, such as dry wallers, painters or machinists.

More recently there has been a dramatic increase in incidence in computer users who also are experiencing nerve compression, pain complaints and loss of function throughout the UE. These clients can be more complex to diagnose and to treat based on their multiple symptoms and complexity related to postural asymmetries. Ergonomic factors, as well as the demands that our society is placing on interfacing with computers for work, social networking and entertainment, add to the complexity of finding a long-term solution to this growing problem.

The anatomy involved in TOS classically includes the anterior and middle scalenes, where the neurovascular bundle to the UE lies. This neurovascular bundle houses the nerves, veins and arteries that continue into the UE; the bundle continues distally into the pectoralis minor and then bifurcates into the upper and distal arm. Anywhere along this pathway these nerves can become tractioned, compressed, or a combination of both. Symptoms may include numbness in the fourth and fifth digit, sometimes numbness into the other digits if the middle trunk of the brachial plexus becomes irritated, diminished coordination including frequent dropping of items, loss of dexterity, pain anywhere from the neck, shoulder, axilla, upper arm, forearm and into the hand. If the irritation is severe enough, vascular changes, such as color changes, and lymphatic symptoms, such as swelling of the hand and digits, will be seen.

Usually, the pain starts in a vague, isolated pattern anywhere in the arm, and, if the irritating factors remain, this pain pattern will spread and become more diffuse and increase in intensity. It may disrupt sleep, make home and work duties difficult and interfere with normal daily functioning.

This disorder can be quite frustrating for the client and healthcare provider who may not be well versed in this syndrome. Misdiagnosis is very common, and many times medical interventions, such as surgeries to remove the anterior and middle scalenes, first rib resections, nerve decompression at the elbow, carpal tunnel surgery, Botox and lidocaine injections and pharmacologic treatments will be implemented to no avail in an attempt to alleviate symptoms. Many of our current diagnostic studies, such as nerve conduction studies and clinical examination, do not detect one true source of the nerve compression, thus making diagnosis and intervention even more difficult.

TOS does not respond well to traditional therapeutic interventions such as strengthening. Symptoms can sometimes but not always respond to stretching routines that honour the neural and fascial tension patterns within the system. Current standard therapy programmes performed for TOS clients include the following:

- treatment to the neck, shoulder and shoulder blade

- strengthening

- general conditioning.

Localized treatments such as these often fail to alleviate symptoms because of their reductionist approach, attempting to treat only the symptoms while ignoring the overall postural patterns which lie at the core of this condition.

The majority of TOS origins lie in poor posture, poor ergonomic work practices and overuse. There are a smaller amount of diagnosed cases that are due to an extra cervical rib, enlarged transverse cervical processes, or Pancoast tumours, but they exist in small numbers.

Most often, the TOS pattern starts in the rib cage and its relationship to the pelvis. Because of poor ergonomics, heavy excessive workload, anxiety in the workplace, previous injuries/surgeries, trauma or general deconditioning, changes in pelvic and thorax alignment will be present, and shallow inhalation and exhalation breathing patterns will develop due to poor excursion of the diaphragm. Consequently, the muscles of secondary inhalation, involving the scalenes, levator scapula, upper trapezius, sternocleidomastoid (SCM) muscle and levator costarum, will begin to take over. When this occurs, there will be a narrowing of space between the neck and the shoulders due to the vertical nature of the breathing pattern of the rib cage, instead of the normal three-dimensional expansion present in normal breathing. The yoke, being the region bordered by the clavicle anteriorly, the spine of the scapula posteriorly and the head medially, will become altered and will no longer be positioned horizontally to the floor. The yoke will narrow in width and/or depth and will tilt anteriorly or posteriorly based on the positioning of the thorax. Subsequently, this yoke space, which houses important vascular and nerve structures including the brachial artery and the brachial plexus nerve bundles, will become altered in either compression, tractioning or both. The head will often come forward based on the alignment of the arms and often a posteriorly tilted thorax. The scapula will then be forced into scapular protraction based on the rib cage positioning. This will cause the shoulders and glenohumeral joints to internally rotate.

Due to the load being placed on the secondary inhalation muscles to now become the primary breathers, they will naturally increase in density and strength. Their length will modify to incorporate and meet the demands of primary breathing to sustain the life of the organism. These length and girth changes will then further affect the postural positioning of the surrounding bones, muscles, nerves and lymphatic system, often creating further changes such as nerve compression and/or cervical disc herniation.

These asymmetries in the postural alignment and tension patterns will often translate both proximally and distally, creating imbalances down the whole arm and into the head and neck, further tractioning and disrupting the normal positioning and function of the nerves, blood supply and lymphatic system.

Bowenwork provides a unique, alternative approach to treating TOS, and such a plan may follow:

1. Because Bowenwork provides global three-dimensional input to the body, especially affecting the alignment of the pelvis, thorax and cervical region, the body has the ability to alter the dysfunctional tension patterns of the diaphragm and subsequently begin to normalize the breathing patterns, which will affect the structural alignment of the rib cage, neck, head and UE.

2. The nervous system will be directly affected with Bowen intervention, and the system can resume its balance of normal parasympathetic functioning, allowing the breathing patterns to also normalize and the client to return to more relaxed state of overall functioning.

3. Postural and movement exercises can simultaneously be initiated, reinforcing the individual's ability to restore alignment of the structures.

4. Exercises involving diaphragmatic breathing can be emphasized to ensure the re-patterning and strengthening of the diaphragm will return to normal dominance.

TOS remains a complex medical condition which can be severely debilitating. Strategies affecting the nervous system, structural fascial system and musculoskeletal system to restore alignment and tensegrity are imperative to restoring balance to the whole system and subsequently restoring normal functioning and quality of life to the individual.

CASE STUDY

| *Ros Elliott-Özlek, Izmir, Turkey (www.bowen.web.tr)*

Keziban is a hairdresser in her mid-30s. She has been running her own salon for about ten years now. I met her about three years ago when she had a serious case of carpal tunnel syndrome brought on through the nature of her work. At that time she couldn't even hold a pen in her right hand and therefore couldn't use the handheld hairdryer at all. She dropped things and was in constant severe pain. Doctors had recommended operating, but warned her that this kind of operation would need to be repeated and the maximum number of times it could work effectively was only three. Keziban did not want to have the operation as her work was obviously going to lead to more repetitive starin injury (RSI) and further operations, which would eventually end her career.

We decided to try the Bowen Technique on her, and over the next few weeks she had regular sessions, starting with minimal moves, working up to cover all the basic procedures with specific procedures for the arms and shoulders. From weekly treatments we were able to space out the sessions to two weeks, then three, then a month, and suddenly she was absolutely fine for about six months. I would drop by the salon on my way to work and ask how she'd been since the last session. We would then decide when to arrange another session.

I should perhaps add here that Turkish ladies' hair can be very long, thick and naturally curly, and blow-drying a typical customer's long hair can take a stylist at least half an hour of heavy work using their wrists and hands while holding a heavy and powerful blow-dryer. After the first six months' reprieve (almost like being in 'remission' as she put it) the pain started again, and since then it has had phases when it is severe, moderate (5–7 out of 10) or minimal (0–2 out of 10). Different approaches are needed according to Keziban's pain levels and these are greatly influenced by the following factors:

- previous accidents – some car prangs, which affected her lower back and legs

- dehydration – she never drank water much until she started Bowen, but now tries to have two litres a day minimum

- cigarettes – she was smoking about a packet a day three years ago but gave up after six months

- genetic factors – every female member of her family has this problem to a greater or lesser extent. I have treated her sister, who was not a hairdresser, but had similar RSI through giving injections all day to hospital patients. She responded very quickly to minimal Bowen moves and only needed one session, the effects of which lasted about six months

- physique – Keziban's wrists and those of her family are very thin and small-boned, but the skin around them is thicker and often shows oedema. Her skin in general is tight, with very little 'slack' for Bowen moves. In some places this is because of muscle spasm, but other areas are simply built this way.

In the second year since starting Bowen, Keziban made some big changes in exercise and diet, lost a lot of weight (about 15 kilos) and ran/walked on a treadmill for up to 40 minutes a day. This has not continued and she is now the same weight as when I first met her, and doesn't exercise. We also added a wide range of specific exercises to strengthen her large muscle groups and thus reduce the strain on the small muscles. I can now honestly say that, although all these factors seemed important, the biggest cause of flare-ups in her carpal tunnel syndrome was this next one:

- stress – this seems to be, actually, the largest contributing factor – more important, even, than hectic days working overtime before national holidays (when everyone wants their hair done to look nice for the festive celebrations). At certain times Keziban explained to me about problems with her staff when she was feeling a lack of support from her team, and there were several periods when staff just left without notice, and even tried to persuade regular customers to come to their own new salons. At these times her pain and inability to hold things increased dramatically.

Keziban has said that if she remembers how she was when she started with Bowen, there is now no comparison. In those days the pain was constant. Now it is 'manageable' but flares up now and then. Here is her summary in her own words, translated from the Turkish:

Three years ago my arms and wrists hurt so much that I couldn't work. I couldn't hold things or straighten out my hands and fingers, and they were always half-clenched. I met Ros through a friend and we started the Bowen therapy sessions. I didn't feel anything during the first session but the next day my wrists hurt less and I could work better. I would say that during these three years since that day, I have about 80 per cent less pain than before and can still carry out my work. Thank you Ros and Bowen. (Keziban Özgun, December 2013)

CASE STUDY

| *Jean Hanlin, Glasgow, Scotland*

The client is a 55-year-old woman who has a senior position in a full-time healthcare occupation.

She was referred for Bowen therapy from her employer attendance management service.

The client had a history of right shoulder pain. In August 2013 she experienced an 'acute frozen shoulder episode'. The symptoms were managed by her GP with prescribed analgesia and a referral for physiotherapy. After eight weeks she had some improvement in mobility and some reduction in pain, however pain relief medication caused gastric disturbance and NSAID analgesia was stopped. Physiotherapy consisted of exercise regime and continued during Bowen therapy.

The client attended for Bowen therapy in November 2013, presenting with acute pain in right shoulder, right side neck restriction of movement and with pain radiating down her left upper arm. Her symptoms impacted on all daily tasks at home, work and leisure that involved lifting, gripping, driving, carrying equipment. The client struggled with her daily swim.

The client received a total of five sessions of Bowen, three appointments a week apart, then a 28-day break, and then two appointments weekly.

Assessment

At the first appointment assessment, I identified that the right shoulder's range of movement was very limited (e.g. elevation less than 90 degrees), that there was a slight weak grip in the right hand and poor mobility in her neck area. There was no history of trauma noted by client. On the second appointment the client was aware of changes in and reductions to her pain levels and improved coping with work activities without increase in pain and also improved sleep. The client also reported to remembering sustaining a 'strain' in her upper back when lifting a cushion from the floor a few months earlier, but didn't relate this as causal factor to acute shoulder issue. The basic relaxation work, shoulder, elbow and wrist, was performed during treatment with an ensuing improvement to range of movement.

At the third appointment, the client's pain was now more tender in nature rather than painful, with an improved range of movement. The physiotherapist was also pleased with level of improvement, with the client able to swim breaststroke pain-free. During this session, the three BRMs (basic relaxation moves), pelvic, shoulder procedures were performed and the right shoulder elevation was now over 90 degrees.

By the fourth appointment (following a four-week break, as per shoulder protocol), the client was very impressed with her progress to date. She reported being pain-free most of the time, with only occasional twinges that were no longer debilitating. There was now full range of movement in both shoulders, with some weakness felt in right forearm/hand.

By the fifth appointment the client was delighted with her progress. She was now pain-free, with marked improvement in mobility and range of movement, a general improved wellbeing and now able to cope with most daily activities. There remained a slight weakness in right-hand grip that sometime affected intrinsic finger movements. In the treatment, BRM 1 and 2 stoppers were performed, with procedure to address the pectoralis muscles, and the outcome was that she was pain-free; that she had full range movement in both shoulders, neck and her hand grip showing marked improvement.

Client Comment

After Bowen Therapy: my shoulders/arms have fully recovered and I'm pain free. Back to swimming, shopping, lifting equipment, etc. and practising the fiddle again. Thank you so much for therapy sessions. I'm sure Bowen was key to my recovery. (SM)

References

Myers, T. W. (2009) *Anatomy Trains: Myofascial Meridians for Manual and Movement Therapists* (2nd edition). Edinburgh: Elsevier.

8

Headaches, Migraines and the Temporomandibular Joint

Background

Tom Bowen developed a number of procedures that address the head, neck and jaw. These include what he referred to as the headache, upper respiratory, TMJ (temporomandibular joint), eye, sinus, additional moves to aid vision and additional moves for sinus problems.

My interest in these moves started in 1994 when I observed Oswald Rentsch treating a participant on one of the early Bowen courses in Somerset, UK. During one of the coffee breaks, I was sitting next to a lady who was wearing very thick glasses. Ossie approached her and, with her permission, worked on her head with a series of moves which I had never seen before. The whole process took about a minute and then he walked off. After a couple of minutes, this lady took off her glasses and began to cry. When she had settled down she revealed that she was so short-sighted that she had never been able to see as far as the end of the room before, and now she was able to. I have no idea how long this reaction lasted, but it was impressive enough to get me intrigued.

Whilst most of the upper respiratory work affects the superficial and deep fascia on the front of the body, the moves on the head are done over joints, blood vessels, muscles and sutures. There has been much debate about what type of sensory nerves exist in the sutures and what their role is. John Upledger posited in a short study (Retzlaff *et al.* 1978) that these receptors existed in the cranial sutures to sense movement, an underlying principle of craniosacral therapy. They are similar to the nerves that exist in all joints in the body – in other words, free nerve endings, Golgi, Ruffini and Pacini type endings. Some of these nerve endings are quite insensitive, so it is difficult to know precisely what their function is. Most of the Bowen work on the head was not taught officially until a few years ago, under the banner 'specialized procedures 2', most of which was derived from Ossie Rentsch's original notes from the 1970s when he was still working with Tom Bowen.

Bowen Upper Respiratory and TMJ Work

Most of the deep cervical fascia effectively hangs off the base of the cranium, where much of the Bowen work around the head and neck is done. Specifically, the fascia attaches on to the superior nuchal line of the occiput (where moves 3 and 4 of the neck procedure are done), the mastoid process of the temporal bone (where the drainage moves finish in the upper respiratory work), the inferior border of the mandible (where the upper respiratory moves start), the styloid process of the temporal bone (where we do the moves behind the top of the mandible) and the hyoid (which we address with the moves on the throat). It also attaches on to the sphenomandibular ligament (which we go over when we do the first moves of the TMJ itself).

The Bowen upper respiratory work, which Bowen apparently used for hay fever sufferers, starts by addressing, among other structures, the attachments of the mylohyoid muscles, the submandibular glands, the top of the superficial front line at the sternal attachment of the sternocleidomastoid (SCM) muscle and the pre-tracheal fascia (which blends in with the pericardium). The gentle rocking of the trachea also affects the carotid sheath, which surrounds the carotid artery, internal jugular vein, cervical lymph nodes and vagus nerve. Finally, the gentle massaging movements around the large SCM muscles affect the many lymph nodes in the neck, as well as the vagus nerve itself.

One of the functions of the upper respiratory work seems to be to encourage drainage and flow (particularly lymphatic flow) downwards towards the thoracic outlet. Bowen practitioners are generally taught to do this before going on to the TMJ work as this helps create a passage for outflow from the neck and cranium into the lymphatic ducts which drain into the venous system. A similar principle is used in manual lymphatic drainage and osteopathy.

The TMJ work itself then encourages blood flow both to and from the cranium (particularly outflow through the jugular foramen). Signs that this is happening are that people often report seeing more vivid colours as blood flow improves to the eyes, a feeling of fluid trickling down their throats, a softening of the SCM and trapezius muscles and a desire to swallow because of stimulation of the vagus and glossopharyngeal nerves, both of which travel through the jugular foramen. It is unclear why, but this work seems to create more space generally in the cranium, allowing the hard palate to fall by releasing held patterns in the temporal area and particularly across the sagittal suture at the top of the head. The positive implications of any therapeutic interventions that encourage blood flow to the cranium are discussed in detail in the fascinating book *The Downside of Upright Posture* which blames the onset of Alzheimer's, Parkinson's and MS on the unique problems faced by our bipedal stance of insufficient blood flow to and from the cranium (Flanagan 2010).

Through working on babies, I have seen how powerful the TMJ work is at changing the shape of babies' heads and particularly in lowering the hard palate – something that can cause feeding, speech and dental problems unless it is addressed. The power of this work came home to me when I was teaching in France a few years ago. One of the students related how, when her baby was born, it had a hard ridge of bone at the top of the head where the fontanels normally are. Worried that her baby might have a condition known as craniosynostosis, which means that the sutures are fused, she instinctively did the TMJ work when her baby was only a few hours old. She related, with tears in her eyes, that while she and her husband watched, both the anterior and posterior fontanels gradually opened and the ridge of bone at the sagittal suture began to soften and subside.

Ramifications of Problems with the TMJ

There are many factors that might affect the functioning of the TMJ and most of these are poorly understood (possibly because they are so complex). Although there are many treatment options available for people with TMJ dysfunction (TMJD), there is no widely accepted treatment protocol and a general lack of good evidence for any one treatment approach exists (Bessa-Nogueira, Vasconcelos and Niederman 2008).

Probably the most common and least invasive treatment approach involves the use of occlusal splints of various kinds, pain killers and cognitive behavioural therapy (CBT). Because issues in the TMJ (particularly if this involves long-term inflammation in tissues around the joint) can lead to an increased sensitivity to external stimuli – in other words a stimulation of the sympathetic fight or flight response as outlined in Chapter 6 – this can have an effect on the heart and breathing as well as causing anxiety (Orlando *et al.* 2007). The reason for this is because the TMJ, the ligaments around it, the articular disc and the teeth themselves are innervated by the trigeminal nerve. This nerve is unusual as it has both sensory and motor components, which means that sensitization caused by inflammation in any of those structures can trigger a motor response, leading to a variety of unusual and seemingly unrelated symptoms such as muscle pain or breathing problems. This is particularly the case with inflammation in root canal fillings and it is wise for clients to have these checked out regularly, even if they are asymptomatic (as they often are). This is easy to do by requesting an X-ray, as inflammation will affect the periodontal ligament. Chronic inflammation from any source is a potential risk to health, but specifically there is a proven link between coronary heart disease and periodontitis (Spahr *et al.* 2006).

The relationship between TMJ disorders and posture has been discussed in the chapter in back pain and is something that has been postulated by osteopaths for many years. More recently, a study found a clear relationship between TMJ disorders and head forward posture (Kritsineli and Shim 1991), something that changes visibly after Bowen, with clients standing more upright.

Conditions of the Inner Ear

Conditions that affect the inner ear can be horrible for the sufferer and really affect quality of life. Labyrinthitis, tinnitus, Ménière's disease and vestibular problems are all too common, particularly in the elderly, and can affect people's ability to undertake normal daily activities. Again, it is poorly understood as to why many of these conditions occur and treatment usually involves long courses of drugs such as betahistine and diazepam. In my experience, Bowen can help considerably to lessen some of the symptoms of these conditions, especially dizziness, nausea and pain. A recent case involved a woman who was almost housebound because of Ménière's. She was unable to play the violin (her passion) or sing in the local choir because of her extreme sensitivity to noise. Attempted trips to the theatre or dinner with friends would often result in a hurried return home with symptoms of nausea and extreme dizziness. This particular lady noticed an improvement after only two sessions of Bowen and, whilst the condition was not cured and she needed ongoing sessions, she found she was again able to do the things she loved. Many of her friends reported that her life had been transformed.

Glue Ear

Children can suffer a lot with inner ear problems, especially around teething time. The condition known as glue ear, or otitis media with effusion as it is technically called, is exactly that – fluid in the middle ear. Nobody knows why, but glue ear involves the fluid becoming more sticky, probably due to a lack of drainage via various channels, including the Eustachian tube. Dentists have observed a relationship between TMJ problems, bedwetting and glue ear, something that is also not easy to explain (Youniss 1991). Because so much of Bowen work around the temporal area encourages fluid drainage, many practitioners have reported children avoiding the need for grommets or T-tubes after Bowen sessions. Many Bowen moves around the cranium actually pass over areas where blood vessels and nerves exit the cranium through passageways in the bone (foramen), which is possibly why people with congestion and sinus problems find Bowen helpful. Examples of these types of move are over the supraorbital and infraorbital foramina, which carry branches of the trigeminal nerve as well as various veins and arteries.

Facial Palsy, Bell's Palsy and Trigeminal Neuralgia

There are several major structures that pass close to the temporal bones and the inner ear that are particularly susceptible to pressure, inflammation or entrapment. Some of these structures include the cranial nerves V, VII, IX, X and XI as well as the jugular vein and carotid artery. The two nerves affected in facial palsy and Bell's Palsy are the facial nerve and the trigeminal nerve. If we have a look at various areas where these nerves might get compromised, we realize why Bowen can help in these situations by creating more space in the surrounding connective tissue and improving blood supply to nerves, a crucial factor in their efficient functioning. Some Bowen moves address the facial nerve directly and I have seen myself considerable improvement after Bowen in not only pain but also the facial 'droop' experienced by people with Bell's Palsy.

How Bowen Can Help TMJD

Although the three pairs of muscles involved in closing the mouth (the temporalis, masseter and medial pterygoid) are some of the strongest muscles in the body, the lateral pterygoid (as well as the digastric, mylohyoid and geniohyoid which assist with the initial opening movement) are relatively weak by comparison. The muscles of mastication are controlled by the trigeminal nerve, one of the few cranial nerves to be affected adversely by inflammation and tissue damage because of its dual sensory and motor functions. The superior head of the pterygoid attaches on to the greater wing of the sphenoid (the small indentation just back from the corner of the eye) and the articular disc and fibrous capsule of the TMJ. The inferior lateral pterygoid goes from a plate lower down on the sphenoid to the mandible itself. Bowen work addresses the pterygoid muscles by directly moving over them in both posterior and inferior directions. The pterygoids (Figure 8.1) have interesting functions in terms of coordinated movement of the jaw and any irregularity will create deviation in movement and bite, something that has ramifications for the neck and posture in general.

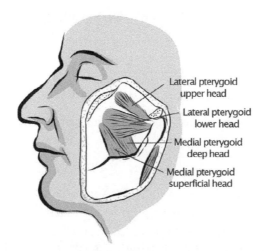

Lateral pterygoid
upper head

Lateral pterygoid
lower head

Medial pterygoid
deep head

Medial pterygoid
superficial head

Figure 8.1 The pterygoid muscles – enlarged view
Source: Martin Gordon

Some of the TMJ moves also affect the sphenoid, which has a very important articulation (a synchondrosis) with the occiput, deep in the base of the cranium. Cranial osteopaths consider the relationship between the sphenoid and the occiput of vital importance in terms of alignment of the body and, certainly, when we work in this area, people often report sensations as if the whole of one side of their body is lengthening or shortening.

In view of the importance of the sphenoid, it is crucial to understand its potential effect on the whole body. These influences will either be bottom-up or top-down. The reason for this is that there are strong dural and fascia attachments at the sphenoid, both of which can create shortening or rotational patterns in the body. The need to look beyond treating local symptoms came home to me recently when treating a woman for TMJ pain and a clicking jaw. Whilst working in the region of her jaw, she experienced a sensation of a pull through the whole left side of her body. As it turned out, the originating cause of her jaw pain came from being thrown off a horse aged eight years old, where her left foot became caught in the stirrup and she was dragged along the ground for a considerable distance. This had affected all the fascia through her left side, pulling into the attachments of the front fascia at the base of her cranium and jaw. Although her pain decreased significantly by working on the TMJ itself, the problem did not resolve completely until I had addressed the pelvic imbalance caused by the accident.

Headaches and Migraines

There are various causative factors in headaches and migraines, which involve one or more of the following:

- irritation of the meninges and their blood supplies (dural arteries and pial arteries)
- some of the large veins such as the temporal artery
- some of the spinal and cranial nerves, particularly the trigeminal
- certain muscles of the head and neck
- intracranial vasodilation and/or vasoconstriction
- neuronal excitability in the cerebral cortex (particularly the occipital cortex) in migraines
- hormonal changes.

The link between the jaw and migraines was supported by a recent study in Israel that discovered a link between chewing gum and headaches (Watemberg *et al.* 2014), but there is still no clear mechanism involved. A small-scale study of 39 participants conducted by Nikke Ariffe in the UK between 2001 and 2002 looked at the impact of Bowen on people with migraines: 31 participants reported a positive change in severity and/or frequency of attacks after Bowen (Ariffe 2002).

One of the most obvious explanations as to why Bowen might help people with headaches and migraines is that the TMJ work directly affects the temporal artery. This artery is known to be a major influence in both migraines and headaches (Tunis and Wolff 1953) and supplies oxygenated blood to the head and neck. Interestingly, when we move over this artery (which lies just above and in front of the top of the ear) practitioners often notice a 'jump' as the artery reacts. In terms of Bowen's effect on migraines, the TMJ work also addresses the operation of the vagus nerve, having a direct effect on some of the unpleasant side effects of migraine such as nausea and vomiting (Wilson-Pauwels, Stewart and Akesson 1997). In addition, the Bowen neck work affects the sub-occipital muscles in the neck and the dural membranes, both factors in headache and migraine.

CASE STUDY

Joanna Austen, the Therapy Room, Bodmin,
Cornwall (www.bowenincornwall.co.uk)

Jane is a lady in her 40s that I met on a visit to her farm. While feeding the cattle, I noticed Jane hanging out the washing. She was moving awkwardly. I was introduced to her and could not help mentioning that she seemed in some discomfort. She then told me the story of her jaw pain. I did a quick assessment with her standing in the yard, noted pelvic misalignment and obvious jaw misalignment. She was unable to talk easily and had trouble opening her mouth, particularly moving the jaw sideways.

I was just about to go away on a two-week holiday, so did a quick TMJ treatment with her standing, plus a move on the medial pterygoid which immediately increased movement. I showed this to her as a self-help move and we arranged that she would see me in clinic in a couple of weeks. When she came in I did Bowen treatment incorporating pelvis and TMJ. This improved her jaw movement and pain levels reduced from 10/10 to 4/10, enabling a reduction in her pain medication. One more treatment, again incorporating pelvic and TMJ, adding moves over the medial pterygoid and lateral pterygoid, improved pain levels so much that Jane felt that she needed no further treatment. This is Jane's story in her own words:

> I first noticed discomfort in the left side of my jaw in the middle of January 2013. I took paracetamol and thought nothing more of it. However, it did not go away. I started to get left-sided headaches and earache. Ibuprofen joined the paracetamol but nothing was touching the increasing pain. Chewing anything large or hard was agony, as was yawning. I started to take stronger pain killer and this had some effect short term.
>
> On seeing my nurse practitioner she was concerned that I might have arteritis as the symptoms were synonymous with this serious condition. Luckily, a blood

test proved that it was not the case. My GP then sent a referral to the oral surgery department. By this time I was taking 2 x Zapain (30 mg codeine phosphate and 500 mg paracetamol) and 2 x 400mg cuprofen tablets four times a day.

During a chance meeting with Joanna Austen, I mentioned that I was having problems with a painful jaw and that it had been suggested that it could be related to a problem in my back. Well, Jo was in her element and quickly confirmed that it was indeed to do with my back. My jaw was also out of alignment. I was shown a technique to relieve the pain and I felt better for a short while. I then made an appointment to visit her in her clinic. Here I received treatment which again brought relief and my analgesia could be reduced. My appointment day at the oral surgery unit arrived and I was given the diagnosis of temporomandibular joint dysfunction (TMJD). What 'a mouth full'. More exercises were advised. Back to see Joanna and finally after six months my pain was resolving. Now I take the occasional paracetamol.

My advice to anyone suffering with this condition is to make an appointment to see your local Bowen practitioner as soon as possible.

CASE STUDY

Joanna Austen, Bodmin and Liskeard, Cornwall, England
(www.bowenincornwall.co.uk)

G.T. of Liskeard writes:

At the age of 40 I started having migraine attacks which were very infrequent but debilitating when they happened, with visual impairment with the typical aura followed by arm and facial numbness and excruciating headaches. Medical advice could offer no obvious cause or solution.

At the age of 60 they started becoming far more frequent, almost monthly, and lasting longer, usually about three days. With increasing frequency the need for a solution became more urgent and over a period of time we thought we had tracked the source to chocolate and so for the last 12 months I have avoided chocolate completely along with all food items that contain it. This reduced the frequency but still they occurred regularly, affecting my ability to work and being self-employed this became more and more debilitating. I tried acupuncture and medication but nothing solved the problem, only masking the symptoms.

When I tried the Bowen Technique, Joanna Austen suggested that there might be a link with dental work I had had done and during which my mouth was open wide for long periods. When I looked back at instances of migraine they had indeed all followed dental treatment (which I have had frequently over the last few years).

Jo followed up this revelation with treatment of the face, neck and jaw to re-align the jaw and neck and sure enough, as history now proves, every time

I had this treatment the migraines stopped until further dental work after which a further treatment solved the problem again. Now I plan to have a Bowen treatment immediately after any future dental works. I'm also planning to start eating chocolate again next year!

I cannot recommend strongly enough the benefit of Bowen treatment for obtaining relief from migraine as there are many ways in which your jaw and neck can become misaligned other than by dentistry and I know only too well the pleasure in the relief of escaping the nightmare of frequent and debilitating migraines.

References

Ariffe, N. (2002) The Bowen Technique National Migraine Research Program. Available at www.bowenmigraineresearch.co.uk, accessed on 13 May 2014.

Bessa-Nogueira, R.V., Vasconcelos, B.C. and Niederman, R. (2008) The methodological quality of systematic reviews comparing temporomandibular joint disorder surgical and non-surgical treatment. *BMC Oral Health* 8 (1), 27.

Flanagan, M.D. (2010) *The Downside of Upright Posture: the Anatomical Causes of Alzheimers, Parkinsons, and Multiple Sclerosis.* Minneapolis, MN: Two Harbors Press.

Kritsineli, M. and Ys, Shim (1991) Malocclusion, body posture, and temporomandibular disorder in children with primary and mixed dentition. *Journal of Clinical Pediatric Dentistry* 16 (2), 86–93.

Orlando, B., Manfredini, D., Salvetti, G. and Bosco, M. (2007) Evaluation of the effectiveness of biobehavioral therapy in the treatment of temporomandibular disorders: a literature review. *Behavioral Medicine* 33 (3), 101–118.

Retzlaff, E., Mitchell, F., Upledger, J. and Biggert, T. (1978) Nerve fibers and endings in cranial sutures. *Journal of the American Osteopathic Association* 77 (6), 474–475.

Spahr, A. *et al.* (2006) Periodontal infections and coronary heart disease: role of periodontal bacteria and importance of total pathogen burden in the coronary event and periodontal disease (corodont) study. *Archives of Internal Medicine* 166 (5), 554–559.

Tunis, M. and Wolff, H. (1953) Studies on headache: long-term observations of the reactivity of the cranial arteries in subjects with vascular headache of the migraine type. *A.M.A. Archives of Neurology and Psychiatry* 70 (5), 551–557.

Watemberg, N., Matar, M., Har-Gil, M. and Mahajnah, M. (2014) The influence of excessive chewing gum use on headache frequency and severity among adolescents. *Pediatric Neurology* 50 (1), 69–72.

Wilson-Pauwels, L., Stewart, P.A. and Akesson, E.J. (1997) *Autonomic Nerves: Basic Science, Clinical Aspects, Case Studies.* Malden, MA: Blackwell Science.

Youniss, S. (1991) The relationship between craniomandibular disorders and otitis media in children. *Cranio: The Journal of Craniomandibular Practice* 9 (2), 169–173.

9

Stress, Anxiety and Depression

Soothing touch, whether it be applied to a ruffled cat, a crying infant or a frightened child, has a universally recognized power to ameliorate the signs of distress. How can it be that we overlook its usefulness on the jangled adult as well? What is it that leads us to assume that the stressed child merely needs 'comforting,' while the stressed adult needs 'medicine'?

Juhan Deane (2003)

Background

We Brits are a touch-deprived nation. A study found that when the average Londoner sits in a cafe with a friend, he/she rarely touches that friend at all beyond an initial peck on the cheek. In Florida the average number of times touch is used over a coffee is two, in Paris 110 and in Puerto Rico a whopping 180 (Field 2003, p.22).

Despite this rather alarming finding, we haven't entirely lost our sensitivity to the nuances of touch. Two studies with participants from the USA and Spain showed that strangers were able to identify emotions from touch alone (without actually seeing the person who was touching them). Participants were touched and usually able to perceive emotions such as anger, fear, disgust, love, gratitude and sympathy. Strangely, men were not able to perceive when women touched them with anger and women were not able to perceive sympathy when touched by men (Keltner 2009, p.192). Another study showed that we are able to differentiate emotions by just observing people touch one another (Hertenstein and Keltner 2006).

What has this got to do with stress? Well, partly because Bowen is all about sensitive touching, and, crucially, touch has the ability to radically change our nervous systems, particularly its response to stress (Keltner 2009, p.185). This is true in an adult, but even more important for the young developing brain. A ground-breaking study looking at rats conclusively showed that baby rats that were licked and groomed by their mother were more resilient to stress, had better immune function, were calmer and, crucially, had reduced receptor levels of stress-related neurons in the brain (Weaver *et al.* 2004). This means that touch has a highly beneficial effect on what is called our hypothalamic-pituitary-adrenal (HPA) axis, a vital element in our stress and immune response.

Stress and Genetics

Although the media like to portray our genetic make-up as a kind of immovable blueprint of tendencies towards particular traits or diseases, what these types of studies show is that the difference between someone who is calm or anxious is not all in the genes; it is what is called 'epigenetic'. What this means for the rat is that her licking and grooming actually programmes her pups' DNA to thrive and succeed, allowing certain information to be passed on to them without having to go through the slow process of natural selection. Both the positive and negative effects of this have been studied extensively by researchers such as Bruce Lipton and the neurobiologist Allan Schore, who explain that the epigenetic code is influenced by all kinds of factors such as nurturing (or lack of it), availability of food (or lack of it) and a variety of psychological and environmental factors (such as exposure to toxins) (Doidge 2008; Lipton 2011).

One of the unexpected findings in relation to Bowen and genetics is the effect of treatments on people (especially children) with genetic conditions. I remember treating a teenager with Williams syndrome, a rare genetic condition which affects the production of elastin, often producing joint pain and stiffness. Treatment resulted in a considerable lessening of pain, more mobility and a lessening of her scoliosis. More recently, treating a baby with a genetic disorder that affects the heart and liver, has resulted in a considerable improvement in her sleep patterns, bowel function, overall happiness and symptoms of itchiness. Other Bowen practitioners have noticed similar improvements with clients with lupus, Sjogren's syndrome, Ehlers-Danlos Syndrome and other conditions with a genetic component.

Lifestyle and Stress

Most people don't like to admit they are stressed, but the unfortunate fact is that most of us are pretty stressed a lot of the time. In fact, some biologists such as the pioneering endocrinologist Hans Selye, who almost single-handedly coined the term stress in the 1930s, suggest that our fight-or-flight response is on high alert most of the time because of the high level of stimulation in our Western culture. This creates an over-active HPA axis which has a cascade of ramifications for our health.

Briefly, the hypothalamus, pituitary and adrenal glands have a complex interactive relationship which is involved in the neurobiology of mood disorders and can be linked to conditions such as anxiety, insomnia, depression, IBS, CFS, alcoholism, attention-deficit hyperactivity disorder (ADHD) and serious conditions such as bipolar and post-traumatic stress disorder (PTSD). One of the chief functions of antidepressant and mood stabilizing drugs is to try to regulate the HPA axis.

When the body perceives stress (which could be an internal or external stressor), signals are sent from the hypothalamus to the pituitary and the adrenals. The adrenals release cortisol and adrenaline (epinephrine). The stress circuit is controlled by special receptors in the hippocampus that detect cortisol levels (GR receptors) which then send signals to the hypothalamus to shut down the stress circuit.

A detailed explanation of why the HPA axis is so important is beyond the scope of this book. There are already many excellent explanations on the subject including the very accessible *Mapping the Mind* by the science writer Rita Carter (1999). The relationship between stress and disease is also a highly complex subject and is covered in depth in other publications such as *Why Zebras Don't Get Ulcers,* by Robert Sapolsky (2004). However, it is important for therapists to understand why it is, for example, that short-term stress stimulates an immune response but long-term stress suppresses it. It is important because even such an apparently beneficial thing as a Bowen treatment can unconsciously be perceived by an already highly stressed individual as a stressful event and can create a flare-up of symptoms for a day or two. This is particularly important to bear in mind when working on people whose immune systems are already compromised, such as those with autoimmune conditions.

Glucocorticoid Receptors (GR) and Cortisol

People with higher levels of GR are better at detecting cortisol and they recover from stress more quickly. Over time, GR receptors can effectively become desensitized. We know that chronic stress not only down-regulates the sensitivity of the glucocorticoid receptors but it also causes atrophy in some of their neurons (Magarinos *et al.* 1996). This atrophy can be temporary, which might explain our tendency towards forgetfulness when we are stressed. The good news is that hippocampal neurons are almost unique in that they are able to regrow – something that happens in response to stimuli such as exercise, learning (Sapolsky 2004, p.218) and, interestingly, pleasurable experience (Leuner *et al.* 2010). The fact that Bowen is a highly pleasurable experience for most people might add some ammunition to the idea that it, too, might aid neurogenesis of hippocampal GRs.

There are several studies that have looked at the beneficial effect of massage on the HPA axis and cortisol levels, one of them after a single session (Rapaport, Schettler and Bresee 2010) and the other as a result of multiple sessions (Rapaport, Schettler and Bresee 2012). The latter study unsurprisingly showed more beneficial effect from multiple massage sessions (twice per week), but only the light touch massage produced a change in corticotrophin (ACTH). This is a hormone released from the pituitary that signals the adrenals to release glucocorticoids. This merits further investigation in terms of the potential benefits of light touch versus stronger touch in cases of severe stress. The other interesting area of potential investigation could be on how the type of touch used in Bowen influences glucocorticoid receptors, which are expressed in almost every cell in the body and have major metabolic influences on skeletal muscle.

Stress and the Body

Because stress is so widespread and because it is apparently so linked to the development of chronic disease, Bowen practitioners are dealing with stressed clients every day. There are some specific procedures which have a beneficial effect on lowering the stress response and making people more centred in their body. One of the most powerful approaches to dealing with stress and trauma, developed by Peter Levine (Levine 1997), involves getting clients more in touch with body sensations in present time. This in itself calms the SNS down, since it is impossible for it to be over-active when the client is in touch with body sensation. Because Bowen sessions involve both touch and sensation, this in itself has a calming effect. Added to this, clients often report a remaining sensation of the therapist's hands on their body long after the therapist has left the room, increasing the felt sense in their bodies. Encouraging a felt sense in the body is nearly always a good thing and why playing music in a therapy room can be unnecessarily distracting.

Doing minimal work and encouraging the client to track bodily sensations is the basis of the work developed by Margaret Spicer and Anne Schubert known as 'Mind Body Bowen'. As Margaret writes:

> Mind Body Bowen (MBB) takes the Bowen move/s and, by utilizing the client's own awareness, mindfulness or 'felt sense', explores the relationship of the sensations arising following the moves to the body's bioelectric fields, muscle/ meridian and fascial links. Sensations lingering after the moves, especially the bottom stoppers, provide indicators to areas related to previous trauma.
>
> MBB recognizes and works directly with the body's innate self-healing intelligence, which uses signs and symptoms as a means of communication and thus access to causative factors underlying the client's condition. In particular it addresses retained 'body' or somatic memory related to sensation, tension, contraction and armoring as a result of residual associated physical, emotional and behavioural stress.
>
> Taking an extensive case history related to the sensations felt, patterns of a lifetime emerge. Enduring effects from birth trauma including pre- and postnatal issues, together with residual long-term patterns of compensation and aspects of post-traumatic stress become more apparent. Once discussed or brought to the surface, very often a relaxation response and changed breathing patterns are seen. The person can then be balanced and the healing process begun.

This kind of work can invoke powerful responses such as trembling or emotional release. These reactions are explained clearly in Peter Levine's work of Somatic Experiencing (1997) and Bessel van der Kolk's seminal essay 'The body keeps the score: memory and the evolving psychobiology of post traumatic stress' (1994) where he eloquently outlines his theory of 'somatic memory'. Reactions such as trembling or feeling cold can be an indication that the nervous system is processing held activation, usually related to a previously traumatic event, which the body has been unable to process. This can be a powerful tool for releasing trauma, something that if not dealt with therapeutically, can be a cause of later anxiety and depression.

Stress and Sleep

One of the most common responses after Bowen is that clients say they feel unusually thirsty for a few days (sometimes they describe it as a 'raging thirst') as well as feeling a need to sleep more than usual. Most importantly, their quality of sleep improves, something which is also seen with babies after they have had Bowen. Sleep has a very beneficial effect on the nervous system and, as we know, allows repair. This is why we naturally need to sleep more when we are ill or recovering from an illness. Lack of sleep is clearly linked to a multitude of ills: forgetfulness, being more prone to accidents, depression, weight gain, chronic illness, lack of libido, etc. (Dement and Vaughan 2000). But it would also appear that the quality of the sleep is more crucial than the actual number of hours.

Specific Bowen Procedures for Stress and Anxiety

The two intrafascial receptors that, when stimulated, have an effect on lowering the stress response in the hypothalamus are the Ruffinis (which respond to slow melting pressure) and the interstitials (which respond to very light touch). As already discussed, most Bowen moves can be adapted in terms of pressure and speed to stimulate these receptors. In the case of the interstitials, the response in the client can be immediate. The work on the colon, for example, which affects our enteric nervous system, one of the major parts of the ANS, and which has as many neurons as we have in our spinal cord, usually results in the client feeling cold and sleepy, a sign that their parasympathetic system is kicking in. The coccyx procedure also has a powerful calming effect on the central nervous system by stimulating the membranes at the filament terminalis. Impulses from these moves travel up through the dural membranes to the pituitary and the hypothalamus, which sit in a little trough (the sella turcica) in the middle of the sphenoid bone, right in the centre of the cranium. This could also be why this work has such a profound effect on the hormonal system. Both the coccyx work and the moves in the mid-back have a powerful calming effect on the sympathetic chain of the SNS. The kidney work can be very useful in addressing the adrenals, particularly in people with adrenal exhaustion caused by long-term stress.

Breathing and Stress

Other Bowen work that helps stress is freeing up breathing by releasing the diaphragm. People often instinctively breathe less frequently and more shallowly when they are suppressing emotions. You can see this with children, who will instinctively hold their breath if feeling strong emotions such as anger. The Bowen respiratory and sternal work affects breathing profoundly, which then has a knock-on effect on all the systems of the body as the diaphragm resumes its important functions. Stress can initiate high blood pressure by inhibiting the excretory function of the kidneys; something that is exacerbated by poor breathing (hypoventilation). Stress seems to be a factor in low frequency of breathing at rest, something that is more marked in women (Anderson and Chesney 2008, p.119). Most clients will report an improvement in breathing immediately following the Bowen respiratory work.

In Bowen work we always try to do moves on the exhalation wherever possible, possibly because inhalation is activated by the sympathetic nervous system and exhalation is activated by the parasympathetic part, thus encouraging a more parasympathetic response. Stephen Porges also points out that long exhalations stimulate the parasympathetic nervous system (PNS), something I had discovered when playing some of the flute obbligato parts by Bach from his church cantatas. These involve playing extremely long lines of melody which means that the player can't take a breath without breaking up the phrasing. Although technically challenging, these pieces have an extremely relaxing effect when you play them.

Bowen and Body Awareness

Certain procedures such as the hamstring and ankle work can help bring a body awareness into the lower part of the body. This can be immensely helpful for people who tend to live too much in their heads. When someone says that their mind is always active and they wish they could 'switch their minds off', this is a clear indicator of an over-active SNS.

The vagus nerve, being the major parasympathetic nerve in the body, is extremely important to address in cases of stress and anxiety, and this is discussed in Carolyn Goh's section below. Stephen Porges's recent book *Clinical Insights from the Polyvagal Theory* (2013) is particularly useful for therapists wanting to understand the implications of the vagal system. The specific Bowen moves that address the vagus are the diaphragm (the lower branches of the vagus travel through the diaphragm next to the oesophagus), the upper respiratory, TMJ work, as well as the powerful vagus procedure itself.

Conventional Treatments for Anxiety and Depression

The discovery that most conventional antidepressants (specifically the selective serotonin re-uptake inhibitors (SSRI) type) appeared to have no better effect on helping depression than a placebo received a lot of press a few years ago, and is still the topic of many an animated conversation. A meta-analysis study done in 2008 (Kirsch *et al.* 2008) that looked at published and unpublished trials failed to show a significant advantage of SSRIs over inert placebo, with exercise and psychotherapy showing benefits at least equal to those of antidepressants.

The documented side effects of many antidepressants give deep cause for concern, particularly as more than 1 in 10 adult Americans take them regularly. Although there is only anecdotal evidence to show that Bowen can be helpful for people with depression, a randomized controlled trial (RCT) study from 1998 showed that electro-acupuncture, with which Bowen has many parallels, was equally as effective as amitriptyline for patients with anxiety (Luo *et al.* 1998).

The Placebo Effect

Kirsch's study also brings up the hot topic of whether some alternative therapies are actually any better than a placebo. I am not going to go into this now, because in relation to Bowen the purpose of this book has been to show clear mechanisms of how Bowen is working in specific situations. It is clear, however, that the placebo effect is a hugely under-used resource in all medicine. Although the main focus of debate about the use of placebos is centred around potential for dishonesty on the part of the physician, the effect of positive statements used in communication with a patient is clearly hugely beneficial. Likewise, the use of negative statements, or so-called 'nocebos', which often accompany a diagnosis, has negative effects on health, something that has not been taken on board by teaching faculties at medical schools. The extreme power of the nocebo came home to me a few years ago when a client of mine had been given (erroneously) a diagnosis of ovarian cancer. Following the diagnosis she went into a spiral of depression from which she never really recovered, despite being given the all-clear after only a couple of weeks.

Giving clear, positive instructions about how a client can become actively involved in their recovery is crucial in a Bowen session. Clients are able to recover much better if they not only understand their condition but are then able to modify their lifestyle to address the underlying causes. Clients can often be left feeling powerless and uninformed about the complex processes going on in their bodies, particularly after a diagnosis such as cancer. Unfortunately, the feeling of powerlessness and a lack of ability to change one's situation, which is also common in high-stress jobs, is the most likely instigator of feelings of hopelessness and depression, all things which are unhelpful when people are trying to recover or deal with a chronic illness.

Stress and the Autonomic Nervous System

ɤ Dr Carolyn Goh

The autonomic nervous system (ANS) is part of the peripheral nervous system and is also known as the involuntary nervous system. It regulates the functions of internal organs (the viscera) such as the stomach and heart, and operates below the level of our consciousness. Some of the functions of the ANS are to regulate heart rate and blood pressure as well as digestion. The ANS is divided into two main subsystems: the sympathetic nervous system (SNS) and the parasympathetic nervous system (PNS).

The SNS is known as the 'quick response mobilizing system'. It exhibits the classic fight or flight response to a perceived harmful event, attack or threat to survival (Cannon 1932). The body goes into a state of heightened awareness (e.g. dilation of pupils) and vasoconstriction occurs to direct blood to vital organs and muscles. There is an increase in blood pressure, heart rate and muscle tension. In this state, less energy is available for other functions such as digestion of food and repair of the body. The body's immune system is suppressed, making it more vulnerable to infection. Long-term heightened sympathetic activity can have detrimental effects on health over time (Carlson 2013).

The PNS is known as the 'rest and digest system'. It is responsible for bringing the body back into homeostasis after activation of the SNS. Some of its functions are to control salivation, lacrimation, urination, defecation and digestion. The PNS works in harmony with the SNS to bring balance to the body. One very important component of the PNS is the tenth cranial nerve called the vagus nerve. *Vagus* is Latin for 'wandering', and it is an accurate description of this nerve. The vagus nerve emerges at the back of the skull and makes its way through the abdomen and branches out to the heart, lungs, voicebox, stomach and ears, among other body parts (Berthoud and Neuhuber 2000). The vagus nerve is command central for the function of the PNS. It is geared to slow the body down, like the brakes on a car, and uses neurotransmitters such as acetylcholine and gamma-aminobutyric acid (GABA) to lower heart rate and blood pressure. Increasing the activity of the vagus nerve (vagal activity) increases PNS activity and brings the body back into homeostasis post activation of the fight-or-flight response. Vagal tone is a measure of how reactive/sensitive the vagal nerve is and how quickly the brakes can be applied.

A high vagal tone indicates a responsive vagal nerve that functions well to bring the body back from an excited, hyper-alert state to a calm relaxed one. An individual with high vagal tone is better able to cope with stressful situations as the body can easily rebalance. They are also more likely to be healthier as their immune systems are less affected by stress and are more resilient (Porges 1995). Low vagal tone on the other hand suggests that the vagus nerve is less reactive and less able to bring the ANS into a state of homeostasis after a stressful encounter. Long-term heightened sympathetic activity (stress) dampens/decreases vagal tone. Individuals with low vagal tone are more sensitive to stress and more prone to illness (Porges 1995). Studies show that in healthy subjects, reduced heart rate variability (HRV) (i.e. low vagal tone) is independently associated with increased inflammatory markers C-reactive protein (CRP) and Interleukin-6 (IL-6) levels (Haensel *et al.* 2008; Sloan *et al.* 2007). Low vagal tone is also reported to be associated with impaired stress recovery of Tumour Necrosis Factor (TNF) levels (Weber *et al.* 2010). Patients with cardiovascular disease report that parasympathetic tone as inferred from HRV is inversely related to inflammatory markers (IL-6 and CRP) (Haensel 2008; Lanzal *et al.* 2006). Finally, increased morbidity and mortality following cardiac surgery, myocardial infarction, sepsis, rheumatoidal arthritis, irritiable bowel disease, Systemic Lupus Erythematosus and sarcoidosis has been reported to be associated with decreased vagus nerve activity (Huston and Tracey 2011).

Vagal Tone

The key to maintaining a balanced autonomic nervous system and optimal health lies to a large degree on vagal tone. By increasing vagal tone and vagus activity, the body is able to strengthen the immune system, reduce inflammation and encourage repair. There are many ways in which the vagus activity can be stimulated. Carotid sinus massage, used in modern medicine, is a way to directly stimulate the vagus nerve via baroreceptors. The carotid sinus sits above the point where the carotid artery divides into its two main branches. Rubbing the carotid sinus stimulates an area in the artery wall that contains baroreceptors. Baroreceptors act as pressure sensors and respond by activating the vagus nerve to slow down heart rate. The negative feedback loop communicating signals to the vagus nerve is called the baroreflex. This method is used to diagnose carotid sinus syncope in patients with hypersensitive carotid baroreflexes (Lagi *et al.* 2012). This method of vagus stimulation makes use of the relationship between baroreceptors and vagal activity.

Baroreflex dependant activation of vagal activity causes a short-term burst in vagus nerve firing as seen in blood pressure control (Levy and Pappano 2007). This increase in vagus nerve activity brings the body into a temporary state of homeostasis until the SNS is reactivated. A long-term increase in vagal tone, however, is the ability of the ANS to increase vagal activity independent of external stimulation of baroreceptors; as soon as sympathetic activity is no longer necessary to return to homeostasis, the body is able to rest and repair.

Bowen and Stimulation of the Vagus Nerve

Case studies on the Bowen Technique (see below) report clients feeling calm, relaxed, balanced and better able to deal with stressful situations for weeks after a Bowen session. Clients also report increases in parasympathetic activity (e.g. rumbling tummy, feeling calm) during the session associated with certain types of move, indicating short-term vagus nerve activity. The short and long-term balancing effects of the Bowen Technique on the body suggest that Bowen acts to activate the vagus nerve using both baroreceptor dependent (short-term) and independent (increase vagal tone) methods. Indeed, research carried out by Kollai *et al.* (1994) shows that cardiac vagal tone (defined by change in R-R interval, see below) can be generated by both baroreflex dependent and independent mechanisms.

The Bowen Technique involves both tactile and kinaesthetic stimulation, which act on both baroreceptors and mechanoreceptors in the body. Research carried out by a group in Korea (Field 2008) measured responses to infant massage (tactile and kinaesthetic stimulation), using baseline vagal activity, heart rate and oxygen saturation. The results showed an increase in vagal activity and oxygen saturation and a decrease in heart rate. Studies indicate that baroreceptors and mechanoreceptors within the dermis are innervated by vagal afferent fibres projecting to the vagal nucleus of the solitary tract (NTS), the predominant source of afferent inputs to the efferent neurons of the nucleus ambiguous (NA) and the dorsal motor nucleus of the vagus (DMN) (Kandel, Schwarz and Jessel 2000). The DMN, in turn, gives rise to most of the efferent fibres that provide parasympathetic control of the gastro-intestinal system in the form of the gastric (stomach, proximal duodenum), hepatic (liver) and celiac (pancreas, spleen, kidneys) branches of the vagus (Chang, Mashimo and Goyal 2003; Kandel *et al.* 2000). Bowen moves stimulate several types of intrafascial mechanoreceptors (Golgi, Ruffini and interstitial receptors) that affect muscle tonus and increase vagal tone (Wilks 2013).

Bowen and Baroreceptor Stimulation of the Vagus

Research carried out on heart rate variability (HRV) and Bowen has shown that the Bowen Technique can cause an increase in HRV (Whitaker, Gilliam and Seba 1997). The increased levels of HRV are indicative of an increase in vagal tone. In order to explain how Bowen can influence vagal tone, it is necessary to go into a little more detail on how the vagal tone is measured and studied.

Vagal tone cannot be directly measured. Other biological processes are measured that represent the functionality of vagal tone. An increase in vagal tone both slows the heart and makes heart rate more variable (i.e. there is more beat-to-beat change between heart beats). This is called heart rate variability (HRV). The most common method of measuring HRV is using the electrocardiogram (ECG) signal. The ECG signal consists of a QRST waveform resembling the electrical activity of the heartbeat. Each individual beat is represented on the ECG as the PQRST complex. Each sequential letter represents a sequential discrete part of the complex and each represents a different portion of the cardiac cycle. The P wave represents the initiation of depolarization in the sinus node and subsequent atrial contraction. The QRS complex represents the conductance and sequential depolarization of the ventricles. The ST segment follows the QRS complex. The ST segment represents the period of time in which the ventricles are isoelectric. Each heartbeat has an R peak (normally the highest point of the QRS waveform) and represents a stage in the depolarization of the right and left ventricles of the human heart. To measure HRV, the difference between R peaks – called the R-R intervals – are measured. These are then plotted to form the HRV signal. The vagal tone can then easily be measured using HRV.

Once the HRV is obtained, it can then be viewed in the frequency domain using the Fast Fourier Transform (FFT). This method is often used to convert data from the time to frequency domain. In the frequency domain, both the PNS and SNS are depicted as different waveforms ranging over different frequencies. The frequency domain analysis yields power spectrum values which represent the sympathetic (LF-low frequency), mixed sympathetic and parasympathetic (MF-mid frequency) and parasympathetic nervous systems (HF-high frequency) respectively. A shift in the spectrums indicates heightened nervous system activity corresponding to the specific frequency range.

The nervous system can be likened to an electrical circuit in the body and the activity of the autonomic nervous system can be charted using HRV analysis in the frequency domain. In 2005 Goh was able to model the baroreflex system in infants using computer modelling (control theory) to access autonomic maturity at different levels of development. The results were compared with real-life models. This study proved that frequency domain analysis is an accurate measure of nervous system activity.

Frequencies can also be thought of in terms of vibrations. Anything that vibrates has a certain frequency. Each nervous system, central, peripheral and autonomic, has its own range of frequencies at which it operates. In fact, cells, subcellular components and molecules all exhibit characteristic vibrational patterns of functional importance. DNA structures containing G-C base pairs, for instance, vibrate at a higher frequency than those containing A-T base pairs (Chou 1984). Recent studies have also shown that variations in vibrational frequency correlate with various types of cell growth (Myrdal and Auersperg 1986). Cancer cells have a vibrational pattern distinct from all normal cells (Mohler, Partin and Coffey 1987; Partin *et al.* 1988).

In view of these findings, it is not unreasonable to consider the possibility that every cell in the body may respond to changes in vibrational frequency coming from the outside environment. A study by McClelland (1979) showed that music can change the pulse rate, circulation and blood pressure. Widespread effects in the body have been demonstrated by another study, which showed that different types of music have different effects on gastric motility, electrical conductivity of the skin, papillary dilation and muscle contraction (Bruya and Seversten 1984). These are all signs of changes in vagal activity.

The Bowen Technique uses a very specific rolling motion that varies in frequency (slower or quicker moves with less or more pressure) at different points on the body.

This rolling motion is thought to send vibrations of specific frequencies through the muscular structure of the body. As with any vibrational energy/force, it can travel and influence the frequency of vibrations within the body.

A well-known and much researched form of meditation, Transcendental Meditation (TM), uses mantras of different vibrational frequencies to calm and rebalance the body (Alexander *et al.* 1989). Likewise, the Bowen Technique uses moves with varying rolling motions that create different vibrational frequencies at certain points in the body. The heightened and prolonged increase in vagal tone during and after Bowen treatments (based on clients' testimonies) suggests that the vibration produced during a Bowen session has a tuning effect on the nervous system. This lasting effect may work by resonance with the nervous system to increase vagal tone.

Bowen practitioners recommend at least five days between Bowen sessions, indicating the effects of the treatment are still evident in this period. This could be used as a marker for further research using HRV to evaluate and document the vagal tone of individuals for a longer time period.

ↁ

CASE STUDY

| *Pierre Saine, Bowen practitioner and instructor, Montreal, Canada*

A woman aged 45 had been suffering from depression for six months, undergoing psychotherapy and taking antidepressants. I saw her three times during the month of February 2013. During the first session she felt a great relaxation after the session. In the afternoon she went into a deep sleep which was unusual as she had described sleeping poorly since her depression had started.

During the second session she had tremors in her limbs which, towards the end of the session, developed into uncontrollable tremors at the jaw and a big emotional reaction. I advised her to not interfere or repress the process of discharge (not to repress what needed to be expressed).

At the beginning of the third session, she described the sensation she had after the previous meeting: she had the sensation of a ball rising from the stomach into the throat. Then came a feeling of wellbeing that she had not felt for a very long time.

CASE STUDY

| *Lorraine Evans, Bowen practitioner, Montreal, Canada*

K, 50 years old, male, has been suffering from anxiety for the last 25 years. During this time K's anxiety has been preventing him from leaving his home town as he has very strong agoraphobia; he never travels more than 2 kilometres from home. His posture portrays his constant anxious state, he has rounded unrelaxed shoulders and his muscles are all very tight. I have treated K four times now. The first time after doing the basic relaxation moves there were only small improvements in his anxiety, whereby he felt slightly calmer directly after the treatment. The second time where I did a bit more, he reported having mild hallucinations – he saw an arch of coloured spectrum lights which overlaid his vision for 20 minutes. This actually made him more anxious briefly! I suggested he try to relax into whatever occurred after a treatment and allow the sensations to pass through. During the third treatment he experienced some disassociation for 20 minutes directly afterwards during which time I allowed him to rest. Dissociation is a clear sign of parasympathetic activation. He then slept for two hours and it was gone. The fourth treatment bought some positive news. He reported feeling completely anxiety-free for the first time in 25 years.

CASE STUDY

| *Pierre Saine, Bowen practitioner and instructor, Montreal, Canada*

A woman aged 45, and a university teacher. Day 1: Procedures done are the basic relaxation moves along with the head procedure with long pauses, creating lasting body sensations. She finishes with an uncontrollable continuous euphoric laughing for more than 30 minutes. The next day, she writes: 'I am still surfing on joy...this evening, I had to confront a family dispute that would, usually, make me sick and I came out of it better than usual: I stayed positive, calm and effervescent. It is nothing but marvellous. I think I am in a dream and I do not want to sleep, fearing that tomorrow morning life returns as it was before. I wonder if I have ever experienced such calm and intense happiness. Maybe once, but I am not sure. One thing is certain: it is really good to be illuminated. I doubted it, now I know. Thanks a million.'

Day 17: 'I am relatively well, I am back to work this morning. I would really have liked that the extraordinary effects of the last session would stay eternally, but it took them about one week to gradually fade. Nevertheless, I have not fallen back as low as before the Bowen session. When can I make next appointment?'

CASE STUDY

| *Anne Schubert, Bowen practitioner and instructor,*
| *Forster, New South Wales, Australia*

A local employment agency directed Roxanne, a middle-aged lady, to my Bowen Clinic to see if there could be some assistance with her extreme anxiety which was inhibiting her ability to cope with job interviews. Even as she approached my door I could sense her nervousness so I took extra care to make her feel comfortable and welcome. I explained how gentle Bowen work was, showing her Tom Bowen's photograph working with a young child and showing her my charts so she could have some understanding of the process.

My Bowen bed is wide and comfortable and I covered her lightly with a sarong to enable her to feel cared for and secure. After the first lower back moves I encouraged her to take note of any subtle feelings that might flow and told her I would leave her to quietly consider. On returning, Roxanne said she couldn't feel anything; however, she felt like she wanted to go to sleep, she was so relaxed. With that I told her I would simply move in and out of the room after doing gentle moves around her body and if by any chance she did feel anything she could tell me. And so for the rest of the basic work, Roxanne became more and more relaxed and the session concluded with her gently smiling and keen to see me in a week. I suggested a walk on the beach would be a perfect conclusion for her first Bowen experience.

A smiling Roxanne eagerly began her second treatment. Her only feeling was a gentle all over body warmth and I included the respiratory work as I had noted some tension in her upper back. I also chose to conclude with the head procedure as it always has a very pleasant response when anxiety and nervousness are indicated. As I held Roxanne's head, an amazing thing happened. Her head and neck began to strongly arch back towards me six or seven times. Then her head began vibrating, getting stronger and stronger as I gently cradled her skull.

'Oh!' she said. 'Oh my goodness!' not fearfully but in sheer amazement. I calmly explained to her it was a trauma her body was releasing and after several minutes I asked if she had had any traumas in the past. No, there were none she remembered, so I enquired about her birth. Sure enough there was the answer, first born, 48-hour labour and a recognition that for her entire life she had felt anxious when doing things for the first time. Gradually the vibrations calmed and I left her for a few more minutes 'Wow!' she said. 'That was amazing! I feel so free and relaxed.'

References

Alexander, C.N., Langer, E.J., Newman, R.I., Chandler, H.M. and Davies, J.L. (1989) Transcendental Meditation, mindfulness, and longevity: an experimental study with the elderly. *Journal of Personality and Social Psychology* 57 (6), 950–964.

Anderson, D.E., McNeely, J.D., Chesney, M.A. and Windham, B.G. (2008) Breathing variability at rest is positively associated with 24-h blood pressure level. *American Journal of Hypertension* 21 (12), 1324–1329.

Berthoud, H.R. and Neuhuber, W.L. (2000) Functional and chemical anatomy of the afferent vagal system. *Autonomic Neuroscience: Basic and Clinical* 85 (1–3), 1–17.

Bruya, M.A. and Severtsen, B. (1984) Evaluating the effects of music on electroencephalogram patterns of normal subject. *Journal of Neurosurgical Nursing* 16 (2), 96–100.

Cannon, W.B. (1932) *The Wisdom of the Body*. New York: Norton.

Carlson, N.R. (2013) *Physiology of Behavior*. Harlow: Pearson.

Carter, R. 2010. *Mapping the Mind*. London: Phoenix.

Chang, H.Y., Mashimo, H. and Goyal, R.K. (2003) Musings on the wanderer: what's new in our understanding of vago-vagal reflex? IV: current concepts of vagal efferent projections to the gut. *American Journal of Physiology. Gastrointestinal and Liver Physiology* 284 (3), G357–366.

Chou, K.C. (1984) Low-frequency vibrations of DNA molecules. *Biochemical Journal* 221 (1), 27–31.

Dement, W.C. and Vaughan, C. (2000) *The Promise of Sleep: A Pioneer in Sleep Medicine Explores the Vital Connection between Health, Happiness, and a Good Night's Sleep*. New York: Dell.

Doidge, N. 2008. *The Brain that Changes Itself: Stories of Personal Triumph from the Frontiers of Brain Science*. London: Penguin Books.

Field, T. (2003) *Touch*. Cambridge, MA: MIT Press.

Field, T. and Diego, M. (2008) Vagal activity, early growth and emotional development. *Infant Behavior and Development 31* (3), 361–373.

Goh, C. (2005) *A Systems Approach to Cardio-Respiratory Analysis in the Infant*. PhD thesis, Imperial College, University of London.

Haensel, A., Mills, P.J., Nelesen, R.A., Ziegler, M.G. and Dimsdale, J.E. (2008) The relationship between heart rate variability and inflammatory markers in cardiovascular diseases. *Psychoneuroendocrinology 33* (10), 1305–1312.

Hertenstien, M. and Keltner, D. (2006) Touch communicates distinct emotions. *Emotion 6* (3), 528–533.

Huston, J.M. and Tracey, K.J. (2011) The pulse of inflammation: heart rate variability, the cholinergic anti-inflammatory pathway and implications for therapy. *Journal of Internal Medicine 269* (1), 45–53.

Juhan, D. (2003) *Job's Body: A Handbook for Bodywork* (3rd edition). Barrytown, NY: Barrytown/Station Hill.

Kandel, E., Schwartz, J. and Jessell, T. (2000) *Principles of Neural Science* (4th edition). New York: McGraw-Hill.

Keltner, D. (2009) *Born to Be Good: The Science of a Meaningful Life*. New York: W.W. Norton.

Kirsch, I., Deacon, B.J., Huedo-Medina, T.B., Scoboria, A., Moore, T.J. and Johnson, B.T. (2008) Initial severity and antidepressant benefits: a meta-analysis of data submitted to the Food and Drug Administration. *PLos Medicine 5* (2), e45.

Kollai, M., Jokkel, G., Bonyhay, I., Tomcsanyi, J. and Naszlady, A. (1994) Relation between baroreflex sensitivity and cardiac vagal tone in humans. *American Journal of Physiology 266* (1, Pt 2), H21–27.

Lagi, A., Cerisano, S. and Cencetti, S. (2012) Recurrent syncope in patients with carotid sinus hypersensitivity. *ISRN Cardiology*, Epub 10 September 2012.

Lanza, G.A., Cianflone, D., Rebuzzi, A.G., Angeloni, G. et al. (2006) Prognostic value of ventricular arrhythmias and heart rate variability in patients with unstable angina. *Heart 92*, 1055–1063.

Leuner, B., Glasper, E.R. and Gould, E. (2010) Sexual experience promotes adult neurogenesis in the hippocampus despite an initial elevation in stress hormones. *PLoS One 5* (7), e11597.

Levine, P.A. (1997) *Waking the Tiger: Healing Trauma – The Innate Capacity to Transform Overwhelming Experiences*. Berkeley, CA: North Atlantic Books.

Levy, M. and Pappano, A. (2007) *Cardiovascular Physiology* (9th edition). New York: Mosby Elsevier.

Lipton, B.H. (2011) *The Biology of Belief: Unleashing the Power of Consciousness, Matter and Miracles*. London: Hay House.

Luo, H., Meng, F., Jia, Y. and Zhao, X. (1998) Clinical research on the therapeutic effect of the electro-acupuncture treatment in patients with depression. *Psychiatry and Clinical Neurosciences 52*, S338–40.

Magariños, A.M., McEwen, B.S., Flügge, G. and Fuchs, E. (1996) Chronic psychosocial stress causes apical dendritic atrophy of hippocampal CA3 pyramidal neurons in subordinate tree shrews. *Journal of Neuroscience 16* (10), 3534–3540.

McClelland, D.C. (1979) Music in the operating room. *Journal of the Association of Operating Room Nurses 29* (2), 252–260.

Mohler, J.L., Partin, A.W. and Coffey, D.S. (1987) Prediction of metastatic potential by a new grading system of cell motility: validation in the Dunning R-3327 prostatic adenocarcinoma model. *Journal of Urology* 138 (1), 168–170.

Myrdal, S.E. and Auersperg, N. (1986) An agent or agents produced by virus-transformed cells cause unregulated ruffling in untransformed cells. *Journal of Cell Biology* 102 (4), 1224–1229.

Partin, A.W., Isaacs, J.T., Treiger, B. and Coffey, D.S. (1988) Early cell motility changes associated with an increase in metastatic ability in rat prostatic cancer cells transfected with the v-Harvey-Ras oncogene. *Cancer Research* 48 (21), 6050–6053.

Porges, S.W. (1995) Cardiac vagal tone: a physiological index of stress. *Neuroscience and Biobehavioral Reviews* 19 (2), 225–233.

Porges, S.W. (2011) *The Polyvagal Theory: Neurophysiological Foundations of Emotions, Attachment, Communication, and Self-Regulation.* New York: W.W. Norton.

Porges, S.W. (2013) *Clinical Insights from the Polyvagal Theory: The Transformative Power of Feeling Safe.* New York: W.W. Norton.

Rapaport, M.H., Schettler, P. and Bresee, C. (2010) A preliminary study of the effects of a single session of Swedish massage on hypothalamic-pituitary-adrenal and immune function in normal individuals. *Journal of Alternative and Complementary Medicine* 16 (10), 1–10.

Rapaport, M.H, Schettler, P. and Bresee, C. (2012) A preliminary study of the effects of repeated massage on hypothalamic-pituitary-adrenal and immune function in healthy individuals: a study of mechanisms of action and dosage. *Journal of Alternative and Complementary Medicine* 18 (8), 789–797.

Sapolsky, R.M. (2004) *Why Zebras Don't Get Ulcers: An Updated Guide to Stress, Stress-Related Diseases, and Coping.* New York: Owl.

Sloan, R.P., McCreath, H., Tracey, K.J., Sidney, S., Liu, K. and Seeman, T. (2007) RR interval variability is inversely related to inflammatory markers: the CARDIA study. *Molecular Medicine* 13 (3–4), 178–184.

van der Kolk, B. (1994) The body keeps the score: memory and the evolving psychobiology of post traumatic stress. *Harvard Review of Psychiatry* 1 (5), 253–265.

Watt, M.C. and Stewart, S.H. (2008) *Overcoming the Fear of Fear: How to Reduce Anxiety Sensitivity.* Oakland, CA: New Harbinger Publications.

Weaver, I.C.G., Cervoni, N., Champagne, F.A., D'Alessio, A.C. *et al.* (2004) Epigenetic programming by maternal behavior. *Nature Neuroscience* 7 (8), 847–854.

Weber, C.S., Thayer, J.F., Rudat, M., Wirtz, P.H. *et al.* (2010) Low vagal tone is associated with impaired post stress recovery of cardiovascular, endocrine, and immune markers. *European Journal of Applied Physiology* 109 (2), 201–211.

Whitaker, J.A., Gilliam, P.P. and Seba, D.B. (1997) The Bowen Technique: a gentle hands-on method that effects the autonomic nervous system as measured by heart rate variability and clinical assessment. Abstract presentation, American Academy of Environmental Medicine 32nd Annual Conference, La Jolla, California.

Wilks, J. (2013) The Bowen Technique – mechanisms for action. *Journal of the Australian Traditional-Medicine Society* 19 (1), 33.

10

Asthma and Other Respiratory Conditions

Overview

Asthma can have a devastating effect on people, often affecting a child's schooling or an adult's ability to hold down a job, as well as limiting families' abilities to do normal enjoyable activities. It can be a source of constant stress for both the individual and the family, affecting over 5 million people in the UK, with 1.1 million of those being children (that is 1 in 11 children). The cost of treatment is huge – over £1 billion is spent anually by the NHS alone on treating asthma and in 2008/9 over a million working days were lost due to breathing or lung problems (Asthma UK 2013). In the USA asthma is on the increase with nearly 19 million adults and more than 7 million children suffering from it (NCHS 2011). In 2007 asthma cost the US about $56 billion in medical costs, lost school and work days and early deaths (CDC 2011).

The History

Tom Bowen's interest in treating asthma came from his desire to help his wife Jessie, who was frequently hospitalized with asthma. His regime of regular treatments along with dietary changes pretty much halted her attacks and, according to his daughters, she never had to go to hospital again. It is difficult to know precisely where Tom got his moves that address the respiratory area, but they are ingenious to say the least.

A full treatment involves starting at the upper back with moves over the erector spinae muscles at around T7 followed by gentle moves that work the trapezius, rhomboids and the levator scapulae muscles. The lateral moves around the erector spinae muscles seem to have a very energetic effect on the lungs, possibly because they go close to the sympathetic viscero-somatic reflex areas which span T1–T4 bi-laterally (these moves address the sympathetic nerve supply to the lungs as well as affecting other muscles involved in respiration). The real work that affects the diaphragm (the main structure involved in breathing) happens with the moves on the front of the body. This part of the procedure involves the practitioner using their finger as a gentle holding point right at the attachment of the diaphragm, just beneath the cartilaginous xiphoid process. This holding point serves to keep the impulses focused in the diaphragm whilst the moves themselves go directly over the attachment sites of the anterior part of the diaphragm and the transverse abdominis muscle that sit beneath the ribs. These moves also affect the transverse thoracis and, to a certain extent, the internal intercostal muscles, both of which aid expiration by decreasing the diameter of the rib cage. This is crucial as the ability to exhale is often one of the major problems in asthmatic attacks. The moves also go over the stomach, hepatic and splenic flexures of the large intestine as well as the liver, which is why this work can also be so useful for digestive complaints.

The final move (which ideally needs to be done on the full exhalation) is fascinating, as it affects so many structures at the same time. It goes over some strong attachments of the diaphragm and the rectus abdominis on to the xyphoid, the linea alba (a tough band of ligament and fascia which travels all the way down to the pubis) and the falciform ligament (a remnant of the umbilical vein), which goes through the liver. This could be why this move can have such a strong emotional effect on people, as it touches on deep tissue memories to do with connection, our first breath and coming into the world. This move on its own can also be a lifesaver for anyone suffering an asthmatic attack (having first called for an ambulance, of course). This is described below.

The treatment usually finishes with moves at the neck as the scalene muscles assist breathing by helping to move the chest wall in inhalation. When treating people with respiratory issues, it is sometimes also necessary to look further afield as the diaphragm has close connections above with the pericardium of the heart and below with the psoas major muscles.

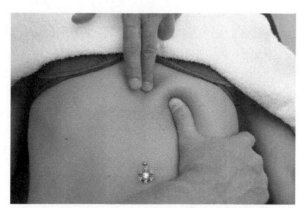

Figure 10.1 Bowen moves at the diaphragm
Source: image courtesy of Karel Aerssens, Bowen Netherlands

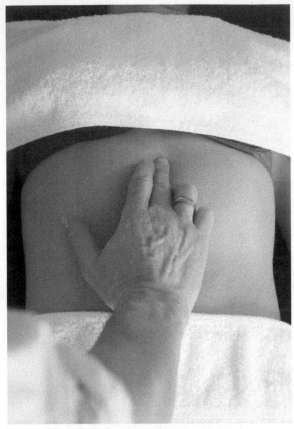

Figure 10.2 The Bowen Emergency Moves or Bowen Release Moves
Source: image courtesy of Karel Aerssens, Bowen Netherlands

The Bowen Emergency Moves (Bowen Release Moves)

It is important to stress that these moves are not designed to take the place of proper medical intervention, which is vital in the case of an asthmatic attack or conditions such as chronic obstructive pulmonary disease (COPD). Some of the features of a severe asthmatic attack, which need immediate medical attention, are:

- too breathless to feed or talk
- chest recession (chest wall collapsing inwards)
- use of accessory muscles of respiration
- respiratory rate above 50 per minute
- peak flow 50 per cent of expected best.

Symptoms of life-threatening bronchial asthma are:

- conscious level depressed/child agitated
- exhaustion

- poor respiratory effort

- cyanosis (e.g. lips going blue)

- peak flow reading 33 per cent of expected best

- silent chest (e.g. no wheezing).

With the above caveats in mind, many parents and sufferers have described these simple moves as lifesavers in their own right. As well as being useful in an emergency, many people have also found these simple moves to be life enhancing. In most cases it relieves a tight chest long before the asthma attack has become an emergency. It is also excellent for anxiety of any sort, panic attacks, hiccups and coughing. It can be useful for children to use it before taking exams, in other stressful situations, such as performing in public, and later before interviews. You might find it easiest to find the locations on your own body before trying this on someone else.

Find the base of the breast bone (the sternum). Just beneath it you should feel a small softer structure, which might feel like a small spring-board, about the length of the last joint on your little finger (smaller on a child or baby). This is often quite sensitive to the touch and usually prominent in young children. With your finger placed on the skin just beneath this, gently take some slack up to the base of this structure (it is called the xiphoid process). If they are breathing, then wait for an out-breath and move the skin down towards their feet with your finger. This move is not firm but it is definite and fairly fast. If they are having an attack, then do this move as soon as possible, having first called for help.

Other moves that people find helpful are moves on the back, level with the bottom of the shoulder blades (the scapulae). These moves tend to have a very calming effect on people suffering an attack or who are in shock. Locate the bottom of the shoulder blades (these are about a third of the way down the back). Find the muscles that run all the way up the back close to the spine (the erector spinae muscles). Place your fingers on these muscles level with the bottom of the shoulder blade on the left hand side of their body. Gently take some skin slack out towards the shoulder blade, then gently do a rolling type move with your fingers towards the spine, repeating the same thing on the right. If they are breathing, then try to co-ordinate these moves with their out-breath.

Diet

There are many potential triggers for an asthmatic attack, occasionally dietary but often environmental, and some of these are listed below. When Bowen was developing his work in the 1960s, it was very unusual for someone to change their diet in order to treat an illness. Nevertheless, he was convinced that diet had a big part to play in recovery, particularly in respiratory conditions. When he testified to the state inquiry in 1973, he said that he thought that about 90 per cent of his asthma clients had obtained relief through a combination of his work and dietary changes. Specifically, he recommended asthmatics avoid 'sago, rice, spaghetti, fried foods, potatoes or onions, milk or chocolate milk drinks, chocolate or pastry, peanuts or peanut butter, strawberries or passion fruit' (Ward 1973). Most nutritionists nowadays advise an elimination diet which involves removing suspected triggers entirely for between two and eight weeks rather than cutting out groups of foods wholesale, particularly with children where a balanced nutritious diet is so essential.

Other triggers known to induce an asthmatic attack include:

- cold, viral infection or illness, bronchitis

- cats, dogs, horses, furry animals, feathers

- smoking and cigarette smoke

- anxiety

- alcohol in excess

- aspirin and ibuprofen

- some foods and colourings

- dust mites and pollen

- perfume, chemicals, household cleaners, car exhaust

- mould

- exercise

- cold air or rapid change of temperature

- dust (e.g. from building work)

- dairy (only in some cases).

Asthma Study

ও Alastair Rattray and Carolyn Goh

In 1999 a remarkable event led to a study of the effects Bowen had on asthma cases. Alastair treated a two-year-old girl who had severe asthma attacks every ten days. She had had a severe reaction to increased steroid treatment which so alarmed her parents that they had stopped all medication. The child arrived at Alastair's clinic wheezing heavily. Shortly after she had received a short Bowen session, the wheezing stopped and she did not have another asthma attack for six years. She did, however, have occasional Bowen sessions over the first few months.

This was such a profound indicator that Bowen may help other asthmatics that Alastair set out to find out whether this was simply a 'one-off' or whether there was a more consistent set of indications that Bowen could help improve the quality of life of asthmatics. At first he thought this generally applied only to children. However, it soon became apparent that it seemed to work well on all asthmatics, whatever the doses of medication they were on.

While this was not a rigorous scientific study, the Bowen 'fingerprints' soon became obvious and consistent. It did not seem to change whether the asthmatic had been diagnosed with severe or mild asthma. The quality of life enjoyed by almost all asthmatics treated by him was significantly improved. A number had been hospitalized several times in weeks leading up to their first Bowen session. None of them needed hospitalization after they started Bowen. The study, however, did highlight one condition where this was not the case. Where the asthma sufferer also suffered pneumonia attacks frequently, Bowen did not seem to prevent that from happening.

As the study progressed, so a new aspect was introduced which led to a dramatic reduction in the need for the asthmatics resorting to their reliever inhalers (Ventolin/Salbutamol). Alastair asked the asthmatics to use a simple, but very effective, Bowen procedure, which is taught on all basic Bowen courses, that causes the diaphragm to release in the same way that the inhaler did. However, he emphasized to all his cases that they should use the inhaler if their doctor or asthma nurse had directed them to do so for a fixed period. Typically, this was after a spell in hospital when they might well be directed to use the inhaler several times a day for up to ten days in order to rehydrate the lungs. But, for the majority of cases, this procedure, a gentle but sharp move downwards below the bottom of the breast bone, encourages the diaphragm, which starts to spasm more and more in an asthma attack, to release – in the worst cases, immediately, but usually in about the same time that the reliever spray causes it to do.

A typical result was a woman of 27, whose medication had to be increased more and more, yet was using her reliever inhaler 20 times a day. As a comparison, five times a week is regarded as sufficient for asthma being under control. She stopped using her reliever medication immediately and used the Bowen move instead. This she found might be needed a few times a week as she worked in an environment where stress and dust were problems for her. Although she had been convinced she would have to give up her career, this one Bowen move gave her back control of her life.

The Bowen Release Move is a very gentle signal to the nervous system to get it to release any tension in the diaphragm. It is done starting at about 1 inch below the bottom of the sternum or breast bone. Initially, only the skin is taken up, slight pressure applied, and then a sharp but gentle downwards move towards the feet (not inwards) is made, rather like switching on a light. If done heavily and inwards (in other words, towards the back) it would have the opposite effect of tightening the diaphragm. Children even as young as five have been able to use this move on themselves successfully. It is also very effective when someone is suffering from an anxiety/panic attack as the diaphragm reacts in the same way.

Treating babies with breathing difficulties is very simple and can be highly effective. What the study discovered was that babies who were secreting excess mucus, which can take some months to release, will respond overnight and the mucus simply pours out of them. Five cases of this have all responded in the same way. All the babies were pre-term. As the lungs are the last part of the body to develop, they were the most at risk of problems such as this. The procedure used only took 30 seconds to do and was not only very gentle but took far less action than a parent did changing the baby's nappy.

Conventional medical treatment of preventers (steroids) and relievers (beta agonists bronchodilators) work to decrease inflammation and thereby increase gas exchange, but this is only targeting one small area of the problem. Without any air being drawn in by the diaphragm, there will be no gas exchange!

At the beginning, relievers and preventers (steroids) will help asthmatics increase gas exchange and breathe. But if the tightness in the diaphragm and intercostal muscles is not addressed, the muscles will remain tight and the tension will only increase with each further asthma attack. This is why medication does not seem to work and why even the slightest trigger can set off an asthma attack.

When the muscles are very tense, almost any stressor such as a change in temperature (cold) or a respiratory infection can cause an asthma attack. The more dangerous and scary prospect is that the puffers and steroids will soon work much less effectively, if at all. Typically, the patient will then be given a higher dose of steroids and increase the use of their puffers.

Anything that calls for extra strain by the breathing muscles will cause them to seize up and go into a spasm, thus causing an asthma attack. This is true of all muscles in the body. Example: if you get a cramp in your calf muscle whilst out running, the first thing you do is massage the muscle or rest it. If you continue running or walking at a fast pace, it will cramp again and this time the cramp will be more severe and last longer. If the muscles involved in breathing are treated and relaxed after an asthma attack, they will be much less likely to go into a spasm and, if they do, it can be treated again very easily. It does not mean that a person will be cured of their allergies but it does mean that it is possible to prevent asthma symptoms from escalating into asthma attacks.

Asthma Triggers

The most common trigger for an asthma attack in children, 95 per cent of whom suffer from 'allergic' asthma, is the common cold. For some, they never seem to recover before another cold starts. Many have to be admitted to hospital, some frequently. Quite a few families reported that the child was often given antibiotics. However, this does not seem to work well with them. Most parents reported that the child developed what seemed like a chest infection as soon as they started a cold and that they often needed medical help such as the use of steroids, antibiotics and nebulizers. This trigger was confirmed by several senior consultants as being the trigger most commonly seen. This informal study has, over the years, seen a large number of children with this common start to an asthma attack. What the study has highlighted is that almost all did not have a 'chest infection' condition when they developed colds after they had started receiving Bowen sessions. This suggests that Bowen may have caused the immune system to improve its response to the common cold. As highlighted earlier, this did not apply to children who regularly suffered from pneumonia attacks. What was also observed was that, if either an adult or child was starting a common cold, and they received Bowen on the first day or so, most colds did not develop, which again suggests that the immune system might be enhanced by having Bowen treatments.

Allergies and Asthma

There are too many allergies to be able to study directly whether Bowen has the ability to reduce the effects on a sufferer. What has been observed is that cat allergy can seem to be reduced in its effect on many of those affected. A typical example was a 13-year-old boy who was badly affected by cats. When he visited his grandmother, who owned several cats, he would need to dose himself well with Ventolin before, during and after his visit. Soon after starting Bowen sessions, however, he found he could cope without additional medication. Some four years after no longer needing Bowen, he stayed with a friend who allowed cats on their beds overnight. This led to a very severe asthma attack, so the effects may not last without occasional Bowen sessions.

The inflammatory response of the body to allergens is a sympathetic nervous system response to a foreign object. Pharmaceutical drugs act by blocking receptors on the lungs to stop this inflammatory process. This, as you can probably imagine, is only a means of treating the symptoms and not the cause.

Asthma and the Stress Response

Allergies are strange things. We can grow up without any and slowly acquire them or we can stop being allergic to what we used to be. Why does this happen?

This may be because the body changes depending on the state of the nervous system. Think of the nervous system as the central processing unit (CPU) of the body. If there is an imbalance, this affects every system in the body, including the inflammatory response, which is what causes an allergic reaction.

The sympathetic nervous system is responsible for getting the body ready for a potentially dangerous situation and plays a huge role in promoting a strong inflammatory response when exposed to stress (during the first hour of exposure to a physical or psychological stress). However, long-term exposure to stress has the opposite effect of actually suppressing the immune system. This is probably why, when there is an imbalance in the nervous system and the sympathetic nervous system keeps the body in a state of constant alertness, the inflammatory response is affected, particularly by sudden exposure to some kind of environmental, physical or psychological stress or the triggers mentioned above (Sapolsky 2004, p.154).

If the parasympathetic nervous system, responsible for creating calm, is not tapped into, then the body remains in this highly strung state of an overzealous inflammatory response system and starts to become allergic to triggers that were never previously bothersome. Things can then go from bad to worse.

Bowen treatments are able to reduce the effects of allergies on sufferers and in some cases cure them completely. This leads to the suggestion that Bowen can tone down the inflammatory response of the body, possibly by rebalancing the autonomic nervous system. Mechanisms for how this happens are described in Chapter 1.

Both asthma and allergies may be linked through the nervous system. An imbalance in the nervous system can cause breathing difficulties, which can lead to allergies or vice versa. When the central nervous system perceives the threat of restricted oxygen uptake and carbon dioxide extraction during an asthma attack, it instructs the accessory breathing muscles to activate. The body is then placed in a fight-or-flight situation through strong activation of the sympathetic nervous system. The fight-or-flight response prepares you for a stressful situation by initiating breathing through the mouth rather than your nose (to get more air in) and using your accessory muscles of breathing to aid your primary muscles, such as the diaphragm. Because the diaphragm is restricted in its movement, there is little movement in the abdominal region during breathing. This is called 'chest breathing' as opposed to 'stomach/diaphragm breathing'. Chest breathers are essentially using their secondary respiratory muscles all the time and often lose the ability to use their diaphragm at all. This can have undesired knock-on effects in the body because the respiratory diaphragm is so important to the efficient functioning of the lymphatic system.

Chest breathing is not a normal breathing pattern but is commonly found in asthmatics and other respiratory conditions. Without a means of relaxing the breathing muscles after an asthma attack, the nervous system is triggered to stay in the sympathetic mode. The body is then in a constant state of stress and alertness which can alter chemical and hormonal states. Inverted breathing pattern symptoms are well documented and include increased anxiety levels, increased allergic response, changes to the pH levels of the blood to more alkaline, increased stress hormone production, not to mention the knock-on effect on posture and movement dysfunction causing tension and pain (Chaitow 2004).

Some of the case studies will illustrate that having Bowen sessions can lead to an overall improvement in the quality of life for asthma sufferers. This is partly due to the treatment effect of rebalancing of the body's systems. While this is difficult to measure scientifically, observations suggest that a change in symptoms clearly take place.

Take the case of a six-year-old who was sensitive to so many things that she rarely completed a week at school. Her mother could not work as she was called in to school so frequently. The child could not play outside, nor stay in another house longer than an hour and would have an attack if she got into or out of a car or ran more than about 20 yards. The family were virtually housebound. On the day she received her first Bowen session, she had not had any medication, even though she was clearly wheezing and starting yet another cold. The wheezing stopped immediately at the end of a five-minute session which entailed a few gentle moves. Later that day, she ran home all the way from school. Her parents were astonished when she not only did not have an attack, but did not have an attack for some years. Her mother was able to take on a job, they were able to go out to play areas and even went abroad for holidays with no further problems.

One child who was very allergic to many triggers, including visiting the woods or a farm, was able to tolerate them perfectly well after having a few Bowen sessions. Her case is more fully documented in the case studies section. She had suffered a nearly catastrophic attack and had her first Bowen session, while still very unwell, some 12 days afterwards. Over the next several years, she had not needed an unscheduled visit her doctor. Such significant changes to the quality of life experienced by asthmatics have often been seen.

Often, asthmatics are encouraged to check their breathing twice a day using a peak flow meter. This measures the strength of an out-breath done as strongly as possible. The result of such a puff is measured on a scale between 0 and 1000. There is no standard measurement, only the individual's, as this can vary enormously from person to person, age, sex and origin. A specialist will suggest a target and the asthmatic will try to maintain this target. If the measurement declines by more than 20 per cent, then medication is usually increased as it is a sign of a potential asthma attack.

There was a case of a lady in her 60s who had been a severe asthmatic all her life, and indeed had needed to retire early because of it: 'lived at the doctors', as she put it. She would become ill if the weather changed, and rarely achieved her target of 350. She kept daily records of her peak flow as well as all her 11 medications for many years. She had four sessions of Bowen, which led to her increasing her peak flow to 400 with very few dips below 350 and maintained this level for a year. Then her health declined again due to family stress. Bowen was restarted after eight months. Her peak flow immediately responded and moved up to an average of 400 where it stayed for some years, illustrated by the charts in Figure 10.3.

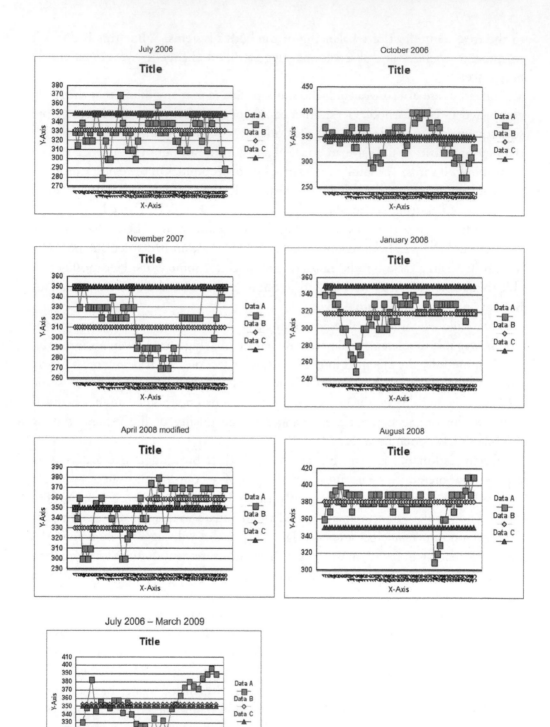

Figure 10.3 Peak flow charts

COPD

Chronic obstructive pulmonary disease (COPD) is a general term which includes the conditions chronic bronchitis and emphysema. Asthma and COPD are very different diseases that may sometimes present with similar symptoms such as breathlessness and coughing. In COPD, however, there is permanent damage to the airways. The narrowed airways are fixed, and so symptoms are chronic and persistent. Treatment to open up the airways as used for asthma rarely works for COPD patients. The main symptoms of COPD are a chronic cough with phlegm accompanied by breathlessness.

COPD is most commonly caused by smoking. Air pollution, irritants and genetics also play a part; long-term exposure to these irritants causes an inflammatory response in the lungs which causes a narrowing of the small airways and breakdown of lung tissue resulting in emphysema.

Emphysema is a disease marked by destruction of the alveoli in the lung. The walls of the alveoli become inflamed and damaged and lose their elasticity. Pockets of dead air (called bullae) form. These pockets then cause narrowing of the airways, trapping air and mucus, and making exhalation more difficult.

In chronic bronchitis, inflammation of the bronchial tubes (from smoking, air pollution, etc.) causes the production of mucus which clogs the airways and makes breathing difficult. The mucus is cleared through coughing but constant coughing and inflammation can damage the bronchial tubes. The tubes swell and thicken, leaving less room for air flow.

How Can Bowen Help in COPD?

Patients suffering from COPD typically present with increasing breathlessness together with a productive, chronic cough. Damage to the lung tissue itself is irreversible. The feeling of breathlessness is not due just to damage to the lung tissue (reducing gas exchange) but also to a tightness in the breathing muscles that restrict inhalation and exhalation. A chronic cough and the resultant extra work needed to breathe will cause tension in the muscles and these muscles can be relaxed using Bowen therapy. Clients report the ability to 'breathe again' immediately after a Bowen treatment.

Another interesting factor is that clients feel a 'shift' in their lungs and are able to cough up more mucus and sputum than before. They also report getting fewer colds that go straight to their chest, possibly as a result of a stronger immune system.

Stress and anxiety play a large role in COPD. Breathlessness activates the SNS which then causes a release of stress hormones. The nervous system is always in a heightened sympathetic mode as the body tries to bring in more air to the lungs. This is a vicious cycle that can bring about feelings of depression and hopelessness. Ironically, many patients smoke more to handle the stress. Bowen can aid in rebalancing the nervous system and in the longer term strengthen the immune system to prevent against chest infections.

CASE STUDY

Lesley, aged 40, developed severe asthma in 1996. When she first came for treatment, she needed to rest twice climbing the stairs. Within three weekly treatments, she was able to climb the stairs without stopping. Her usage of Ventolin went down from 14 times a day (as the school she worked at was on hilly ground), to just four 'Bowen Release Moves'. After a year, her consultant reduced her medication. She felt she could last ten days between treatments to remain stable.

Hay Fever

One of the main problems with the body's response to an allergen is that the production of histamine causes extra mucus to be produced to trap the allergen, and the mucus builds up in and around the sinuses and eyes. Unfortunately, the drainage channels have often become clogged so that the mucus cannot get away, causing the congestion to build up, blocking the nose and creating bulging eyes. The Bowen moves for this condition unblock the channels, which allow the mucus to drain. Keeping the channels clear from time to time relieves much of the misery.

CASE STUDY

Susannah, aged nearly six, had been allergic to a wide range of foods and colorings since birth. When she was two years old, she was diagnosed as asthmatic. She responded to many different triggers ranging from animals, colds or virus attacks and foods, all of which would induce an asthma attack. Additionally, she could have an incident if she visited the woods for any length of time, as well as any change of location, such as a visit to her grandparents or sudden changes of temperature. Her mother was a trained nurse who was meticulous in administering the prescribed drugs and in preparing all her foods. Susannah was on Beclomethasone (a steroid) twice a day and Ventolin as required. Asthma attacks were frequent with a number of admissions to hospital being needed. As the situation was becoming more worrying, the family asked for her to have Bowen Therapy to see whether that might help stop the decline in her health.

Before the first treatment could be given, Susannah suffered a major asthma attack, having caught a virus from her brother who also had respiratory problems. Her mother summarized the development of the attack as follows:

> Susannah had had three days of oral Prednisolone (a powerful steroid) prior to admission for wheezing. On the early morning of the fourth day, she was admitted into hospital via ambulance for a severe asthma attack. She worsened

on admission and did not respond to oral steroids and nebulizers (Atrovent and Salbutamol). Intravenous steroids were then given without effect. An infusion of Aminophylline (a bronchodilator) was commenced along with intravenous fluids and potassium; nebulizers continued. After 48 hours she began to improve. She had a temperature on admission which worsened and persisted. Antibiotics were administered for one week.

When Alastair saw Susannah for the first time on 10 March 2004, some 12 days after the attack, she looked a very sick child with dark rings under her eyes. She was still wheezing with a little 'grunt' at the end of each breath. Her mother was, naturally, very anxious and worried as to whether there could be any sort of reaction to the treatment. He assured her that he did very little and that there had never been a reaction with a case like this. Susannah was still in such a delicate state that anything could have induced a further attack. Treatment was very simple. When she got off the couch, the wheezing and grunt had stopped. Her mother was shown how to administer the Bowen emergency move very gently, should she become wheezy or have another asthma attack.

In week 4 of the Bowen sessions, Susannah's mother reported the following:

I have noticed some significant changes relating to Susannah's long standing asthma this week. On Friday (2 April 2004) she awoke with a cold. Prior to this she had had no wheezing or temperature, both of which she normally exhibits prior to any episode of ill health. During Friday night, she coughed continuously for just under two hours. It is unprecedented for her not to have developed asthma under these circumstances. During the next 24 hours, she continued to cough in varying degrees. It is now 4.00pm on Sunday 4 April 2004 and she has not, so far, had an asthma attack associated with this cold.

(Note: Nor did one develop. This is a very common 'fingerprint' of Bowen, often after just one treatment.)

Just over two months after the attack, on 5 May 2004, her mother wrote the following summary:

I have noticed some considerable change in Susannah over the last two to three weeks. She has not had a day off sick from school for some time. On 24 April (end of week 8) we went to a wedding. It was a long day and the reception was on a farm; the meal was in a marquee. These are all normally things that would result in wheezing at least, an asthma attack at worst. Susannah was fine until about 7.30pm – much longer than she would normally have coped with in such a situation. I could hear a small squeaking in her breathing at 7.30pm and took her home. She had a settled night. This is also significant – normally she would have been coughing and unsettled.

After this tiring weekend with a lot of travelling and change of places to stay, she then did a full week at school with no problems (she had a Bowen session on the Wednesday of that week). The following weekend (end of week 9), she went to ballet on Saturday morning and a party on Saturday afternoon where everyone was smoking. On Sunday, she had a very long day spent outside in damp conditions with a high pollen count. She was running around, playing on the trampoline and very excited. The following day (week 10) we were out for the whole day in a high pollen count in damp weather. Yesterday, she attended a full day at school with no problem.

The above illustrates an unprecedented lifestyle for Susannah. Any one of the days mentioned would have resulted in an exacerbation of her asthma and time off school. To have had several days of the type mentioned in close proximity has not been possible for her in her life so far. The fact that, as yet, she has had no adverse reaction to her activities over the last three weeks leads me to the conclusion that Bowen has benefited her enormously. It is particularly significant that she has coped as well as she has following the worst asthmatic episode of her life so far.

Susannah has continued to receive Bowen treatments when required. In August her mother called to say that she was wheezing quite badly but that she could not identify any trigger. However, by the following day it became obvious there was a trigger, which turned out to be dust from building work which had just started next door. As it was very hot it was impossible not to open windows. She immediately had a Bowen session, which reduced the wheezing. This had to be repeated as she was still receiving plenty of building dust from next door. Once she had been removed during the day from that environment, her situation improved.

Susannah is an interesting case because of the way she has responded to Bowen since her very serious attack at the end of February 2004. She has responded to Bowen in the same way as many other children have done. When she caught another virus a few weeks later, it did not produce an asthma attack, just as the cold did not. She continues to have Bowen sessions as and when required now.

She had an attack where she became very wheezy to the point where she would not have been able to avoid going to hospital by the end of the night. She immediately had a Bowen session to which she responded well. She then began a course of Seretide, a combination drug with a lower dose of steroid but including bronchodilator medication. She has now been on this medication once a day and has remained well for some months.

When reviewing the case, her mother commented that all the things that Susannah has been able to do since she started Bowen remain valid today.

CASE STUDY

Olivia was six and had been on steroids since she was a baby. She could not run more than 20 yards without needing her inhaler and would often have difficulty speaking without taking many breaths. She could not sing more than a line at a time without gasping for breath, though she loves singing with her sister. Breathing was always laboured with her shoulders rising up and down in a typical fashion and wheezing constantly. Any cold would lead to a chest infection needing antibiotics. She was on Becotide morning and evening and Ventolin when needed both during the day and night. She was starting a cold when she had her first Bowen session. Her mother had not given her any medication that day 'so we can see what happens!'

At the end of her first Bowen session, the wheezing virtually stopped. Later that day she ran all the way home from school, and has not stopped running around ever since. She was starting a chesty cough the day she had her third treatment. That cold also stopped by the following day. Her medication halved from the start and by mid January she had no Ventolin at all, all week. She caught the flu from her mother recently but managed well, without any wheezing. Interestingly, her breathing was totally normal with no sign of the laboured breath we started with just before Christmas and she was back to school the day after her Bowen session. She is often singing whole verses with her sister now.

Her mother commented about Christmas Day, 2004: 'I had to note all this because previously I would not have opted to go out, especially for a day, as this would have been a worse case scenario for Olivia's health and my stress levels. What actually happened was so rare, I had to note it down. Olivia was just one of four very happy, very healthy, excited children. Today no pump, no allergic reactions, no need for Mum to act like a neurotic nurse! Lovely day, a mini miracle!' This was after just two Bowen sessions.

After 40 days (and nights) Olivia had not used her Ventolin until she visited an aquarium attraction with the school. The strong chemicals caused a little wheezing needing Ventolin once. So she had another Bowen session and was fine and still running… When she caught a virus recently, she did not develop a chest infection and her chest was clear, so antibiotics were not needed. She is full-time at school. After a five-month gap, Olivia had another Bowen session having been a little wheezy over the previous two days. During the whole of this time, she had not had an infection, something which happened all the time before she had Bowen. She has a normal life, is often playing outside, which again she was always unable to do, and is fully integrated at school.

Olivia is still very well generally and attends school regularly, probably over 90 per cent of the time. Her mother commented during an interview about Olivia's case that the day she had her first Bowen treatment 'everything changed' in their lives. Olivia has been able to go to many places she could not visit in the past, and can take part in many events which were just unthinkable before she had that all-important first treatment lasting only a very few minutes. The family was even able to travel abroad without incident.

CASE STUDY

Jacob was born just over one month prematurely and, like most babies at this stage, was full of mucus which he had great difficulty expelling. At night, his breathing sounded 'like Darth Vader', according to his parents, and was a deep, rattling wheeze. Both eyelids were a deep, bright red and were described by the doctor as being probable birthmarks. He had some breathing difficulty all the time, often suffered from hiccups and his nose was severely congested since birth. The hospital consultant advised the parents that it would take six months for the mucus to clear.

The parents were told to use a saline drip up his nose four times a day to help clear the mucus as the doctor was concerned about his condition. They were also told to give him Ventolin before sleeping up to four times a day. This they found very difficult to do. Jacob was then brought for his first Bowen session at three months old, which took only a few moments of gentle treatment.

That night, mucus poured out of him from every part – his nappy, mouth and nose. It was green and thick and looked infected. The bright red eyelids mostly cleared (probably caused by the mucus congestion). Straight after the Bowen session Jacob 'chilled out' and relaxed to such an extent that his parents had to check on him throughout the night. They could no longer hear his noisy breathing.

On the fourth day Jacob was brought in to a Bowen class to show the effect of Bowen on a case like this. What we all saw was a very cheerful, happy, well-looking baby with no mucus around his nose, breathing normally without any sign of wheeze or rattle. Jacob continued to make excellent progress, still occasionally bringing up some mucus, though it then looked yellow or clear and no longer looked infected. Apparently Jacob's first words were 'My Mum and Dad think Bowen is fantastic!'

CASE STUDY

Alex is a competitive swimmer. He trains for three hours a day, four times a week. Alex was diagnosed with asthma as a child at the age of eight. By the age of ten he no longer used his inhalers and did not have any symptoms of asthma.

In recent months he had become breathless and wheezy during training sessions in the pool. As a swimmer, he feared the worst: a chlorine allergy. He needed to use his Salbutamol inhalers at least three times during a training session and would sometimes have to miss sessions. Any slight change in chlorine levels or pool temperature would affect his breathing. He would begin to feel tightness in his chest and start wheezing. The doctors increased the dosage of his steroids and changed his medication. However, this had little effect.

After two bad asthma attacks in one week in 2010, Alex came for a Bowen treatment. The first thing I noticed during the treatment was the tightness of the muscles in the upper back and diaphragm. During the session, Alex reported the feeling of his lungs expanding. The very next day, he used the Bowen release move both before his training session and after. He did not feel wheezy or breathless throughout the entire session. Alex had two follow-up Bowen sessions. In between these sessions he had a cough and cold, which caused some breathlessness and wheezing but never developed into anything more severe. Alex also reported that his peak flow values were much better and more consistent after the treatments. Since then, Alex has gone on to compete in a number of county championships and performing very well.

CASE STUDY

Prashanth, aged 30, was diagnosed with acute allergic rhinitis. He is sensitive to the change in temperature, deodorants and perfumes. When exposed to any of these triggers, his eyes become very itchy and watery and he starts sneezing profusely. At his worst he sneezes up to 50 times in a row and needs a large number of handkerchiefs with him at all times. Apart from the symptoms mentioned, he also feels as though he is constantly having to swallow and feels his sinuses are very blocked up.

Despite being on antihistamines and nasal decongestants, his symptoms did not improve. These symptoms affect his ability to perform at work and also affect his sleep. This is a vicious cycle as he realized that lack of sleep was also one of his triggers. After his first Bowen treatment, Prashanth reported that his swallowing and sneezing had improved by 50 per cent and he could feel his nostrils unblocking immediately. By his third treatment he had not experienced any sneezing or sniffing for the past week despite being exposed to the same triggers. His swallowing feels normal and his eyes are much less itchy. He also mentions that he is much more alert mentally and more able to cope with stressful situations. His body feels balanced, calm and relaxed and not as highly strung. Prashanth continues to have regular follow-up treatments every four to six weeks.

ℰⱱ

References

ASTHMA UK (2013) Asthma facts and FAQs. Available at www.asthma.org.uk/asthma-facts-and-statistics, accessed on 14 May 2014.

CDC (2011) *Asthma in the US*. Washington, DC: Centers for Disease Control and Prevention.

Chaitow, L. (2004) Breathing pattern disorders, motor control and low back pain. *Journal of Osteopathic Medicine* 7 (1), 33–40.

NCHS (2011) *Asthma*. Hyattsville, MD: National Center for Health Statistics. Available at www.cdc.gov/nchs/fastats/asthma.htm, accessed on 14 May 2014.

Sapolsky, R. (2004) *Why Zebras Don't Get Ulcers* (3rd edition). New York: St Martin's Griffin.

Ward, H. (1973) Transcript of Proceedings before the Osteopathic, Chiropractic and Naturopathy Committee Geelong, 8 October.

Resources

Using the Bowen Technique to Relieve Asthma
www.bowen-for-asthma.com

Relieve Childhood Asthma with the Bowen Technique
www.relieve-childhood-asthma.com

11

Women's Health

Introduction

A part of our Bowen Client Assessment involves a set of questions pertaining to women's health. These include questions on whether periods are absent, regular, irregular, heavy, painful, whether the woman might be pregnant and then whether they consider themselves to be peri-menopausal, menopausal or post-menopausal. We also ask for other comments pertaining to the menstrual cycle such as whether there are long/short cycles, pre-menstrual syndrome (PMS) and an opportunity to note whether they might have something like endometriosis or polycystic ovarian syndrome (PCOS) and perhaps any other abnormalities such as ovarian cysts, fibroids, any problems in relation to the cervix and any abnormal smear test results and, of course, cancer in any part of the reproductive system.

How Bowen Works for Menstrual/Women's Health

Both the Bowen coccyx and the coccyx oblique moves affect the end of the sympathetic chain which has a ganglion just in front of the coccyx (this is part of the sympathetic nerve supply to the reproductive organs) (Figure 11.1). There are also parasympathetic nerves around the coccyx that innervate the lower bowel and reproductive organs. The way that Bowen affects nerve supply is basically because it frees up the fascia through which the nerves and their blood supply travel. Nerves are supplied with blood via the vasa nervorum. When blood supply is compromised by restrictions in the fascia (something that can be seen clearly in the images of Dr Guimberteau), this has an immediate effect on the ability of nerve axons to transmit action potential.

The coccyx move itself goes right over the attachment of the dura, arachnoid and pia membranes at the filum terminale (or coccygeal ligament), affecting the nervous system directly. The impulses seem to travel up these membranes (called meningeal fascia) as they attach on to the top of the neck and then up to the cranium where the pituitary and hypothalamus sit in a trough (the sella turcica) in the sphenoid bone completely encased in these membranes. (This is a similar mechanism to the way the coccyx–neck procedure works as the impulses travel straight up the spine without the influence of the bottom stopper moves.)

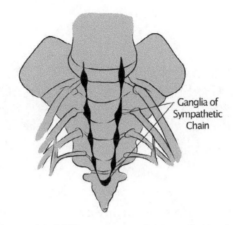

Figure 11.1 The coccyx and sympathetic chain
Source: Martin Gordon

The Menstrual Cycle

The average age of menarche in the Western world is 12.9 years (Hamilton-Fairley 2004) and coincides with the secretion of androgens to stimulate oestrogens, the pubertal growth spurt and female sexual characteristics of growth of axillary and pubic hair, and breast development, usually at Tanner Stage 3 (Hamilton-Fairley 2004).

The pituitary gland is responsible for the release of growth hormone and luteinizing hormones. Luteinizing hormones in turn stimulate the ovaries to increase androgen production and start the maturation of oocytes (eggs) in the ovary so that menstruation can begin (Hamilton-Fairley 2004). It is estimated that a woman will have approximately 400 menstrual periods during her lifetime, so it is not a surprise that a woman's period holds great significance to her health during her reproductive phase (and beyond).

For some reason, most of the medical literature points to the menstrual cycle being 28 days and this is what is shown in all the diagrams, but of course there is some deviation, with some women having shorter or longer cycles. If we allow for the 28-day model, the first five days of the cycle are counted as the actual 'bleed' or menstrual period. Luteinizing hormone levels reduce, causing the lining of the uterus to break down and the onset of menstrual bleeding (Hamilton-Fairley 2004). Over the next 7–14 days, the follicle stimulating hormone (FSH), stimulated by the pituitary gland, stimulates oestrogen levels to rise and the uterine lining to grow in anticipation for the ova to be released and potentially fertilized during ovulation, or the women's most fertile period between days 12 and 14. Following that, levels of the hormone progesterone increase and continue to thicken the uterine lining in response to a potential pregnancy. If the egg is not fertilized or embedded, hormone levels drop, causing the lining of the uterus to shed, the menstrual period to take place and the cycle to start again (Hamilton-Fairley 2004). It should be noted that the surge in progesterone levels can make the breast tissue more sensitive and women might experience what is commonly known as pre-menstrual tension or PMS, as they also feel more 'swollen' in response to the hormonal activity taking place during the days leading up to menstruation.

Oligomenorrhea: Infrequent/Absent Periods

As noted in Hamilton-Fairley (2004, p.29), a girl's weight needs to reach about 45 kg before menstruation can begin. Common reasons for a delay in starting menstruation can be related to low body weight, perhaps because of sporting pursuits or serious ballet training which require the girl to retain a very slim, pre-pubertal figure. Often, once the weight has increased, menstruation will occur. Indeed, Hamilton-Fairley suggests that investigations for absence of menarche may not begin until the girl is about 16 years of age (Hamilton-Fairley 2004).

Other young women might have irregular periods to start with and/or irregular or even absent periods. One obvious explanation is pregnancy, but, that aside, low weight might be to blame or hormonal imbalances (Tucker 2000), which may need further investigation.

Many clients report that their periods become more regular after Bowen. This could be due to the balancing and calming effect of Bowen sessions, but it could also be because the pituitary is specifically targeted in some Bowen procedures such as the TMJ and coccyx work.

CASE STUDY

Angela is a yoga teacher in her mid-20s. She had not had a period for a year and her energy levels were low. The first thing that happened the day after Angela's treatment was that she had a period. Although she may have not been overjoyed to have a period as such, she fully understood how important restarting her menses was for the protection of bone health, and certainly for any future plans for having children. Her diet was largely vegan, so we discussed the importance of iron and ensuring her weight remained high enough to sustain a regular menstrual cycle.

Metrorrhagia: Irregular Periods

Some women have irregular periods. This is often a nuisance for them because they do not know when they are going to menstruate and this can cause problems, particularly if they are trying to conceive, when there is no regular cycle or therefore determined ovulation.

Bowen can be helpful in regulating the menstrual cycle due to its influence on the pituitary gland, both through rebalancing the body via the basic relaxation procedures and through doing work on the coccyx, which is one of the main Bowen procedures for menstrual problems. In addition, women might wish to consider dietary, naturopathic and nutritional aspects of their reproductive health.

Maggie Chambers (homeopath and nutritionist) and Sandra Gustafson (registered nurse, integrative healthcare and Bowenwork practitioner) suggest ways below to improve these conditions naturally, using diet, herbs, homeopathy and physical therapies, all approaches that can support Bowen work.

Nutritional and Natural Approaches

NUTRITION

- If a sluggish thyroid is causing lack of menstruation, add *kelp* to the diet.

- Drink sufficient *water*.

- Avoid weight fluctuations and maintain a *healthy balanced diet*.

- *Celery juice* promotes menstruation.

SUPPLEMENTS

- *Green foods* supplements such as *chlorella* and *spirulina* detoxify the system and regulate the menstrual cycle.

- Take an *evening primrose oil* supplement.

- *Vitamin B* is necessary for the production of sex hormones.

- *Vitamin E* will help to restore the cycle.

- *Zinc* will increase the flow and regulate the periods.

HERBAL REMEDIES

- *Chaste tree* (*Vitex agnus castus*) is the main herb to assist in regulating the menstrual cycle via its action on the HPA axis (Bone 2003).

- *Paeonia* (*Paeonia lactiflora*), improves follicle formation and corpus luteum function in the ovaries and supports progesterone production (Bone 2003).

- *Dong quai* (*Angelica sinensis*) is a good female tonic that regulates the cycle and nourishes the blood (Bone 2003).

- *Black cohosh* (*Cimicifuga racemosa*) modulates oestrogen activity, is a uterine tonic and promotes menstruation.

- *Turmeric* (*Curcuma longa*) moves stagnant blood and supports healthy liver function (Bone 2003).

HOMEOPATHY

- *Aconite* is useful for menstruation that has stopped due to physical or emotional shock.

- *Pulsatilla* can help normalize irregular menses in women who are anxious, teary and prone to feeling cold.

Physical Treatments

- Ensure plenty of *rest* and *relaxation*.

- Take gentle *exercise*.

- *Hot compresses* on the abdomen increase the blood supply and relax the muscles.

- *Hot* and *cold water* applied alternately to the pelvic region provides an increased blood flow and detoxification.

- *Marjoram oil* massaged into the lower abdomen can have a stabilizing effect on the menstrual cycle.

Dysmenorrhea: Painful Periods

Dysmenorrhea means painful periods. Primary dysmenorrhea is pain that happens in young women, and is classed as 'primary' before they consider childbirth, or has an unknown cause (Dawood 2006). Secondary dysmenorrhea is that which follows childbirth or has secondary and underlying pathology, such as endometriosis (Proctor and Farquhar 2006). Either way, painful periods can be very distressing for women and can result in absenteeism from school or work (Dawood 2006) when they become severely affected.

Dysmenorrhea is caused by excessive uterine contractions that cause cramping-type pain (Dawood 2006). It is thought that prostaglandin levels that cause the uterine lining to shed are higher in women with more severe dysmenorrhea (Proctor and Farquhar 2006). Typical medical management of dysmenorrhea is usually painkillers such as NSAIDS, paracetamol and then possibly trialling oral contraceptives that seem to 'significantly' reduce pain. Tricycling contraceptives, taking three packets of the contraceptive pill back-to-back, with no breaks so that women have fewer periods, may be suggested since there is not 'strictly' a need for a monthly bleed (Dawood 2006; Hamilton-Fairley 2004; Proctor and Farquhar 2006). Both Dawood and Proctor and Farquar suggest the use of TENS machines to block the nerve receptors and the same authors also advocate for dietary supplements (see below) such as magnesium, calcium, vitamins B and E and herbs. Finally, the authors discussed in this section advocate the use of alternative therapies, in particular acupuncture, which have shown good results (Dawood 2006; Proctor and Farquhar 2006). Bowen might also be considered a useful adjunct, and research and clinical trials would be worthwhile contemplating in addition to the evidence we have from our female clients that Bowen improves their pain symptoms.

Endometriosis

Endometriosis is a condition in which the endometrial tissue (the lining of the uterus) escapes into the surrounding pelvis and elsewhere (Henderson and Wood 2000). It is a condition that is so far poorly understood. The displaced endometrial tissues cause pain and inflammation as the cells attach themselves to other parts of the pelvis and grow in response to the women's menstrual cycle hormones. One of the likeliest reasons for endometriosis was discovered by Dr Sampson in the 1920s; he developed the theory of 'retrograde menstruation' (Mills and Vernon 1999). More recent arguments to explain the causes of endometriosis include immune factors, blood and lymph transportation theories, genetic and pollutant factors (Henderson and Wood 2000).

Endometriosis can be found in any area of the pelvis including the bladder and bowels. It can also be found (rarely) in the lungs, kidney and diaphragm (Hamilton-Fairley 2004).

Symptoms of endometriosis are:

- period pain (dysmenorrhoea)

- painful intercourse (dyspareunia)

- painful ovulation

- infertility

- painful urination

- painful bowel movements

- back pain

- digestive complaints

- fatigue

- depression

- psychological – poor memory and concentration.

(Mears 1996)

Some women will experience only one or two symptoms where others will experience a whole spectrum of symptoms depending on the severity of the condition.

Medical Management

Some women might find that they experience less pain after a laparoscopic surgery (Ballweg 2003). They might even be able to conceive. For other women, the symptoms of endometriosis can reappear again even quite a short time after surgery. This is because, whilst normal menstruation continues, any remaining endometriosis or new endometrial sites continue to be fed by the woman's hormones during the natural menstrual cycle.

There are a few well-known methods and established drug therapies that can be used to medically manage endometriosis, many approaches being similar to treating dysmenorrhoea. One is through using the oral contraceptive pill, sometimes tricycling packets (combining three months medication at a time) so that a woman has fewer episodes of menstruation (Proctor and Farquhar 2006). Another method is through use of Danazol, which results in some unpleasant side effects. Some women are treated using Depo-Provera, a form of progesterone, but this also causes side effects and is less commonly used these days. Last, a group of drugs known as GnRH analogues is often used in the treatment of endometriosis. These work by reducing the FS (follicle stimulating) and LH (luteinizing) hormones and lead to lower levels of oestrogen. Since it is the oestrogen that 'feeds' the endometriosis, this means that its growth is inhibited. HRT is given in the form of 'add-back' therapy to minimize the pseudo-menopausal symptoms incurred by this drug regime and to ensure that bone density is retained, as far as possible.

One of the problems with any of these drug regimes is that they cannot be used for indefinite periods. In particular the use of GnRH analogues is not usually recommended for longer than 6–12 months because of concerns about osteoporosis and decreasing bone density. The long-term usage (continuous usage over many years) of GnRH analogues requires further investigation.

This all means that medical treatments for endometriosis are fairly short term, so that even if a woman is experiencing good pain relief and improvement in her symptoms, just as she starts to possibly feel well again the drugs are often stopped. This can be very frustrating, especially if the treatment has been successful.

Pain Management

Pain management for endometriosis is difficult because of the wide range of symptoms that it encompasses, and many approaches are similar to the management of dysmenorrhea. A range of analgesia may be used including paracetamol, aspirin, NSAIDs and codeine-related products. Some women who are in severe pain are occasionally hospitalized and offered morphine-related drugs.

The use of a TENS machine is helpful for some women with chronic pelvic pain and endometriosis. Electrical stimulation on the skin via a TENS machine distracts or alters the nerve pain signals and can provide temporary relief. A nutritious diet is also important. One high in fish oils and vitamins B and E, zinc and magnesium can help with the inflammation of endometriosis (Mills and Vernon 1999). Some women also find complementary medicine can be helpful in their management of endometriosis – for example herbal medicine, homeopathy and acupuncture. Again, Bowen has been shown to be helpful for this condition, but larger research trials are needed.

Nutritional and Natural Approaches

Maggie Chambers suggests ways the practioner can advise the patient to improve these conditions naturally, using diet, herbs, homeopathy and physical therapies.

NUTRITION

- Avoid wheat and dairy in order to calm inflammation and strengthen the immune system.

- Foods which may aggravate the symptoms of endometriosis are coffee, tea, fried foods, processed foods, salt, sugar and chocolate.

- Eliminate alcohol intake as it can lead to raised oestrogen levels.

- Cut out meat if possible, to avoid ingesting excess artificial hormones.

- *Phyto-oestrogens* are found in soya foods, beans, lentils and chickpeas.

- *Shiitake mushrooms* help regulate the immune system and inflammatory pathways and inhibit the growth of endometrial tissue.

- *Bitter salad leaves* such as rocket and watercress may help to clear pelvic lymphatic congestion.

- *Seaweed* and other sea vegetables contain iodine, which is beneficial to thyroid hormone regulation. Other iodine-rich foods are watercress, pineapple, pears, artichokes, egg yolks, seafood and citrus fruits.

- Increase omega 3 essential fatty acids in oily fish, nuts and seeds to reduce the inflammatory reaction.

- Increase foods high in beta-carotenes to promote healing, such as carrots, apricots, squash and sweet potatoes.

- Eat fruit and vegetables that are rich in alkalizing minerals.

SUPPLEMENTS

- Take a good quality *multi-vitamin* and *mineral* supplement.

- Take *flax seed oil* and *evening primrose oil.*

- Include *bromelain* (pineapple enzyme) for its anti-inflammatory action and to promote absorption.

- *Vitamin C* with *bioflavonoids* can support healing.

- Add an *antioxidant* such as *pycnogenol* to calm the inflammation in the endometrial cells.

- Take *Swedish bitters* after meals to optimize digestion and absorption of nutrients from your food.

HERBAL REMEDIES

- *Agnus castus* is recommended as a hormone balancer.

- *Wild yam* is anti-inflammatory, anti-spasmodic and has a mild progesterone action.

- *Black cohosh* strengthens the uterus and may help to dissolve adhesions.

- *Milk thistle* helps the liver to metabolize excess oestrogen.

- *Dong quai* helps relieve the symptoms. Simmer the root to make a tea, or use as a tincture.

- *Dandelion root* tea helps the liver metabolize excess oestrogen.

- *Nettle* tea is useful if excessive bleeding has resulted in anaemia, and is a good anti-inflammatory.

- *Pau d'arco* is an effective herb if taken regularly to strengthen the immune system.

- *Cramp bark* (*Viburnum opulus*), Paeonia, black haw (*Viburnum prunifolium*), chamomile (*Matricaria recutita*) and ginger can help relieve pain and cramping (Romm 2010).

Physical Treatments

- Avoid doing headstands or shoulder stands when menstruating.

- Use *sanitary pads* instead of tampons.

- Avoid IUDs.

- *Regular strenuous exercise* stimulates the circulation and clears toxins.

- *Sunlight* can help regulate the endocrine system.

- Use a *castor oil* pack a couple of times a week to help relieve symptoms of pain and inflammation.

CASE STUDY

Joanna Austen Bodmin and Liskeard, Cornwall, England (www.bowenincornwall.co.uk)

Brenda is a lady in her late 40s who has suffered from the associated pain and discomfort of endometriosis for 20 years. When she first came for Bowen she was suffering with constant abdominal pain at a level of 8/10, struggling with mobility, sleeping for no more than four hours and had difficulty in passing urine unless her bladder was very full. She also had severe gastritis and arm pain associated with her working practices.

Medication was 1000mg diclofenac four times daily, paracetamol daily up to the maximum allowed, as required, and esomeprazole 40 mg daily. She was fitted with a Mirena Coil (IUD) six months prior to starting her Bowen treatment.

Treatment commenced in February and included standard Bowen coccyx and TMJ work. After three treatments the diclofenac dose had been reduced to two daily. Sleep had increased to 5.5 hours, but in herself she was feeling very tired and was suffering symptoms of runny nose and lethargy as with a cold. Her arm pain had increased and she had difficulty with neck rotation. 'Period type' pain had increased to 6/10 and she was feeling bloated. Bowen pelvic and TMJ work was used.

It was decided that Brenda would start on a course of an enzyme called serrapeptase.

The next week Brenda reported that she had had a period for a week, the first since the Mirena Coil had been fitted. She had reduced the Diclofenac to one in the morning and no paracetamol. Her arm and neck were still giving her pain and tingling sensations in the arm. Coccyx and TMJ were again applied.

Two weeks later bleeding had stopped, arm pain had gone and neck had freed up. However sleep was again disturbed and the abdominal pain had not reduced from 6/10. There was a constant discharge.

I then completed a course called Hormonal Balancing, the Bowen Way (see below for details). This encompassed a set of procedures specifically targeting endometriosis. The protocol recommends weekly treatments for a month, which can be completed in about 20 minutes, reducing to fortnightly and further reducing to a monthly treatment until the issues resolve. During this time Brenda was still taking the serrapeptase. However, I noticed a sudden change in Brenda's demeanour. She had colour in her cheeks and a brighter countenance. She was taking no painkillers and all discharge had stopped. As at the time of writing this case study we are now on a monthly 'tune-up' cycle.

Menorrhagia: Heavy Periods

Some women present for treatment of menorrhagia (heavy periods) that can be very disruptive, causing flooding and ensuing embarrassment, as well as risk of low iron, anaemia, and resulting in fatigue. One cause of menorrhagia can be fibroids, benign growths that are found in the uterus, or polyps. It might be possible to manage menorrhagia with contraceptive medication. For example, the Mirena Coil has been found to significantly reduce heavy periods (Albers, Hull and Wesley 2004; Hamilton-Fairley 2004). Some women may also decide to consider hysterectomy and/or other surgery (Albers, Hull and Wesley 2004; Hamilton-Fairley 2004).

CASE STUDY

> Joanna Austen, Bodmin and Liskeard, Cornwall,
> England (www.bowenincornwall.co.uk)

Lyn was a 50-year-old who attended for Bowen treatment hoping for help with back pain. In the course of history-taking it emerged that she had a history of very heavy, painful periods which had worsened in the last year. Her doctor diagnosed fibroids and suggested a hysterectomy. Lyn tried other therapies before Bowen, including regular chiropractic, Chinese medicine and herbs, and acupuncture for six months weekly.

We started a course of Bowen Therapy which included treatment for back pain, but emphasis was placed on treating the abdomen. The coccyx move was used regularly, as was work directly on the abdominal area. Immediate reaction was felt, the abdominal area became hot and started bubbling. Three treatments at weekly intervals were carried out, then a course of monthly visits followed. Each time abdominal work was applied using Bowen moves over the uterine area and on any tense areas found; this was in addition to other Bowen moves that were appropriate on that date.

Gradually the pain and heavy bleeding decreased to the degree they caused no problems. It was a year before the fibroids were no longer causing a problem and normal menstruation recurred until a natural menopause started.

Lyn's story:

> Several years ago before being peri-menopausal I suffered with heavy and painful periods. I went to my GP who referred me to my local hospital to undergo tests. The results showed that I had several fibroids in my womb. My GP advised a hysterectomy, which I was strongly against, saying that I would seek a more holistic approach to the problem. I tried quite a few options, some of which were long term and very expensive, and did not seem to help.
>
> I decided to try Bowen Therapy for other health issues and talked to Jo about the fibroids. We undertook a course of treatment. It took almost a year to eradicate the fibroids, but it immediately helped alleviate the pain and heaviness of the periods.

Maggie Chambers suggests ways the practioner can advise the patient to improve these conditions naturally, using diet, herbs, homeopathy and physical therapies.

Nutritional and Natural Approaches

NUTRITION

- *Vitamin A* supports the immune system. Eat liver, peppers, carrots, apricots and kale.

- *Vitamin C and bioflavonoids* aid the immune system. Eat parsley, broccoli, peppers, watermelon, cherries and sprouts.

- *Iron* is essential to avoid anaemia so eat kelp, blackstrap molasses, wheat bran, pumpkin seeds and wheat germ.

- *Vitamin K* is needed for healthy blood clotting and can be found in broccoli, lettuce, cabbage and spinach.

- *Essential fatty acids* in nuts, seeds and oily fish support healthy hormone balance and regulate dysfunctional bleeding.

- Avoid meat and dairy products produced with artificial hormones.

- Avoid caffeine and fried, processed and refined foods for optimal health.

SUPPLEMENTS

- *Brewer's yeast* is rich in vitamin B complex and supports good health and energy levels.

- *Lecithin* supports healthy fat metabolism.

- *Evening primrose oil* supports healthy hormonal balance.

- Nettles (*Urtica doica*), Alfalfa (*Medicago sativa*), Yellow dock (*Rumex crispus*) and Dandelion root (*Taraxacum officinale*) can help replace iron deficiencies (Romm 2010).

- Milk thistle (*Silybum marianum*) supports optimal liver function and detoxification.

- Yarrow (*Achillea millefolium*), lady's mantle (*Alchemilla vulgaris*), bayberry (*Myrica cerifera*), shepherd's purse (*Capsella bursa-pastoris*) and cinnamon (*Cinnamomum cassia*) can be used as uterine tonics and for excessive menstrual bleeding (Romm 2010).

Physical Treatments

- *Alternate hot and cold water showers* directed at the pelvic area help alleviate symptoms by supporting detoxification and regulating the menstrual cycle.

- *Exercise* is essential for supporting healthy metabolism. Avoid anything strenuous before and during a period which can deplete the body.

- Ensure adequate *rest*.

- *Keep the bowels moving regularly* to remove toxins and prevent pressure in the pelvic region.

Polycystic Ovarian Syndrome (PCOS)

Sandra Gustafson

Polycystic ovary syndrome (PCOS) is a common gynaecological, metabolic and endocrine disorder that can affect women from menarche to menopause. In addition to the presence of multiple ovarian cysts, there are complex hormonal imbalances leading to:

- hyperandrogenism

- amennorhea

- anovulation/oligo-ovulation

- insulin resistance

- hyperlipidaemia

- increased luteinizing hormone (LH)/decreased follicle stimulating hormone (FSH)

- increased oestrogen/decreased progesterone levels

- increased androgen levels (testosterone, androstenedione and dehydroepi androsterone (DHEA))

- decreased sex hormone-binding globulin (SHBG).

(Barber *et al.* 2007; Romm 2010)

Elevated androgens stimulate hirsutism, alopecia and acne, and elevated oestrogen and insulin levels increase fat production and abdominal girth and weight gain. Evidence suggests genetic predispositions, the pregnant mother's health (gestational obesity) and being born post-term (>40 weeks gestation). Chronic stress and prolonged sympathetic nervous system overstimulation can lead to hormonal dysregulation including elevated cortisol and blood sugar levels, pituitary and adrenal gland dysfunction and ovarian cyst development (Pasquali *et al.* 2011).

PCOS essentially starts with a hypothalamic-pituitary-ovarian (HPO) axis imbalance. Increased pituitary LH secretions stimulate ovarian follicular growth, and decreased FSH suppresses follicular maturation, resulting in chronic anovulation and multiple ovarian cyst formation, and stimulates cyclic androgen overproduction in the ovaries and adrenal glands. Stress responses increase adrenocorticotrophic hormone (ACTH) stimulation and androgen levels from the hypothalamic-pituitary-adrenal (HPA) axis, perpetuating the cycle (Pasquali *et al.* 2011).

Insulin resistance increases insulin secretion and impaired glucose tolerance, and abdominal fat deposition, increasing the risk for hypertension, cardiovascular disease and diabetes Type II. High-sugar, high-carbohydrate diets and stress also increase insulin resistance (Pasquali *et al.* 2011; Romm 2010). Additionally, women with PCOS are at risk for hormone-sensitive endometrial and breast cancer (Barber *et al.* 2007; Romm 2010).

PCOS is diagnosed by:

- ovarian ultrasound revealing enlarged ovaries with fluid-filled cysts (Barber *et al.* 2007; Romm 2010)

- menstrual history of oligo-amenorrhea with inter-menstrual intervals > 42 days (Barber *et al.* 2007)

- abnormal hormone levels of LH, FSH, oestradiol, progesterone, prolactin, testosterone, androgens and SBHG, glucose, cholesterol and triglycerides (Romm 2010).

Symptoms include:

- irregular menses (< 8 cycles per year)

- hirsutism

- androgenic alopecia

- obesity

- infertility

- dysfunctional uterine bleeding

- multiple miscarriages

- acne

- mood disorders (e.g. depression, irritability).

(Barber *et al.* 2007; Romm 2010)

Conventional medical treatment involves:

- regulating androgens, unopposed oestrogens and menstrual irregularity with glucocorticoids, spirinolactones and contraceptives

- increasing fertility with, for example, clomiphene

- controlling blood sugar levels with hypoglycaemics (e.g. metformin)

- weight-loss and exercise regimes.

Complementary treatment is aimed at reducing and managing stress reactivity, restoring HPO- and HPA-axis function and hormonal balance, dietary changes and encouraging physical activity. Ways of restoring balance in the HPA axis are discussed in Chapter 9.

Exercise and weight loss contribute to increased self-esteem and mood elevation, decreased cardiovascular, diabetes and hyperinsulinaemia risks. Obese women who lose 5–10 per cent of bodyweight through gradual and steady weight loss and consistent daily exercise experience decreased PCOS symptoms and more regular menstrual cycles. Low-glycaemic diets and supplementary chromium and fish oil can help improve glucose and lipid profiles and support weight loss (Romm 2010). Bowen work supports deep relaxation and reduces sympathetic nervous system over-stimulation of the HPA and HPO axes. Procedures such as coccyx, TMJ, kidney, navel and pelvis can help to improve optimal function of the pituitary, adrenal and ovarian glands, restore hormonal balance and improve fertility.

CASE STUDY

Alice, a 37-year-old woman, presented at my clinic with a longstanding history of irregular menses, hypothyroidism (treated with levothyroxine), overweight despite eating carefully (body mass index 30), gastro-oesophageal reflux disorder (GORD) and infertility. Blood tests revealed abnormal LH/FSH and elevated fasting glucose levels, all likely indications of PCOS. She had a stressful job caring for elderly people, was recently married and wanted to start a family. Using Bowen work on a weekly basis for about three months, where I mostly used core relaxation and coccyx procedures, Alice's menses became more regular and she could track her ovulation cycle using body temperature and cervical mucus changes. She was feeling less stressed and anxious about her 'biological clock ticking' and more hopeful that she would conceive. She continued to receive Bowen work monthly, using coccyx procedure to support ovulation. After six months of not conceiving, Alice tried invitro-fertilization (IVF), without success. She returned to my office and I suggested weekly Bowen work prior to her next round of IVF. This time it was successful, and Alice is now the proud mother of twin boys.

An informative resource for women with PCOS is PCO Support (www.pcosupport. org).

cs

Menopause

cs *Sandra Gustafson*

Menopause is the cessation of the menstrual cycle for 6–12 months in a woman's life, usually between 45 and 55 years of age, when her ovaries can no longer produce ova. In response to declining ovarian activity, the pituitary gland increases FSH and LH secretion to stimulate the ovaries, which also stimulates androgen and oestrogen production in the adrenal glands (Pizzorno, Murray and Joiner-Bey 2002).

Hormones affect the way women think, sense and act, and diminishing levels during peri-menopause and post-menopause can cause mental and physical changes such as sleep disorders, depression, hot flashes, decreased libido, night-sweats, mood fluctuations, memory dysfunction, hair loss, bone, skin and soft-tissue changes, thyroid and adrenal changes, and weight gain (Hisley 2008).

Oestrogen and progesterone levels drop considerably, affecting the musculo-skeletal system and internal organ integrity, and can lead to osteopaenia, osteoporosis, decreased joint mobility, pelvic organ prolapses, bladder infections and incontinence. Excess oestrogen versus progesterone production after menopause can increase breast and uterine cancer risks. Women who started their periods early and/or go through menopause after 55 years have higher cancer risks due to longer exposure to oestrogen, as do women on post-menopausal hormone replacement therapy (HRT) and using synthetic unopposed-oestrogen long term.

In addition to cancer risks, menopausal women face increased health challenges such as heart disease, fibromyalgia, migraine, adult onset diabetes, dysfunctional bleeding, atrophic vaginitis and vulvodynia. Cardiovascular disease is the number one killer and cancer is the second highest cause of death in women over 55 years of age in the USA (US Centers for Disease Control and Prevention 2013).

Stress factors contribute greatly towards how a woman transitions into menopause. Many of the symptoms menopausal women experience result from hypothalamic dysfunction, altering brain and endocrine function. Overstimulation of the sympathetic nervous system and HPA axis can aggravate many of the common menopausal symptoms. Often, middle-aged women find themselves in the 'Sandwich Generation' – still raising children and having to take care of ageing, increasingly dependent parents, which can cause mental and emotional strain.

Conventional treatment often includes HRT (which delays inevitable menopause but potentially increases cancer risks), bisphosphonate drugs for osteoporosis, thyroid medication (if indicated), and antidepressant and anxiolytic drugs. Coming off HRT can, however, produce side effects of muscle stiffness and joint pain in some women.

Complementary treatment aims to support a women's physiology by optimizing her diet with phytoestrogen-rich foods, essential fatty acids and fresh fruit and vegetables. Women are encouraged to do regular weight-bearing exercise 3–5 days a week. Regular Bowen sessions can support women by inducing deep relaxation to reset the autonomic nervous system from sympathetic overdrive to a more balanced state. The core relaxation, kidney, respiratory and TMJ procedures can improve HPA function, helping to reduce many menopausal symptoms, including fatigue, hot flashes and sleep dysfunction. Bowen work can also address joint and soft-tissue problems and improve a woman's capacity to exercise.

CASE STUDY

Leena was 56 years old when she came to see me. She had been menopausal for four years, and was suffering from sleep disturbances due to having to urinate three to four times a night, in addition to having night-sweats. She was extremely fatigued, felt stiff in her joints and had difficulty concentrating at work. She was a divorcee, was concerned about her financial future and worked long hours running her own marketing business. I determined that she did not have a bladder infection, but was experiencing hormonal imbalances and the effects of long-term stress.

I recommended weekly Bowen work for a month, and then an evaluation of her progress. I used the core relaxation and kidney procedures in the first session to address her general symptoms. The following day, she called to let me know that she'd had the best sleep in a long time, only getting up once to urinate and fell back asleep till morning – she was elated! She continued with three more weekly Bowen sessions where I used kidney, coccyx, respiratory and TMJ (not all in the same session!) and she noticed that her hot flushes and sense of fatigue were diminishing. From then on, Leena came back for tune-up sessions when she noticed her symptoms creeping back. She recently remarked: 'I finally feel like myself again, not that fuzzy-brained, sweaty lady I used to be!'

Maggie Chambers suggests advice practitioners can give:

Nutritional and Natural Approaches

NUTRITION

- Try not to drink out of *plastic containers*. Xenoestrogens (oestrogen-mimicking compounds) are found in pesticides and some plastics and have a detrimental effect on the hormonal system.

- Avoid *fizzy drinks, sugar, caffeine, alcohol and excess salt* as they contribute to calcium loss.

- Avoid *spicy foods and alcohol* which can trigger hot flushes by increasing circulation and vasodilation.

- *Excessive meat, processed cheese and sugar* can contribute to hot flushes.

- Eat *plenty of organic fruit and vegetables* to ensure a good intake of vitamins and minerals and avoid pesticides.

- *Phytoestrogens* help to regulate oestrogen levels. Eat plenty of cabbage and fennel.

- *Essential fatty acids* help balance hormones.

- *Oats* act as a tonic for the nervous system and help relieve stress.

- Eat *calcium-rich foods* such as broccoli, sesame seeds and green leafy vegetables.

- *Drink plenty of water* to support healthy kidney function.

SUPPLEMENTS

- *Vitamin E* regulates oestrogen production and can help relieve hot flushes.

- *B vitamins* help to relieve stress and tension and are necessary for a healthy nervous system.

- *Bioflavonoids* slow the breakdown of oestrogen in the body. If they are combined with *vitamin C*, they effectively reduce hot flushes (Smith 1964).

- *Calcium* and *magnesium*, taken together, are necessary in the case of osteoporosis, as they guard against bone loss.

- *Bee pollen* and *royal jelly* are helpful for menopausal symptoms, especially hot flushes.

HERBAL REMEDIES

- *Agnus castus* helps regulate the hormones and relieve hot flushes via the hypothalamus and pituitary gland (Bone 2003).

- *Sage* (*Salvia officinalis*) is an astringent herb and one of the most useful to relieve hot flushes (Bone 2003).

- *Dong quai* is a Chinese herbal tonic, which balances oestrogen in the body. It can help reduce hot flushes, vaginal dryness and depression (Romm 2010).

- *Black cohosh* is a uterine tonic and modulates the effects of oestrogen (Bone 2003).

- *Partridge berry* (*Mitchella repens*) tincture is a uterine tonic and hormonal regulator, and can relieve hot flushes (Romm 2010).

- *Ginseng* (*Panax ginseng*), *Ashwaganda* (*Withania somnifera*), *Rhemannia* (*Rehmannia glutinosa*) and *Rhodiola* (*Rhodiola rosea*) support the adrenal glands and may decrease the occurrence and severity of flushes, and help improve energy and mood levels (Romm 2010).

- *Liquorice root* tea helps to support the adrenal glands.

- *Motherwort* (*Leonurus cardiaca*), valerian (*Valeriana officinalis*), blue vervain (*Verbana officinalis*) and lemon balm (*Melissa officinalis*) help to calm the nerves and reduce anxiety.

Physical Treatments

- Regular exercise is beneficial, ideally a weight-training regime alongside aerobic exercise.

- Alternating hot and cold showers, or footbaths, dry skin brushing and deep breathing all increase circulation to the abdominal area, and deep breathing can help alleviate hot flushes.

- Vitamin E oil can be used to prevent vaginal dryness.

- Cooling peppermint oil can be used as an inhalant.

- Walk in sunlight to absorb plentiful vitamin D for bone health.

- Kegel exercises tone and supply blood to the vaginal walls and reduce symptoms of incontinence.

Breast Health
Breast Diseases and Conditions
ᥫ *Sandra Gustafson*

Breast cysts, *fibroadenomas* and *fibrocystic breasts* are usually benign disorders; however, they can become very tender and inflamed, particularly in the latter part of the menstrual cycle. Women may also develop breast lipomas (fatty tumours).

Mastitis is inflammation of the breast tissue, most commonly due to an infection caused by bacteria entering via the nipple during breast-feeding. The breasts can become very inflamed and tender, and the axillary lymph nodes are usually swollen too. In conventional medicine, mastitis is treated with antibiotics. An effective natural therapy approach is to make a poultice with cabbage leaves and apply it directly to the breast/s with mastitis. Cabbage contains natural anti-inflammatory compounds. Using the darkest of the cabbage leaves lightly pound one or two leaves to break the cell walls and then place them within a whole cabbage leaf. Secure the poultice either within a loosely fitting bra, sports bra or bandage to keep it in place for about 4–6 hours twice a day until symptoms subside.

Breast cancer is the most common cancer in women, and the second leading cause of cancer deaths in women (lung cancer is the first) in both developed and developing countries (World Health Organization 2013). In the USA the likelihood of a woman under the age of 45 developing invasive breast cancer (carcinoma in situ) is 1 in 8 (12%) (American Cancer Society 2013) and two-thirds of women diagnosed with breast cancer are over 55 years of age. The increasing survival rate of women with breast cancer is attributable to earlier detection, greater awareness and improved treatment options. Breast cancer treatment can involve chemotherapy, radiation therapy, hormonal therapy and/or surgery (lumpectomy or mastectomy).

A woman's breast cancer risk depends on a number of factors, including her family history, reproductive history, race/ethnicity and other factors not yet fully understood.

Mammography and clinical breast examinations are the officially recognized breast cancer screening methods (World Health Organization 2013). From the medical standpoint, thermography (see below) and self-breast examination (SBE) (discussed later) are not encouraged as reliable screening measures, yet many women who do regular self-breast examinations are able to detect changes in the tissues long before scheduled mammography or clinical examinations, and seek medical help for breast lumps that they discover themselves, often not detected by mammography.

ↁↃ

Bowen Hormonal Work

Developed by Trevor Rose, an Australian Bowen practitioner, Bowen Hormonal Work introduces specific moves that were described to him by clients treated by Tom Bowen himself. Trevor's wife, Athalie, was diagnosed with breast cancer in 1999, but had an adverse reaction to Tamoxifen so, together with her oncologist and a local gynaecologist, Trevor developed a treatment to stimulate specific hormones. This treatment was very successful for Athalie and led him to develop other treatment moves for varying conditions.

From 2001 Trevor very successfully worked in conjunction with some local practitioners and developed the technique to include procedures for a variety of hormonal issues based on client information and applying the principles of Tom Bowen's technique.

Infrared Digital Imaging (Thermography)

ᘒ *Jean Nortje, Cape Town, South Africa*

Infrared radiation was discovered in 1900 by astronomer William Herschel. There are various wavelengths of infrared radiation. Long infrared wavelength is called thermal infrared as it targets warm blooded animals and humans. Infrared Digital Imaging contributes to early diagnosis and disease prevention with its safe, radiation-free, client-friendly technology. It reveals asymmetries and variations in body infrared radiation patterns and can help identify the cause of existing or potential problems. It can also provide justification for ordering more expensive tests and diagnostic procedures.

Whilst other imaging procedures such as mammograms, X-rays, MRI and CT scans show changes in skeletal or anatomical structures of the body, infrared imaging reflects soft-tissue physiological changes in the body. Thermal imaging is a misnomer in some ways, because when one hears the word *thermal*, one immediately associates the image with heat. When someone suffers from an aching back and the painful area feels warmer than the surrounding area, the practitioner knows a certain amount of inflammation is present, so theoretically it should show heat on the infrared image. An object's surface emits radiation in various wavelengths and forms.

There are three main types of radiation:

- Visible light radiation which can be seen with the naked eye. So we see colours, trees, animals and people, etc.

- Infrared radiation (longer wavelength in particular). This indicates how 'living' something is. It does not differentiate between hot and cold.

- X-rays are highly penetrating and used to diagnose mainly skeletal abnormalities.

When looking through an infrared digital imaging camera, different colours are seen depending on what radiation is emitted from the surface. For example, sunlight on a wall will look red; without sunlight the wall will look blue. If a hand is placed in front of the sunny wall, the shadow will be blue. The wavelength of the radiation is different. The temperature of the wall is the same. This can be useful for medical purposes. For example, tumours have the same temperature as the surrounding tissue, but they have a different consistency and they are made up of cells that have a different density to the surrounding tissue so they radiate a different wavelength of infrared radiation. They appear blue on the image. This is not because they are cold. They have established a good blood supply and are the same temperature as the surrounding tissue. When examining an infrared image, one looks for *symmetry*. Non-symmetry indicates a change in the tissues. For instance, fractures appear white, not because they are hot, but because the fracture now has a crack or a new edge which emits a different wavelength of radiation. When there is inflammation, the cells swell with extra fluid, giving off a different radiation wavelength.

When seeing a practitioner for an infrared imaging session, there are certain conditions that should be met before the session. The practitioner will advise these conditions when the booking is made. Infrared imaging can be a reliable diagnostic tool for assessing the following:

- Examining breast tissue. Many younger women develop breast tumours, and regular mammograms are not usually recommended until they are 50 years old. For peace of mind, an infrared image can pinpoint areas of concern and be followed up with further medical investigations. Infrared imaging also has the advantage over mammograms in that the whole breast area and the axilla are examined. Infrared imaging can pinpoint a problematic area many months before changes show on a mammogram.

- Inflammatory conditions, infections, tissue injury and arthritis.

- Vascular disorders, deep vein thrombosis, neuropathy.

- Changes such as new blood vessels associated with tumour development.

- Nerve entrapment/impingement and the origin of pain.

The Breast Angel, a self-examination device, can be used in conjunction with the infrared camera. A strong light is directed into the whole breast area including the axilla. Blood vessels are clearly seen and when a tumour is present there will be many small blood vessels forming and surrounding the growth. In a normal breast the blood vessels are larger and spread out.

෴

Self-Breast Examination (SBE)

෴ *Sandra Gustafson*

The author is a strong advocate for monthly SBE and performing the Bowen Chest procedure (see below) as ways of detecting changes in the breast tissue early and to stimulate the circulation and lymphatic drainage of the breast and surrounding lymphatic tissues for optimal breast health. The Bowen Chest procedure can also help relieve symptoms of swelling and tenderness from mastitis, fibrocystic breasts and premenstrual syndrome.

TIP: BREAST HEALTH CARE AND BREAST CANCER RESOURCES

- Learn to perform and teach SBE and Bowen Chest procedure.

- Feel your boobies! Visit www.feelyourboobies.com.

- Make healthy diet choices and consider supplementation of essential fatty acids, vitamin E and vitamin D.

- Check thyroid hormone and iodine levels.

- Seek professional healthcare for clinical breast examination and screening.

- Read *Breast Cancer? Breast Health! – The Wise Woman Way* by Susun S. Weed.

- Educational services and information resources for breast cancer include: Breast Cancer Online (www.bco.org) and the Dr Susan Love Research Foundation (www.dslrf.org/breastcancer).

TIP: PAY ATTENTION TO WHAT YOU PUT INTO YOUR BODY

- Quit smoking NOW! Cigarette smoke contains carcinogens and smoking has been linked to increased risk of breast cancer (Xue *et al.* 2011).

- Limit alcohol consumption to two drinks per day or fewer. Cumulative drinking of > 6 alcoholic beverages per week over an adult life-span is associated with increased risk of breast cancer (Chen *et al.* 2011).

- Buy organic foods to avoid pesticides and chemical exposure.

- Eat a variety of multicoloured vegetables and fruits every day, especially broccoli, kale and Brussels sprouts. Greens are high in vitamins and minerals and help to alkalinize your body. Cruciferous vegetables are high in diindolymethane (DIM), a compound that helps to maintain healthy levels of oestrogen (2/16 hydroxyoestrogen ratio) via liver and kidney excretory pathways, and decreases the risk of breast cancer (Morrison *et al.* 2009).

- Reduce or eliminate your consumption of sugar and white flour products. They promote inflammation and can suppress your immune system.

- Eat a diet low in animal fat and high in omega 3 oils found in salmon, sardines, flax seeds and walnuts.

- Avoid constipation as this allows harmful toxins and hormone products, which have been processed by the liver, to be reabsorbed back into your body instead of being eliminated.

- Incorporate small amounts of seaweed (sea vegetables) into your diet, which contain trace minerals including iodine and are very important for breast health.

- Filter your water from chlorine, fluoride and other toxins. Use a stainless steel canteen to store your drinking water in, and avoid exposure to xeno-oestrogenic compounds found in plastic containers.

- For fibrocystic breast disorders, eliminate the intake of caffeine and methylxanthines in the diet, such as coffee, black tea and chocolate.

TIP: PAY ATTENTION TO WHAT YOU WEAR AND WHAT YOU DO

- Avoid tight and under-wire bras, which can constrict the flow of lymphatic fluid in and around your breasts.

- Exercise, exercise…it lowers your risk of breast cancer.

- Keep your weight within a normal range for your height and body type (BMI – body mass index). Obesity can cause increased inflammation and oestrogen production, which increases cancer risk.

- Breast massage: do regular breast massage in the shower with soap or massage oil to improve circulation and lymph flow around your breasts and underarms.

- Breast thermography: find a resource in your area that offers this simple non-invasive breast scan. Abnormal areas can show up years before seen on a mammogram.

- When possible, get out in the sun every day, for 20 minutes.

- Maintain good dental health. Avoid mercury-containing fillings, and have root canals checked regularly for hidden infections.

TIP: EMOTIONS AND STRESS

- Stress and suppression of feelings play a major role in physical health. Not only is this ancient wisdom, but also it has been proven in numerous scientific studies, documenting how unresolved emotions and stress suppress immune system function. The Bowen practitioner can advise.

- Stress contributes to inflammation and toxicity, which can lead to abnormal tissue growth. Find a regular stress-reduction practice that you enjoy and make it a habit – for example, meditation, yoga, Qigong, Tai Chi, jogging, walking.

- Simplify and quiet your daily life; take time for yourself.

- Express yourself in healthy ways and learn to practise good communication skills.

- Get a Bowen session on a regular basis.

TIP: TAKE A LOOK AT YOUR SURROUNDINGS

- 'Green' your home and yard by replacing chemical cleansers and other household and garden chemicals with safe, natural biodegradable versions.

- Evaluate your workplace for exposure to toxins and create a cleaner, greener work environment.

- Learn more about how exposure to electro-magnetic frequency radiation in your home or work environment may be harmful for your health and how to mitigate its effect (www.powerwatch.org.uk; White 2010).

TIP: WHEN TO DO SELF-BREAST EXAMINATION (SBE): ONCE A MONTH

- For women who are still menstruating, perform SBE at the end of the menstrual cycle, when the breasts are least likely to be tender and swollen. Create a regular habit of doing SBE and then perform the Bowen Chest procedure to enhance the circulation and lymphatic drainage. The Chest procedure can also be performed as needed during the rest of the menstrual cycle.

- For women who have reached menopause or had a hysterectomy, and don't menstruate, choose a significant day or date of the month (e.g. the date of their birthday), then put a pink dot on the calendar on the same date of each month to do SBE followed by Bowen Chest procedure.

TIP: HOW TO PERFORM SELF-BREAST EXAMINATION (SBE)

- While standing in front of a mirror with your hands pressing firmly down on your hips, look at your breasts for any changes of size, shape, contour or dimpling, or redness or scaliness of the nipple or breast skin. (Pressing down on the hips contracts the chest wall muscles and enhances any breast changes.)

- Lie down and place your right arm behind your head. The exam is done while lying down, not standing up. This is because when lying down the breast tissue spreads evenly over the chest wall and is as thin as possible, making it much easier to feel all the breast tissue.

- Use the finger pads of the three middle fingers on your left hand to feel for lumps in the right breast.

- Use three different levels of pressure to feel all the breast tissue. Light pressure is needed to feel the tissue closest to the skin, medium pressure to feel a little deeper and firm pressure to feel the tissue closest to the chest and ribs. It is normal to feel a firm ridge in the lower curve of each breast, but you should tell your doctor if you feel anything else out of the ordinary. If you're not sure how hard to press, talk with your doctor or nurse. Use each pressure level to feel the breast tissue before moving on to the next spot.

- Move around the breast in an 'up-and-down' pattern, starting at an imaginary line drawn straight down your side from the underarm and moving across the breast to the middle of the chest bone (sternum or breastbone). Be sure to check the entire breast area going down, until you feel only ribs, and up to the neck or collarbone (clavicle).

- Use overlapping circular motions of the finger pads to feel the breast tissue.

- Repeat the exam on your left breast, putting your left arm behind your head and using the finger pads of your right hand to do the exam.

- Examine each underarm while sitting up or standing and with your arm only slightly raised so you can easily feel in this area. Raising your arm straight up tightens the tissue in this area and makes it harder to examine.

ↄ

Bowen Chest Procedure

ↄ *Sandra Gustafson*

This procedure aims to increase lymph drainage and reduce swelling in the upper chest area, including breast tissue. It is beneficial for both males and females, especially if lymphatic congestion has been a health concern. For women, it is highly recommended to do as part of an ongoing self-care practice after doing SBE.

If the tenderness or swelling is acute, perform the procedure every 4–5 days until all tenderness is gone, and then perform it monthly for maintenance. The chest procedure may be done sitting, standing or lying down.

The Bowen Chest moves are performed above and below the breast tissue, over the pectoralis muscles and superficial lymphatic vessels on the upper chest. Start on the less tender side first (or, if there is no difference, do the left side first).

Level with midway down the length of the left upper arm: use your left hand to gently displace the breast tissue downward, off the pectoralis muscle. Then, using the side of the right index finger, place the length of the index finger above the left hand, in line with the centre of the breast (horizontally and vertically). Lightly 'glue' your index finger to the skin and, using light pressure, move the skin back towards the outside of the body to take the slack over the underlying tissues without your finger 'slipping' on the skin, as described below.

1. *Move 1:* Beathe in and, at the end of exhalation, using light pressure, move your index finger (glued to the skin) toward your left side following the outer curve

of your body and, keeping both hands together, then apply just a bit more pressure to the deeper tissues (within your comfort) and move both hands back toward your midline, following the curve of your body, moving skin over the underlying tissues. This move is illustrated by arrow 1 in Figure 11.2.

2. *Move 2:* With your left hand, lift your left breast up from the rib cage. In line with the centre of the breast (horizontally and vertically), place the pad of your right index finger below the base of the breast on the rib and muscle tissue. Take a deep breath and let it out. With the lightest of pressure, move your index finger (glued to the skin) toward the midline of the body, and then apply just a bit more pressure to the deeper tissues (within your comfort) and move both hands back towards your left side (arrow 2).

Now perform Moves 1 and 2 on the opposite side.

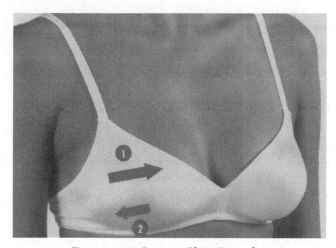

Figure 11.2 Bowen Chest Procedure

෴

Conclusion

As can be seen from this chapter, the Bowen Technique has much to offer in the support and management of women's health. Unfortunately, only after researchers are motivated to conduct larger randomized clinical trials will we have a more serious case in convincing the medical profession at large to suggest Bowen Technique as an excellent form of treatment to support the conditions mentioned in this chapter. There was a Bowen practitioner working at University College Hospital, London, in the endometriosis clinic who was a notable source of support and improvement for women with endometriosis. However, her services were stopped following NHS cut-backs. The authors are hopeful that medical and allied healthcare professionals reading this information will seriously consider recommending Bowen for women's health.

References

Albers, J., Hull, S and, Wesley, R. (2004) Abnormal uterine bleeding. *American Academy of Family Physicians* 69 (8), 1915–1926.

American Cancer Society (2013) What are the key statistics about breast cancer? Available at www.cancer.org/cancer/breastcancer/detailedguide/breast-cancer-key-statistics, accessed on 14 May 2014.

Ballweg, M. (2003) *Endometriosis – Taking Charge of Your Life.* Endometriosis Society of the USA. New York: McGraw Hill.

Barber, T.M., Wass, J.A.H., McCarthy, M.I. and Franks, S. (2007) Metabolic characteristics of women with polycystic ovaries and oligo-amenorrhea but normal androgen levels: implications for the management of polycystic ovary syndrome. *Clinical Endocrinology* 66, 513–517.

Bone, K. (2003) *A Clinical Guide to Blending Liquid Herbs.* St Louis, MO: Churchill Livingstone.

Chen, W.Y., Rosner, B., Hankinson, S.E., Colditz., G.A. and Willett, W.C. (2011) Moderate alcohol consumption during adult life, drinking patterns, and breast cancer risk. *Journal of the American Medical Association* 306 (17), 1884–1890.

Dawood, Y. (2006) Primary dysmenorrhea – advances in pathogenesis and management. *Obstetrics and Gynecology* 108 (2), 428–441.

Guimberteau, J.-C. (2005) *Strolling under the Skin.* DVD, EndoVivo Productions.

Hamilton-Fairley, D. (2004) *Lecture Notes Obstetrics and Gynaecology* (2nd edition). Oxford: Blackwell.

Henderson, L. and Wood, R. (2000) *Explaining Endometriosis.* London: Allen and Unwin.

Hisley, S.M. (2008) *Women's Health: Contemporary Advances and Trends* (3rd edition). Brockton, MA: Western Schools.

Mears, J. (1996) *Coping with Endometriosis.* London: Sheldon Press.

Mills, D. and Vernon, M. (1999) *Endometriosis – a Key to Healing through Nutrition.* Rockport, MA: Element Books.

Morrison, J., Mutell, D., Pollock, T.A., Redmond, E., Bralley, J.A. and Lord, R.S. (2009) Efficacy of dried cruciferous powder for raising the 2/16 hydroxyestrogen ratio. *Alternative Therapies* 15 (2), 52–53.

Pasquali, R., Stener-Victorin, E., Yildiz, B.O., Duleba, A.J. *et al.* (2011) PCOS Forum: research in polycystic ovary syndrome today and tomorrow. *Clinical Endocrinology* 74, 424–433.

Pizzorno, J.E., Murray, M.T. and Joiner-Bey, H. (2002) *The Clinician's Handbook of Natural Medicine.* London: Churchill Livingstone/Harcourt.

Proctor, M. and Farquhar, C. (2006) Diagnosis and management of dysmenorrhea – clinical review. *British Medical Journal* 332, 1134–1138.

Romm, A. (2010). *Botanical Medicine for Women's Health.* St Louis, MO: Churchill Livingstone.

Smith, C.J. (1964) Non-hormonal control of vaso-motor flushing in menopausal patients. *Chicago Medicine* 67, 193–195.

US Centers for Disease Control and Prevention (2013) *Preventing and Managing Chronic Disease to Improve the Health of Women and Infants.* Available at www.cdc.gov/reproductivehealth/WomensRH/ChronicDiseaseandReproductiveHealth.htm, accessed on 15 May 2014.

Weed, S.S (1996) *Breast Cancer? Breast Health! The Wise Woman Way.* Woodstock, NY: Ash Tree Publishing.

White, P. (2010) Are your gadgets killing you? *Boulder Weekly*, 22 April. Available at www.boulderweekly.com/article-2351-are-your-gadgets-killing-you.html, accessed on 19 May 2014.

World Health Organization (2013) *Breast Cancer and Control*. Available at www.who.int/cancer/detection/breastcancer/en, accessed on 15 May 2014.

Xue, F., Willett, W.C., Rosner, B.A., Hankinson, S.E. and Michels, K.B. (2011) Cigarette smoking and the incidence of breast cancer. *Archives of Internal Medicine* 171 (2), 125–133.

12

Pregnancy and Birth

John Wilks and Lina Clerke

Background

Over the last 100 years or so pregnancy and birth have both become increasingly managed with a high degree of medical intervention. It is rare nowadays to hear a mother say that she sailed through her pregnancy with no complications and no interventions at birth.

This need for increasing levels of intervention possibly stems from our sedentary lifestyle, which is not at all conducive to a healthy pregnancy or an easy birth. Midwives who have worked in the field of natural birth for many years have said that birth has become more prone to complications in the last ten years or so. Specifically, they report that many babies are ending up 'back to back' (posterior) in the womb – a particularly problematic position for the baby to be born naturally, and something that seems to be more common with first-time mums.

Conventional Approaches to Pregnancy and Birth

The term 'conventional approaches' is rather arbitrary in the case of pregnancy and birth, as policies, driven by the need for best practice and evidence-based medicine, change constantly. However, even best practice varies from hospital to hospital (particularly in the USA) and country to country. Hence the vast variations in the rates of caesarian sections – 45 per cent for first-time mums in London, but variations between 7 and 70 per cent at hospitals across the USA (Kozhimannil, Law and Vernig 2013).

Some things are definitely improving – skin-to-skin contact between mother and newborn is usually encouraged after birth, and cutting the cord is now usually delayed until it has stopped pulsating. Having the mother lying on her back has been discovered to hinder the progress of the baby down the birth canal as it narrows the gap between the sacrum and the pubis, making birth more difficult for both mum and baby. Mums are now encouraged to stand, squat and move around, and, according to a report by the National Childbirth Trust (NCT), the routine practice of episiotomy declined from 54 per cent in 1978 to 14 per cent by 2003, as it was found to have caused more harm than good (NCT 2003).

Interventions

Commentators and midwives often talk about the 'cascade of intervention' that occurs once the need for an oxytocic intravenous drip to start or speed up contractions is established. Induction is now very common practice – in France around 25 per cent of mothers are induced and a staggering 75 per cent are given an epidural. If a mother is induced, then she is 45 per cent more likely to need an epidural. If she has an epidural, she is much more likely to need some other kind of obstetric intervention such as forceps, suction or caesarian (Donna 2011, p.11). Making the experience safe, pain-free and as comfortable for the mother as possible is the main objective of obstetrics. This is a laudable goal but the need for interventions can often overlook the ramifications for the later health of the baby. This is discussed in the next chapter.

Exercise, Diet and Environmental Considerations

One of the crucial benefits of good posture and appropriate exercise during pregnancy is to encourage what Jean Sutton and Pauline Scott termed 'Optimal Foetal Positioning' (Sutton and Scott 1996). This is the position of the baby in the womb that creates the easiest and most stress-free position for both the mother and the baby to be born. There are many ways this can be achieved through Bowen, appropriate exercise and healthy posture. Most mothers know that sitting too long or slouching on a sofa are not helpful for encouraging the baby to get in the right position in the womb. In most cases simple things such as going around on all fours for a while every day, climbing stairs and swimming (facing downwards 'crawl' rather than breast stroke or swimming on the back) will do the trick.

Using birth balls (or physiotherapy balls) during pregnancy is an excellent way of encouraging good posture and helping to prevent backache, especially if the mother has to sit for long periods. In labour they are wonderful for sitting on or leaning over. After the birth, balls are lovely for rocking the baby and doing tummy exercises.

TIP: Avoid walking in high heels (or any heels) during pregnancy as this exacerbates backache and creates bad posture.

TIP: To help prevent lower back pain in the sacroiliac joint area, make sure when getting out of a car to keep knees and feet close together. Don't put one leg out first so the knees are splayed apart – instead swivel on the seat with the knees touching.

> **TIP**: Walk every day if possible, for at least 30 minutes – and do gentle stretching exercises (for useful suggestions see Spinning Babies a). Swimming is also a lovely activity for pregnant women, especially the crawl.

> **TIP**: It is a good idea for a mother to put her feet up whenever possible if sitting on a chair.

> **TIP**: Wear 100 per cent cotton underwear as this can help reduce the increased likelihood of vaginal thrush during pregnancy.

Certain activities, such as squatting, can be unhelpful if the baby is breech or in a posterior position as this could encourage baby to engage in a less desirable position. There are some excellent books and DVDs on the subject of exercise in pregnancy including *Birth-move-ment* (Berghammer 2008) (produced in Austria, but in English) and the books *Beautiful Birth* by Suzanne Yates (Yates 2008) and the classic *New Active Birth* by Janet Balaskas (Balaskas 1991).

Bowen and Pregnancy

There are many ways that Bowen can help achieve optimal foetal positioning. The ilio-psoas group of muscles has a profound (and often unconscious) effect on posture, something that is discussed at length in Chapter 5. Hydration and fluidity of the psoas is key to a healthy pregnancy and birth as it encourages movement in the whole abdomen and diaphragm as well as creating plenty of space for the baby to expand and grow. A tight or dehydrated psoas has the opposite effect, creating little space for the baby, often forcing it forward or up and under the ribs – uncomfortable for both mum and baby.

For the mother there are a couple of issues that might affect the healthy functioning of the psoas. First, posture plays a big part because any sitting position that involves the knees being higher than the hips will contract the psoas. This obviously happens in the 'couch potato' position, enjoying an evening in front the TV, but it can also be an issue at work. Most office chairs are too low, so it is advisable for pregnant women to sit with their pelvis a good six inches above the level of their knees – in other words, get a cushion under their bottom. In fact, this is a good position for anyone sitting for long periods at a desk. Even men can get tight psoas muscles! This is also where the physiotherapy exercise ball may be used, while sitting at a desk.

The second scenario is where the psoas gets triggered into its 'protection mode'. This is a contraction of the psoas which is designed to create a protective curling action – an instinctive posture that animals adopt when threatened. This contraction can be triggered by small things too, particularly where it can resonate with an earlier trauma. What this means for many women is that if they have been through a particularly difficult birth before, or even if their own birth was traumatic or they have had a car accident, then their psoas is more likely to become contracted the nearer the birth date comes (and therefore the nearer the perceived threat of danger), particularly if some complication has been discovered. This is partly why it is so important for any practitioner to encourage a positive view of birth and not one that stresses the dangers and complications.

Bowen practitioners can do a lot to help the health of the psoas and can vary treatment approaches depending on whether the psoas is just underused (and therefore dehydrated, when it tends to shorten) or contracted due to some trauma such as whiplash, accidents or operations. There are both direct and indirect ways of accessing the psoas via Bowen moves at the diaphragm, pelvis, kidney area and the lesser trochanter. There are also some excellent exercises that women can do to release and 'get in touch' with the psoas which have been developed by Liz Koch in the USA. These are immensely useful for creating a healthy womb and an easeful birth (Koch 1981). Since writing about ways of addressing the psoas in my book (Wilks 2007), many practitioners have contacted me via email and via social networking groups reporting that babies have successfully changed position in the womb following a particular Bowen protocol which involves working around the pelvis, diaphragm and lower back using the Kidney, Respiratory and Pelvic procedures. Similar results have also been reported through the use of acupuncture and reflexology.

Positive Attitudes

The key way that therapists of all kinds can help during pregnancy is through inducing relaxation and above all a positive view of birth – one that encourages feelings of safety and positivity. The more a mother can imbibe positive images of birth, the more likely she is to have a positive experience herself. This is why it is important for anyone working with pregnant women and babies to look at their own issues regarding birth and to work towards healing them, so that strong unconscious negative feelings don't get activated or passed on to their pregnant clients.

Posture

Specifically, as well as aiding relaxation and wellbeing, Bowen can help in pregnancy by improving the mother's posture and encouraging good blood and nerve supply to the uterus. Creating more hydration and fluidity in the fascia, as we do with Bowen, will result in increased blood and nerve supply (Guimberteau 2010). This is particularly important in structures such as the internal iliac artery, which supplies the placenta and muscles in the lower back such as the psoas major and quadratus lumborum.

Posture has as much to do with environmental factors such as how we sit at a desk or drive the car, as with more unconscious influences such as stress or poor eyesight where we might have a tendency to strain forward to read properly. Therapists have an important role in educating mothers about good posture, particularly relaxation postures which will encourage optimal foetal positioning. As the pregnancy progresses and the baby grows, then the centre of gravity changes for the mother and this can put undue strain on areas such as the lower back and sacrum.

Therapists can mirror observations about how mothers are standing and sitting and it's always a good idea for therapists to adopt those postures themselves (briefly!) so they can actually feel where the stresses and strains are for the mother. A useful tool produced by Birth International (a fantastic source of all things related to pregnancy and birth) is their 'pregnancy belly', which mimics the feeling of being pregnant.

Sciatic Pain and Pubic Symphysis Dysfunction (SPD)

Tom Bowen himself worked on women during pregnancy whenever they requested it, particularly if they were suffering from sciatic-type pain. Procedures that release the sacroiliac joints can be helpful during pregnancy and childbirth itself. Because the ligaments around the pelvis and sacrum become more lax during the last two months to allow more space for the baby to come down, this can lead to an aggravation of the sciatic nerve as it exits the sacrum, resulting in pain and discomfort.

The front of the pelvis at the pubic symphysis can also open during this time, resulting in severe pain at the pubic area, making it very difficult to walk and do everyday activities. Bowen work around the pelvis and the muscles that attach on to the pubis, such as the gracilis, seems to be very helpful with this, both before and after birth.

The Pelvic Floor

The sling of the pelvic floor runs as a muscular diaphragm across the area beneath the pelvis, attaching at various places including the pubic bone, sacrum, coccyx and ischial tuberosities (the sit bones). It contains within it the sphincters of urethra and anus, and in women also the vagina. Above it is the pelvic cavity, containing the pelvic organs such as the bladder and intestines, and in women also the uterus.

The pelvic floor is vital in maintaining urinary and foecal continence – the world would be very messy and smelly if we did not have pelvic floors! In women it also plays an important role in facilitating the descent and rotation of babies during the birth process.

During pregnancy the weight of the growing baby increases pressure on the muscles of the pelvic floor so that the more pregnancies a woman has, the harder her pelvic floor must work to maintain its strength and function. This means that the more often she carries a baby (or multiple babies), the more she is at risk of developing various incontinence issues over time if she does not maintain her pelvic floor tone.

Regardless of the kind of birth she has (vaginal or caesarian), her pelvic floor works harder and harder to carry the increasing weight of the growing baby, placenta, uterus and amniotic fluid during pregnancy. Thus it is advisable for all pregnant and postnatal women to do regular pelvic floor exercises in order to strengthen the pubococcygeus muscles of the pelvic floor. There are a few Bowen moves that address the pelvic floor directly, such as the coccyx oblique move which addresses the sacrospinous ligament, the sacrotuberous ligament and the lateral sacrocyccygeal ligament. This can be very helpful in regaining integrity in the pelvic floor after birth and also in addressing malalignments in the coccyx that might be created by the birth process itself; as a way to address vaginal, uterine and even anal prolapse, it can be invaluable.

> **TIP**: The simplest way to do pelvic floor exercises is to squeeze upwards from within, as if stopping yourself from going to the toilet (both urination and defecation). You should be able to feel the sling of the pelvic floor moving upwards toward the belly button as you squeeze. You may also notice that you are squeezing harder more toward the front or to the back, so the aim is to try to make the pressure even. Although other muscles throughout the body do tighten a little when you do pelvic floor tightening, you should not actively tighten the buttocks, belly or inner thighs as this is an internal muscular exercise for the pelvic floor.

> **TIP**: One way to *test* your pelvic floor strength is when going to the toilet – see if you can stop the urinary flow. If you can, your pelvic floor muscles are in good condition. So just maintain their strength by squeezing whenever you can remember. If you *cannot* stop the flow of urine, you need to do some serious and regular pelvic floor work. It is always a good idea to get specific exercises for your situation and check that you are doing them correctly, especially if you have incontinence issues when laughing or coughing, urine leaks, or flatulence or foecal incontinence, etc. However it is important *never* to use stopping urination as a form of regular exercise in itself as this could lead to a urinary tract infection. This exercise is just to occasionally *test* the condition of your pelvic floor muscles.

> **TIP**: When tightening the pelvic floor muscles, one way to help you to squeeze more effectively is to suck hard on your thumb at the same time – go ahead, try it and see how, when your mouth is tight, you feel the pelvic floor tighten up much more efficiently when you squeeze down there.
>
> It is especially important to do these pelvic squeezes *after* the birth, starting whenever it feels comfortable to do so. For some women this will be days, for others it may be a week or more after the birth. One possible suggestion is to do five long squeezes (tighten and count to five and release for ten) followed by five short sharp squeezes. This sequence should be done five times a day, although realistically most people simply forget to do pelvic floor exercises altogether. A simple way to maintain tone is just to squeeze whenever you remember!

TIP: You can have a few 'reminders' – whenever you turn a door handle, squeeze the pelvic floor muscles. Whenever you turn on a tap, stop at a red light, go to pick up the phone, stand in the shower – squeeze! Some women put little red dots or star stickers here and there to remind them to squeeze when they see them. (So now you know what is going on when you see a woman sucking her thumb at a red traffic light!)

It is best not to overdo pelvic floor toning before birth – sometimes 'overly toned' women can have difficulty letting their babies out because they are so tight within. So midwife Lina Clerke recommends that apart from pelvic floor-tightening exercises, women also consciously practice letting go of the pelvic floor. After all, the baby needs to come out at birth. A good way to feel the releasing of the pelvic floor is to make a gentle fist with your hand and gently blow into it, while loosening everything 'down below' as if you are gently 'blowing' out of the vagina, allowing the perineum to 'bulge'.

TIP: Notice how when you are 'loose up above', you are looser down below, and when you are 'tight up above', you can tighten more easily down below. In fact, most people find it really hard to make a very *tight* face and mouth, and still be *loose* down below, or vice versa. Try it and see for yourself. If you squeeze hard down below, it is difficult to have a very relaxed, loose, floppy mouth. It is easier to notice this connection when you are not actually sitting on your bottom, so kneel or stand when you try this.

TIP: I suggest that when pregnant women go to the toilet, they practise having a very loose mouth and 'breathing out their poo' rather than straining. In this way they prepare themselves for 'breathing their baby out' at birth. You can even make a horsey 'brrrrrrr' sound to make for very, very loose lips, and at same time let everything go down below. I have helped hundreds of women 'breathe their babies out' at the 'crowning' phase of birth – this greatly reduces the need for stitches.

An excellent birth motto is 'Loose up above = loose down below' or 'Loose mouth = loose vagina'.

TIP: When a woman is very pregnant it may be more difficult to tighten the pelvic floor when she is standing upright, as there is the maximum weight of the baby on her pelvic floor. If this is the case, she can do her exercises side-lying, on all fours or semi-reclined.

Maintaining a healthy pelvic floor is a great way to support pregnancy and prepare for birth, and it is in fact something everyone needs to do for their whole life. Happy squeezing!

Posterior (Back to Back) Babies

The preferred position for baby in labour is ideally head down, chin well tucked in, with baby's spine toward the front (most optimum is spine toward the left front of her belly – left occipito anterior position or LOA). The baby's spine will likely be palpable to the right front or left front of mum's belly with movements felt on the opposite side of her belly. Posterior position means baby's back is facing mother's back, so her belly may look a little concave when she lies on her back, and she will feel most of the baby's movements at the front of her tummy. Posterior position can cause uncoordinated contractions, and make it longer for baby to find its way through the pelvis. It can also cause a lot of back pain, all of which may lead to exhaustion and subsequent requests for epidural pain relief, and synthetic hormonal drip to speed up labour. If the baby cannot turn around or cannot come out posteriorly, forceps, ventouse or caesarian section will be needed.

Having said all that, it is important not to scare women by the prospect of 'posterior labour' as some pelvises lend themselves well to posterior babies who find their way out just fine. However, because of the increased chance of long difficult labour with posterior-positioned babies, it is recommended that women do whatever possible to encourage baby into anterior position. Here are some recommendations.

TIP: FROM AT LEAST SIX MONTHS INTO PREGNANCY, PREFERABLY SOONER...

- Avoid leaning back when seated – as in a bucket chair, deep sofa/armchair. Especially avoid sitting leaning back with knees higher than hips. Instead sit forward – that is, straddle the back of a chair and place pillows beneath your folded arms (over chair back) for comfort. In this position your knees should be slightly lower than your hips.

- If sitting on sofa, have an extra pillow beneath you so knees are slightly lower than hips (and pillow behind back so your spine is straighter).

- Sit on a birth ball – making sure that knees are slightly lower than hips. Make sure ball is blown up enough to do this and it is the correct size for you. Birth balls make excellent chairs, encouraging gentle movements to stabilize the body, and assisting abdominal muscles to gently work – this not only tones the abdomen, it helps support the back.

- Crawl daily for a few minutes – this encourages baby's heaviest part, the spine – to fall forward so that baby is more likely to be in an anterior position. It also gets Mum familiar with the all fours position which she is likely to adopt in instinctive labour. All fours is a great position to practice rocking/tilting the pelvis back and forth, which helps release the back and pelvic floor. Making circular movements in both directions with the tail is also excellent to keep the whole area supple and mobile. If crawling is not an option, lean forward over chair or sofa and wag tail a lot with spine parallel to the floor.

- Avoid squatting in last trimester (if baby *is* posterior, squatting could encourage baby to descend deeper in pelvis in that position, and to 'engage' in a posterior position).

- If baby *is* posterior in last month or so, crawl often, and even get on floor in knee–chest position and wag tail – this may help give more room to baby to move around if baby is deeper into pelvis in a posterior position.

- Doing forward-leaning inversions can also help to encourage baby into optimum position. It is important to do these properly and to know when to avoid doing them. For details see Spinning Babies (b).

- A rebozo can be used too with good effect to turn posterior babies (Spinning Babies c).

Labour and Induction

There are other very important factors in pregnancy that will encourage a good outcome for the baby. Nutrition is widely discussed in the media and in birth books, but avoiding refined foods during the later stages of pregnancy is also important as this inhibits the synthesis of certain types of prostaglandin (E2) that are essential in preparing the uterus for birth.

In the UK and USA, labour is normally induced if the mother is more than 10–14 days overdue. The use of artificial induction has severe ramifications not only for the baby (Carter 2003) but also for the mother, as it usually makes contractions strong and uncomfortable, often resulting in the need for an epidural and the associated 'cascade of interventions'. For the baby it increases the chance of developing ADHD and other social issues (Kurth and Haussmann 2011). Dr Gowri Motha's book *Gentle Birth Method* (Motha and Macleod 2004) discusses the use of Bowen and other therapies during pregnancy, but there is not much in the literature about what mothers can do if a baby is late. This is where Bowen and other therapies really come into their own. Working around the pelvis, diaphragm, lower back and sacrum can all create the right environment for labour to start. Specifically, working the area around the inside of the ankle (where Bowen practitioners do the peroneal move) can stimulate labour. Treatments can be performed every day if necessary and it is one of those situations where the 'wait a week' rule can be ignored. And if Bowen doesn't do it, then reflexology, aromatherapy or acupuncture almost certainly will.

A Cautionary Tail

The question that I often get asked is: What can you do if a client wants to avoid induction? The answer is emphatically that we are not qualified to induce a baby and to do so would be potentially dangerous. Both Motha and Baker advise the use of the coccyx procedure in pregnancy (Baker 2013, p.79; Motha and Macleod 2004, p.181) but this is contra-indicated in most Bowen training courses. Many

Bowen practitioners have related that when they have done the coccyx work because the baby is overdue, it has nearly always resulted in contractions starting and the baby coming very fast. In fact, one Bowen instructor relates how she performed the coccyx work on her daughter because she was already two weeks overdue and she hardly made it to the hospital! So, for a Bowen practitioner it can be a question of which is the lesser of two evils, given the ramifications for both mother and baby if induction is used.

There is a lot that parents themselves can do to help the onset of labour. Birth educators such as Sheila Kitzinger and Ina May Gaskin have argued for years that things such as nipple stimulation should be encouraged if a woman is overdue as it aids the production of oxytocin. Even some midwifery textbooks have questioned why sexual expression is not more encouraged in labour care (Walsh 2007). Certainly, the prostaglandins in seminal fluid that are released during sex can help soften the cervix and bring on labour as it contains relaxin amongst other hormones. Other vigorous activities such as dancing and walking can also help. Taking castor oil, eating spicy food, pineapple, raspberry leaf tea or homeopathic remedies such as pulsatilla have traditionally been found to be helpful (though probably not advisable all at the same time!). Exploring the mother's fears is often useful, and holding and smelling very new babies is a wonderful way to get those 'clucky' hormones going. Bowen work on a daily basis can be used to prepare the mother and baby for birth, bearing in mind, of course, that the baby will not come until it is ready.

Breech Births

Although in most countries these days breech babies are born by caesarian section, vaginal breech birth is possible with good, experienced support. It is most easily achieved with minimal interference and patience and mother in an upright position such as squatting or kneeling on all fours so that gravity can assist the baby's journey around the curve of the pubic bone. There are plenty of positive stories of women's experience of giving birth to breech babies available online.

Attitudes to Birth

In our culture we rarely discuss the importance of the parents', and particularly the mother's, attitude to the pregnancy and the idea of having a child. Some parents might be ambivalent or nervous about the arrival of a new one into their lives – how it might affect the parents' relationship or how it might affect them financially, for example. The other emotional aspect that can have a profound impact on the ease of birth for the mother is her own anxiety about the forthcoming experience of giving birth. This might be affected by things such as past emotional or sexual trauma in her life, her own experience of giving birth before, or maybe even more unconscious memories of when she herself was born. Midwives have noticed, for example, that often, as the baby's head descends around the pubic arch, many mothers will instinctively mimic the baby's position by arching their heads back, or wanting to push their heads into a firm surface, as though the experience triggers a somatic memory of their own birth.

Although a relaxed and positive attitude to birth is more conducive to an easy birth, the way that giving birth is portrayed in the media is unfortunately the opposite of relaxed. The trouble is that many TV programmes and educational DVDs tend to focus on what can go wrong at birth rather than what can go right, and downplay the ramifications of medical interventions. They also create a cultural anxiety in mothers, which has the effect of increasing the stress hormones, just at a time when they need calming down.

Michel Odent, the natural birth pioneer and author of many books on the subject, discusses at length the need to avoid stimulation of the stress hormones in the mother if she is to have a good chance of giving birth easily and naturally (e.g. Odent 1994). It would seem fairly obvious that putting women in a strange environment (i.e. hospital) where they are surrounded by people they don't know and subjected to procedures which are way outside their control adds untold stress into the situation. When certain areas of the brain are activated in a mother about to give birth, then natural processes tend to shut down and the production of oxytocin becomes inhibited. This is why you will always see animals seeking out places that are away from interference to give birth. Even domesticated animals do this – dogs, cats and even pigs if they are allowed to. Mammals instinctively give birth where and when they feel safe.

An analogy would be of a couple wanting to make love and being told they have to go into a brightly lit room with people coming in every few minutes to check on how they are getting on. Hormones such as oxytocin that are released during birth are in fact very similar to the hormones that are stimulated during sex and orgasm. As we all know, to achieve this people need peace, safety, relaxation and intimacy. It is not for nothing that oxytocin is called the love hormone! Denis Walsh, in his fascinating critique of current birth practice, cites as an example the paper called 'You'll feel me touching you, sweetie' (Bergstrom *et al*. 1992), which is highly critical of the ritualistic and unnecessary over-use of vaginal examinations at the second stage of labour, which he points out would be 'totally unacceptable in any other circumstance except in an intimate sexual context between consenting adults' (Walsh 2007, p.38). Like all mammals, women need to feel safe in order to give birth. Choosing the right environment, caregivers and birth partners is a critical part of good birth preparation.

It is very important to understand that although a new mother will always put her baby first, she may herself have found the whole experience traumatic both physically and emotionally. Bowen can play a big part in recovery for both mothers and babies, as is discussed in the next chapter. Sheila Kitzinger has set up a special website to support mothers who have been traumatized by their birth experience. See Birth Crisis in the Resources list at the end of the chapter for more details. For more information on caesarian birth and vaginal birth after caesarian, see VBAC.

CASE STUDY

| *Enys Evans, Caerwys, North Wales*

Susy, aged 37, is a full-time mother of two young daughters, who suffered with a bad back, shoulder, ankle and symphysis pubis dysfunction (SPD). She had slight scoliosis originating in her lower back deviating to the left. Her SPD started from 11 weeks of pregnancy with both her children, and was so bad she couldn't walk or sleep and would cry in agonizing pain. She would have liked to do more Pilates teaching and exercising in general but her back and the SPD prevented this. She wanted to have another child but was wary because of the possibility of SPD and her bad back. She felt that she has a lot of unresolved feelings regarding her alcoholic mother, who left her when she was 11 years old, and that she has a great deal of stress which she sometimes took out on the children.

After two Bowen treatments her stress, back pain, shoulder and SPD improved. After her third appointment she reported that she had abseiled down a lighthouse and run 5 km in under 30 minutes! She continued to come for monthly Bowen sessions and noted improvements in her mood and stress levels and she reported feeling calmer emotionally. She also reported that she had come to terms with her resentment towards her mother, doesn't feel a victim now and only remembers the happy times.

She is now 24 weeks pregnant on her third pregnancy and has a pain-free pregnancy for the first time.

Susy said, 'I think that Bowen is a miracle! I was in pain most days and would cry with the pain. After being in constant pain for five years I am now pain-free and I can't recommend Bowen enough. It has changed my life!'

CASE STUDY

| *Alastair McLoughlin, Skipton, North Yorkshire, England*
| *(www.MobileTherapyService.com)*

In my years of experience as a Bowen practitioner I have lost count of the times that I've helped women with Bowen to assist conception, cope with back pain during their pregnancies and to help the newborn infants who struggle feeding. However, the personal expectation of a new baby in your own family means much more.

Bowen assisted my daughter, Jaimie, throughout her pregnancy for the low, dragging pain that is often a feature of the third trimester of pregnancy. In fact she had regular Bowen sessions during the whole term – even the impromptu 'tweaks' of her low back and sacrum whilst we were at the supermarket!

Just a few days before she gave birth, Jaimie was examined by her midwife and was informed that the baby was lying posterior, and she should expect a long and difficult labour. The day after this examination I did some Bowen on my daughter in the hope of helping the baby turn. I did another Bowen treatment three days later and within a few hours her labour pains commenced.

Far from it being a long and difficult birth, Jaimie couldn't even make it to hospital in time as the contractions came quick and strong. Baby Georgia was born even before the paramedics arrived. She was delivered at home by her dad, with myself and my wife assisting in the delivery. Georgia arrived quickly and without complications and had indeed turned around into the optimum position.

Immediately after the delivery, whilst my daughter was still on her hands and knees, I put in a couple of Bowen moves in her lower back and within about 90 seconds the placenta just dropped out intact – no pushing involved. Granddaughter Georgia has some Bowen from me occasionally to assist her feeding. An exciting, personal experience that I shall never forget.

References

Balaskas, J. (1991) *New Active Birth: A Concise Guide to Natural Childbirth*. London: Thorsons.

Baker, J. (2013) *Bowen Unravelled*. Chichester: Lotus Publishing.

Berghammer, K. (2008) *Birth-move-ment*. DVD, Filmproduktion. Available from www.birthinternational.com.

Bergstrom, L., Roberts, J., Skillman, L. and Seidel, J. (1992) 'You'll feel me touching you, sweetie': vaginal examinations during the second stage of labor. *Birth* 19 (1), 10–18; discussion 19–20.

Carter, C.S. (2003) Developmental consequences of oxytocin. *Physiology and Behaviour 79*, 383–397.

Donna, S. (2011) *Promoting Normal Birth: Research, Reflections and Guidelines*. Chester-le-Street: Fresh Heart Publishing.

Guimberteau, J.-C. (2010) *Muscle Attitudes* DVD. Pessac, France: EndoVivo Productions.

Koch, L. (1981) *The Psoas Book*. Ashford: Guinea Pig Productions.

Kozhimannil, K., Law, M. and Virnig, B. (2013) Caesarian deliveries vary tenfold among US hospitals, *Health Affairs 32* (3), 527–535.

Kurth, L. and Haussmann, R. (2011) Perinatal pitocin as an early ADHD biomarker: neurodevelopmental risk? *Journal of Attention Disorders 15* (5), 423–431.

Motha, G. and Macleod, K.S. (2004) *Gentle Birth Method: The Month-By-Month Programme to Help You*. London: Thorsons.

NCT (2003) NCT Evidence Based Briefing: Episiotomy and the Perineum. Available at www.nct.org.uk/sites/default/files/related_documents/Episiotomy%20and%20the%20Perineum-pdf.pdf, accessed on 24 June 2014.

Odent, M. (1994) *Birth Reborn: What Childbirth Should Be*. London: Souvenir Press.

Spinning Babies (a) Daily activities. Available at http://spinningbabies.com/more-info/for-pregnancy/daily-activities, accessed on 19 May 2014.

Spinning Babies (b) The inversion. Available at http://spinningbabies.com/techniques/the-inversion, accessed on 19 May 2014.

Spinning Babies (c) Activities for fetal positioning/rebozo sifting. Available at http://spinningbabies.com/techniques/activities-for-fetal-positioning/rebozo-sifting, accessed on 19 May 2014.

Sutton, J. and Scott, P. (1996) *Understanding and Teaching Optimal Foetal Positioning.* Tauranga, NZ: Birth Concepts.

Walsh, D. (2007) *Evidence-Based Care for Normal Labour and Birth.* London: Routledge.

Wilks, J. (2007) *The Bowen Technique, the Inside Story.* Sherborne: CYMA.

Yates, S. (2008) *Beautiful Birth.* New York: Carroll and Brown.

Resources
Further Reading

Blasco, T.M. (2003) *How to Make a Difference for Your Baby if Birth Was Traumatic.* Santa Barbara, CA: Building and Enhancing Bonding and Attachment.

Buckley, S.J. (2009) *Gentle Birth, Gentle Mothering: The Wisdom and Science of Gentle Choices in Pregnancy, Birth, and Parenting.* Berkeley, CA: Celestial Arts.

Cassidy, T. (2007) *Birth.* London: Chatto & Windus.

Central Intelligence Agency (2012) The World Factbook: Infant Mortality Rate. Archived from the original on 18 December 2012. Available at www.cia.gov/library/publications/the-world-factbook/rankorder/2091rank.html, accessed on 24 June 2014.

Chamberlain, D.B. (1998) *The Mind of Your Newborn Baby.* Berkeley, CA: North Atlantic Books.

Chamberlain, D.B. (2013) *Windows to the Womb: Revealing the Conscious Baby from Conception to Birth.* Berkeley, CA: North Atlantic Books.

Davis, E. and Pascali-Bonaro, D. (2010) *Orgasmic Birth: Your Guide to a Safe, Satisfying, and Pleasurable Birth Experience.* New York: Rodale.

England, P. and Horowitz, R.I. (2007) *Birthing from Within.* London: Souvenir.

Gaskin, I.M. (2008) *Ina May's Guide to Childbirth.* London: Vermilion.

Gerhardt, S. (2004) *Why Love Matters: How Affection Shapes a Baby's Brain.* Hove and New York: Brunner-Routledge.

Goddard, S. (2005) *Reflexes, Learning and Behavior: a Window into the Child's Mind.* Eugene, OR: Fern Ridge Press.

Goer, H. (1999) *The Thinking Woman's Guide to a Better Birth.* New York: Berkley.

Kitzinger, S. (2005) *The Politics of Birth.* Oxford: Elsevier.

Kitzinger, S. (2011) *Rediscovering Birth* (2nd edition). London: Pinter & Martin.

Levine, P.A. (1997) *Waking The Tiger: Healing Trauma – The Innate Capacity to Transform Overwhelming Experiences.* Berkeley, CA: North Atlantic Books.

Odent, M. (2005) *Birth Reborn.* London: Souvenir.

Owl Productions (2005) *The Psychology of Birth* (DVD).

Porges, S.W. (2001) The polyvagal theory: phylogenetic substrates of a social nervous system. *International Journal of Psychophysiology* 42 (2), 123–146.

Romm, A.J. (2003) *The Natural Pregnancy Book: Herbs, Nutrition, and Other Holistic Choices.* Berkeley, CA: Celestial Arts.

Schore, A.N. (2003) *Affect Dysregulation and Disorders of the Self.* New York: W.W. Norton.

Siegel, D.J. and Hartzell, M. (2014) *Parenting from the Inside Out: How a Deeper Self-Understanding Can Help You Raise Children Who Thrive* (10th anniversary edition). New York: Jeremy P. Tarcher.

Wambach, H. (1979) *Life before Life.* New York: Bantam Books.

Websites

Alliance for Transforming the Lives of Children
www.atlc.org

BirthChoiceUK
www.birthchoiceuk.com

Birth Crisis
www.sheilakitzinger.com/birthcrisis.htm

Birth International
https://www.birthinternational.com

Birth Psychology
http://birthpsychology.com

Birthworks International
www.birthworks.org/site/primal-health-research.html

Building and Enhancing Bonding and Attachment
www.beba.org

Conscious Embodiment Trainings
www.conscious-embodiment.co.uk

CYMA
www.cyma.org.uk

The Origins of Peace and Violence
www.violence.de

Sarah Buckley
www.sarahjbuckley.com

VBAC
www.vbac.com

Wonderful Birth
www.wonderfulbirth.com

Womb Ecology
www.wombecology.com

CDs

Clerke, L. *Joyful Pregnancy, Birth and Beyond*. Available from: www.wonderfulbirth.com.

DVDs

There are many good DVDs available on yoga and exercise in pregnancy available through www.birthinternational.com. One of the most positive and informative DVDs on natural birth is *Birth as We Know It* (2006), directed and produced by Elena Tonetti-Vladimirova.

13

Babies, Toddlers and Children

In the previous chapter we looked at how to create the best possible outcome for both the mother and baby in pregnancy and birth. This is probably one of the most important areas a therapist can help with. If the pregnancy is as good as possible in terms of positive emotional attitude, diet, correct exercise and good posture, then the birth is likely to be easier and the baby is more likely to thrive.

This last statement might seem controversial, but in the last 30 years there has been an explosion of books and research papers examining the effect of birth on later physical and emotional health. There is now a rapidly expanding field of psychology dealing with the effect of pre- and perinatal experience (see www.birthpsychology. com). Authors such as Thomas Verny, Frank Lake, William Emerson, Michel Odent, Allan Schore, Joseph Chilton Pearce and Ludwig Janus have all contributed hugely to this rich field of exploration. Wendy Anne McCarty's book *Welcoming Consciousness* provides an excellent overview of current thinking in this very complex area. For the therapist it can be hugely enriching to explore how early experience shapes one's view of the world and our place in it, and understanding this territory undoubtedly allows a much deeper therapeutic process to take place when treating both babies and adults.

Physical Imprinting at Birth

I want to start by looking at some of the more physical ramifications of how we are born, how these affect our future growth and physical tendencies (such as posture) and how we can work with them. It would be an exaggeration to say that all early postural imbalances come from birth; there are many other factors – such as accidents, what kind of seat or sling the parents use, what position the baby sleeps in and the development of the oral cavity through feeding – that affect later posture. The unfortunate fact is that none of us are born straight. Even in the womb we are shaped by what is termed 'birth lie'; in other words, whether we are posterior (back towards our mother's back), side-lying, squashed up under the ribs, etc. All these various positions involve a degree of lengthening through one side of the body which later in life can often be seen in certain facial characteristics such as a slightly lower eye on one side as well as asymmetry in the pelvis and leg length discrepancy. There has been a long-running debate amongst osteopaths about why in the population there is a significant tendency towards a short right leg (Juhl 2004) combined with pelvic rotation to the right, creating more likelihood of back pain. This may well be down to the prevalence of the most common birth lie which involves a lengthening through the whole right side of the body. That kind of pelvic rotation also mirrors the rotation of the pelvis in birth itself. (Yet another reason to blame our mothers for all our ills!)

We are the only mammals that rotate as we come down the birth canal. In evolutionary terms, this is because our heads are too large for the mother's pelvis. You could say that we are born nine months early compared to other mammals. This need for rotation causes torsion in the various articulations of the baby's cranium and the neck, which has additional sutures and fontanels compared to the adult. Osteopaths and chiropractors have observed that the majority of us also have a degree of imbalance at the junction between the axis, atlas and the occiput (the top of the neck) resulting from this anomaly of rotation. Rotational forces from birth also affect the jaw and the temporomandibular joint (TMJ). In the opinion of many health professionals, imbalance in either of these two relationships (the occipito-atlanteal joint or the TMJ) can lead to distortions elsewhere in the body and specifically have a marked effect on posture (Sakaguchi 2007), with a more general knock-on effect on efficient functioning of the organism (Cuccia and Caradonna 2009). Indeed, some paediatric dentists work extensively with the relationship between posture and bite (Levinkind 2008), helping conditions such as scoliosis and kyphosis by adjusting a child's bite. The rotational effect of descent down the birth canal can be more pronounced with posterior births, common with first-time mothers, which either lead to a longer rotation or, in some cases, interventions such as epidurals or caesarians. If you add into this evolutionary mix the effect of obstetric interventions, it is clear that the potential for further pressures on the baby's head and body is extreme.

How Bowen Can Help

The process of birth is a complex one and has many potential ramifications for the baby both on a physical and psychological level. In many ways it is much less about what a therapist *does* to a baby and much more how a therapist can create a safe therapeutic environment for it to resolve whatever it needs to resolve, whether that is physical or emotional. Babies' nervous systems work far more slowly than adults, and they tend to find anything that happens too fast upsetting. Hence a fast delivery, although possibly easier for the mother, may not be such a good thing from the baby's point of view.

It is therefore a good idea for the therapist to slow down their movements and speech when treating babies, avoid bright lights in the treatment room and have the temperature nice and warm. Babies who have experienced a quick delivery, especially if they have been induced, can feel quite 'jangled' and may even be in pain as they have had to negotiate the bony parts of the sacrum and pelvis fast, and sometimes roughly. They may be difficult to settle and may over-exhibit the Moro reflex (primitive startle reflex) when their body arches back and their arms fling upwards. Some babies do this as they are about to go to sleep, almost as if relaxing and letting their guard down is somehow dangerous for them. Such babies' nervous systems can be constantly on alert, making it difficult for them to feel comfortable and settled. There are specific ways that Bowen can help with calming babies down, and most of these involve miminal but light touch. Fractious babies can be quite difficult to treat and in my experience will need a few sessions before they begin to feel to settle – specifically in later treatments The psoas, coccyx, kidney or the TMJ procedures can be help in this situation.

Bowen Work for Babies

It is, of course, quite possible to perform any Bowen moves on a baby. The basic Bowen work for babies consists of the top stoppers and a variation on the lower respiratory work. For many babies this is enough to have a profound effect on their mood and wellbeing as well as being highly beneficial for colicky babies. I have lost count of the number of exasperated parents who have said to me after a first Bowen session of doing absolutely minimal work, 'I don't know what you did to him, but he's a completely different baby.'

Body Language

Babies have very clear body language and will often show the perceptive therapist exactly what stages of their birth were difficult. They will do this by making repeated hand contact with areas of their body (often specific areas of their head or belly) and will even grasp the therapist's hand and guide it to the place that they want contact. I have had this happen many times. There is a very different quality to therapeutic touch as opposed to the loving touch of a parent, and a baby can feel the therapist's intention as they begin to make contact and intend to work in a particular area of their body.

On the other hand, if they are not happy with a practitioner working in a particular place, babies will make it very clear by turning away, wriggling or even pushing the therapist's hand away. Usually that area will be holding the tissue memory of some trauma related to birth and it is important to respect their boundaries.

Birth patterns can also be held in various areas of the cranium. One of the most sensitive areas that is prone to compressive forces is the temporal bones. There are a lot of structures just beneath and behind them, which are vulnerable to both compression and traction. These structures include the vagus nerve (cranial nerve X), one of the longest nerves in the body, which controls many of our vital functions such as digestion, breathing and heart rate. Also just behind the temporal bones lies the jugular vein through which flows most of the deoxygenated blood from our heads. There are many types of birth which put excessive strain on this area, notably forceps (which applies strong medial compression) and ventouse (which imprints traction and rotational forces on the occiput and parietals which can then feed into the temporals, the jaw, the base of the cranium and top of the neck). Unfortunately, the head and neck are not really designed for these kind of forces, so the baby will counteract any 'pulling' of its head or neck by clamping down the muscles at the back of its head (the deep sub-occipital muscles specifically), as well as instinctively pulling up its legs by contracting the psoas muscles. Both these areas (the back of the head and the belly) will trigger protective reflexes if the baby feels it is in danger and these tendencies will tend to show themselves later on when that baby's adult body feels stressed or under threat. It can be wonderful to work on babies' psoas muscles and it can give almost instantaneous release from symptoms such as colic and reflux. Because the psoas has attachments on to the back of the diaphragm, any tightness here will tend to affect breathing as well as the structures that pass through the diaphragm (such as the oesophagus and lower branches of the vagus).

Interventions

Treating babies can be much more complicated when interventions have been used at birth. The various possibilities are the use of pain-relieving drugs such as pethidine and epidurals and mechanical interventions such as forceps, ventouse (vacuum extraction), caesarean and/or various types of foetal monitoring.

Forceps births are less common these days; they need a lot of skill to be used safely because they put a considerable medial compression around the temporal areas of the baby. The nerves most affected by forceps are the vagus (cranial nerve X), the spinal accessory (XI) and the glossopharangeal (XII). The effect of this might be to cause problems with digestion (e.g. colic or a sluggish digestive tract), hypertonus in the neck muscles, neck restriction (torticollis is quite common) or feeding problems. The neck and TMJ work can be highly beneficial for babies born with forceps, although commonly they won't want a practitioner anywhere near their head or temporal area until levels of trust have been built up over a few sessions.

Suction, Vacuum Extraction and Ventouse

Ventouse, or vacuum extraction as it is called in the USA, only came into use in the 1970s, so it is probable that Tom Bowen didn't come across it in his practice. However, it is being used much more frequently these days with about 10 per cent of all births in the UK now being assisted with suction caps. It can, of course, be a lifesaver for both mum and baby, but it does have ramifications, particularly for the baby. First it is a very strong local pressure to the back of the baby's head (usually the occiput) which is very uncomfortable even for adults to experience. For the baby, birth is the first really strong imprinting of physical sensation that goes on and if one thinks about the whole phenomenon of tissue memory, then ventouse is potentially an extremely strong effect on a tissue level, along with its associated emotional imprinting.

One of the reasons given for using ventouse over forceps is that there is much less potential for intra cranial pressure with ventouse. However, this doesn't account for the fact that ventouse exerts an extraordinary amount of pressure locally which has much more potential for distortion patterns to be fed into the baby's cranium. Usually it is not just a question of attaching the cap and pulling straight down in line with the birth canal. Often the midwife or obstetrician has to pull off-centre to bring the baby down.

Because the baby's occiput is not fused at birth (Figure 13.1), there is potential for distortion patterns to be fed into the base of the occiput around the condyles. This will then affect the occipito-atlanteal joint (the O/A junction) and the ventricles, particularly the fourth ventricle. Ventricles are the fluid-filled spaces in the brain and what tends to happen is that the fourth ventricle, which travels down towards the brain stem, can get pulled up along with the spinal cord towards the foramen magnum.

The major issue with ventouse is the potential for distortion at the condyles and around the temporal area which then has a direct effect on the TMJ, the hard palate and the bite. From what we have seen earlier, this can have implications for postural issues later on, as well as affecting some of the major cranial nerves, including the vagus. Bowen is great at resolving these patterns, but it is also essential to address the whole neck, particularly where the trapezius attaches on to the back of the head (rather than just moves 5 and 6). As with many situations where the whole shape of the head is affected, the TMJ work or referral to a craniosacral therapist or cranial osteopath can be very beneficial.

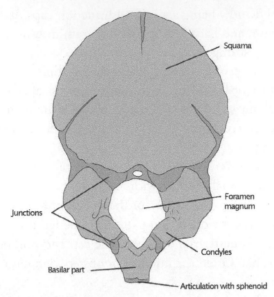

*Figure 13.1 A baby's occiput is in four parts at birth with
significant junctions in the condyles where it articulates with the
atlas, as well as between the basilar part and the squama*
Source: Martin Gordon

Caesarians

There is a generally held perception that a caesarian birth is the least stressful way to give birth for both mum and baby, but this is far from true. There are also some serious health effects of caesarians (C-sections) that are often overlooked. Apart from frequent problems with bonding, Rien Verdult also points out that babies born this way tend to have more respiratory and breathing difficulties and are more at risk of asthma, autism and food allergies (Verdult 2009).

All C-sections have to be performed fast, with some often strong traction and rotation of the baby's neck combined with sudden cutting of the cord. These forces put a lot of strain on the short sensitive muscles and ligaments in the top of the neck, so it can be very beneficial to do some some gentle moves to help address tension held here. In terms of later health problems, there is also the issue of the lack of exposure to the beneficial flora in the vagina that helps colonize the baby's gut. On top of that, they may also be exposed to antibiotics when only a few days old (sometimes through the breast milk if the mother is taking them). The consequences of this are explained in Dr Campbell-McBride's useful book *Gut and Psychology Syndrome* (2010), which also goes into detail about how such effects can be counteracted by clever dietary changes and the use of probiotics. There are several makes of baby probiotics available these days which can be hugely important for creating a healthy gut and lessening the effects of colic.

Cutting the Cord

One of the reasons that work around the diaphragm may be so helpful for babies is that it helps to address the issue of umbilical shock (or umbilical affect as it is termed by psychologists such as Frank Lake). A lot has to happen very quickly right after the baby is born. First it has to go from getting oxygen from the mother to using its lungs for the first time. This involves a small valve in the heart closing over (the foramen ovale) within a few minutes. There also have to be rapid changes in the liver and the bladder at the same time.

If the umbilical cord is cut before it stops pulsating, then these changes have to happen even more quickly and the body is forced into an unnatural situation. One of the consequences of stem cell research has been that some parents store umbilical blood as a kind of 'health insurance' for their children. Unfortunately, this often involves taking blood from the umbilicus immediately the baby is born, necessitating a premature cutting of the cord.

To Crawl or Not to Crawl?

Although there is no hard data on this, colleagues have noticed that many babies born by caesarian are either very slow to crawl or don't crawl at all. They just go from bottom-shuffling to walking. There are many reasons why crawling is important. Apart from helping to develop fine motor skills and what is called cross-lateral integration (encouraging the right and left sides of the brain to work together), crawling develops proprioceptive and visual skills, the muscles of the back and arms, as well as the curves in the spine that are vital for good posture. There also seems to be some correlation between lack of crawling and ADD/ADHD because of a particular primitive reflex that helps us operate our upper and lower body independently. This reflex – the symmetric tonic neck reflex (STNR) – matures between 9 and 12 months by the stimulation of alternate hand and knee crawling and if it doesn't inhibit, it can result in later symptoms such as poor eye–hand coordination and clumsiness (O'Dell and Cook 2004). How Bowen can help in the inhibition of primitive reflexes is discussed in the section by Charlotte Meerman below. There are many sophisticated exercises that help primitive reflexes, which should normally inhibit at a few weeks or months, to be replaced by more complex adult reflexes. Developed by Peter Blythe, these exercises are now taught by teachers trained at his Institute for Neuro-Physiological Psychology (Blythe 2005; www.inpp.org.uk). The controversial programme known as *Brain Gym*, which is used in many schools across the UK and USA, also seems to help address some of these issues.

With babies who are slow to crawl or walk, I have found doing Bowen moves on the lower part of the body (e.g. the pelvic, psoas or even hamstring work) can help hugely with encouraging a sense of mobilization in the pelvis and legs. It is not clear why this might be such an issue with C-section babies, except perhaps that the muscles of the legs are not engaged in pushing during contractions and their psoas muscles can sometimes be frozen into a protective pattern leading to a certain rigidity.

Clumsiness and Proprioception

Working with lack of sensory integration in children is something that was oringally developed by the occupational therapist Jane Ayers at the Institute for Brain Research at UCLA. A child with a lack of proprioceptive awareness will unconsciously exaggerate sensory input by doing things such as slamming doors and generally being noisy and clumsy – activities that tend to drive their long-suffering parents up the wall. Lack of sensory integration can also result in poor bladder and bowel control, which is discussed below and might even extend to biting or head banging in some children. Working with toddlers' and children's sense of proprioception is one of the key things Bowen can help with as it works directly on the nerve pathways that encourage local proprioceptive function.

Plagiocephaly and Brachycephaly

Flat head syndrome has become much more prevalent since 1994 when many national health organizations started advising parents that babies should sleep on their back rather than their front in order to lesson the chance of cot death or sudden infant death syndrome (SIDS). This has halved the incidence of SIDS but has had some inadvertent consequences, one of which is that babies develop less strength and coordination in their upper bodies than they used to, and can therefore be slower to crawl. The other consequence (which has partially been addressed in Sweden by advising parents to use a special pillow) is a flattening of the back of the head, either on one side (plagiocephaly) or both sides (brachycephaly).

Parents can be understandably worried about the shape of their baby's head, but for a therapist, it is often the parts that are not so visible that are important to address. Many health visitors will say that minor distortions in the cranium will subside over the days following birth. This is often true of the cranial vault, which is quite soft. However, many interventions put a strain on areas of the head and neck which are not visible, particularly the cranial base. This is an area of the cranium formed by the more solid parts of the occiput, sphenoid and temporal bones that derive in the embryo from cartilage. For example, the area around the foramen magnum (at the top of the spinal cord) is formed partly by the condyles of the occiput that sit in the concave superior facets of the atlas, allowing for easy flexion and extension of the head. However, in the baby, the occiput is formed by four bones, not just one as in the adult and, more specifically, the condyles which articulate with the atlas are not fused at birth. This means that forces such as traction and/or torsion (inevitable in births that involve caesarian section, forceps or ventouse, but often also occurring in normal vaginal births) will create an imbalance here, with potential effects such as restricted blood flow to the cranium (Flanagan 2010), a pulling up of the brain stem, as well as stress on the short sub-occipital muscles, dural membranes, venous sinuses and ventricles (particularly the fourth ventricle). The potential consequences of poor blood supply to the head are discussed in the cleverly titled *The Downside of Upright Posture* by the chiropractor Michael Flanagan (2010).

Assessing Babies

Tom Bowen used to examine the sclera (the whites) of the eyes in babies who were over three months old to see if they had a neck restriction. One of the reasons for this may be that the vertebral artery, which supplies some of the blood to the brain, passes through foramina in the cervical vertebrae and then does a complicated loop around the base of the occiput before entering the cranium. A restriction in blood supply (which could manifest itself as blueness in the sclera) would result from a neck restriction on either side.

If a baby has a neck restriction, it is common for it to prefer to have its head to one side rather than the other. A mother will have noticed this and one can test it by getting the baby to follow the movement of your finger with its eyes. Babies are naturally inquisitive and will follow any movement with their gaze. You may notice as you bring your finger round that there is some resistance to following your finger. You can ask the mother if they notice that their baby prefers to feed off one breast rather than the other. This can also be indicative of a neck restriction.

An easy way to assess whether or not babies may need the top of their neck attending to is to feel the area around the back of their heads close to where their head naturally makes contact with the mattress. It is common (especially in babies who have had a ventouse delivery) that one side is more anterior to the other or there is some other distortion there. One can also assess this by looking down from the top of the baby's head. If you look at the position of the ears, you may notice that one is anterior to the other. Again, this is not uncommon with ventouse babies and such babies really benefit from the neck and TMJ work.

The Mouth and Jaw

One of the major influences on the development of the hard palate and jaw is breast-feeding. The hard palate in a newborn has the consistency of soft wax, so is very malleable. Research has shown beyond question that bottle-feeding results in more malocclusions as well as affecting the muscles involved in opening and closing the mouth. The strong suck of the baby on the nipple helps mould the whole internal space of the mouth and hence will determine bite and dentition later on. A woman's nipple is perfectly designed to expand in three directions – side to side, top to bottom and front to back; not so an artificial teat, which only expands in two directions (not front to back). The effects of bottle-feeding (and also using a dummy) are therefore extreme in this regard alone, let alone the detrimental affect on the developing immune system.

Premature Babies

The functions of proprioception and interoception involving the myriad of receptors in the joints, skin, muscles and fascia are well developed and very sensitive in the newborn. Research by Professor Stephen Porges (2001) has shown that a baby is born with a highly developed 'social' nervous system and is able to pick up on the emotional nuances of all around it. This 'social nervous system' involves a complex interaction of various cranial nerves that coordinate facial expression, neck and eye movement as well as regulation of the heart and digestion. In the premature baby, certain of these nerve pathways are not yet developed (specifically there is a lack of myelination of the mammalian vagus pathways), meaning that pre-term babies have to rely more on their sympathetic nervous systems to get their needs met. This can mean that such babies not only cry more, but are not necessarily so responsive and interactive. Parents can sometimes feel powerless and inadequate as these babies don't always respond to the normal interactions that soothe full-term babies. Luckily this is something that does not last. There are also specific Bowen moves that address the vagus directly which can be very helpful not just for the premature baby, but all babies where this important nerve is compromised. During birth, a common area for the vagus to become trapped is at the brachial plexus (around the clavicles) as the shoulders are birthed. Bowen moves over the scalenes address this area effectively.

Treating Mums after Birth

Bowen has a unique advantage therapeutically in that the therapist can work on mother and baby at the same time, even if the mum is in a chair holding the baby. In the previous chapter we discussed the use of Bowen in pubic symphysis dysfunction (SPD), a condition that can occur both during and after pregnancy. If the mother has had a caesarian, it can be helpful to work directly on the scar itself. I have noticed many times that scar tissue that is red and raised gets noticeably less inflamed and less fibrotic after gentle Bowen work.

Birth is at best stressful for the mother and sometimes downright traumatic. Allowing the mum to talk about this in a session can be very healing. A new mother will be so focused on the baby that she may not be fully aware of what her body has been through. Gentle therapeutic touch, such as Bowen, can be immensely healing in terms of getting her body back in shape as well as healing some of the more traumatic elements of the birth.

Many Bowen practitioners will advise mums to do pelvic floor exercises after birth (whether they have had a vaginal birth or not) to avoid later problems such as prolapse or incontinence. Bowen moves such as the coccyx oblique influence the muscles and fascia of the pelvic floor directly and can be immensely helpful after birth. The coccyx itself receives considerable stress during a vaginal birth, so for all mums it is a good idea to work here as well. Believe it or not, it is quite possible to address this area even when treating a woman who is seated.

Tissue Memory

The way that the body can hold long-term physical patterns it experiences at birth first struck me 20 years ago when I treated a lady in her mid 20s who was suffering from extreme migraines and headaches. They were so bad that every week she would have to go to bed for at least 24 hours and experienced a background headache all the time. This had a profound effect on her relationship with her husband, her family and her ability to do everyday tasks such as shopping, cooking and going to work.

Whilst I was palpating around the temporal bones (the area around the ears), I felt a very strange pattern emerging, which felt as if her head was being squeezed by a vice, combined with a twisting action which was held in her temporal bones, plus a strong force pulling down towards her feet. To be honest, I had never felt anything like this before, so, as well as being intriguing, it was also slightly alarming.

As I was working, she began to get a slight visual disturbance, as though she was about to get a headache. After a while she began to feel the tightness in her head release, rather like a tightly wound up rubber band slowly letting go.

At the end of the treatment I questioned her about her birth to see if this pattern was related at all. It turned out that she had been born a breech baby – in other words, bottom first. During the birth, they'd also used forceps. The kind of forceps that are used in a breech birth are very specific (they are called Piper's forceps) and attach around the temporal bones, putting a considerable squeeze on the head. The other thing that would have happened during the birth was a dragging down towards the feet in order to get the baby out, along with some rotational forces that I was feeling as I palpated.

When she came back next week, her headaches and migraines had improved dramatically. She no longer had her background headache and had only had a mild migraine during previous week after the treatment. This made me realize that the kind of imprints that we get exposed to at birth have a profound effect on our physicality, and these patterns can stay with us unless they are addressed, causing all kinds of problems for us later in life.

There are various mechanisms by which the body might hold 'memories' of birth apart from the purely mechanical (e.g. inter-osseous or intra-osseous patterns). Hameroff (Hameroff, Rasmussen and Mansson 1998) describes processes that might be at play whereby memories can be held on a tissue level in the cellular microtubules. This is sometimes referred to as 'tissue memory'. James Oschman (Oschman and Oschman 1995, pp.60–74) poses the question:

> Can 'memories' encoded in connective tissue and cytoskeletal structures lead to a conscious mental image of past events? How might such information be 'released' during massage or other kinds of bodywork? And how is such information communicated from the tissue being worked upon to the consciousness of both the client and the practitioner?

Many early feelings and emotions are experienced by the adult as a 'felt sense' of the kind described by Damasio (2010). Perhaps because these felt sensations derive from powerful but pre-verbal experiences they are more difficult for adults to conceptualize and rationalize later in life. This is why early experience can have such a dominating effect on our unconscious desires and emotional outlook throughout our adult life.

Digestive and Bowel Problems in Children

℃ʒ Rosemary MacAllister

According to NICE, constipation is common in childhood, affecting up to 30 per cent of the UK child population. Symptoms can become chronic and constipation is a common reason for referral for secondary care (NICE 2010).

Two years ago, a young mother approached me to see if Bowen therapy would help her ten-year-old daughter who had chronic constipation. The paediatrician had instructed them to increase the medication she was receiving to 'adult' dose. This naturally concerned them both. The mother thought, 'If this is what she's having now, what will she be requiring by the time she is 20?'

When she went for her prescription, the village chemist suggested she try Bowen. This was the start of an amazing journey for myself and several young children aged from just a few months old to 13 and a half. I told her honestly that I did not know if it would help as I had not tried the procedures on children, but they agreed to try.

Family Issues

Bowel problems are disturbing not just for the children but the whole family, including parents and siblings. Only by treating three children on the same day did I realize the real concerns that affect them and everyone around them.

The parent often believes they are the only one trying to cope with the issue. The cost incurred was one concern, having to buy lots of underwear and sheets (if the child is soiling in bed at night) as it is often difficult to clean the article properly. The cost can be quite considerable, especially for parents living on a limited budget. One parent informed me she bought the cheapest of pants and threw them out because of this.

Socializing was also an issue. Many of the older children I treated had never been able to have a sleep-over with friends or go on any school outings that involved an overnight stay. Also siblings did not like to share a room with them if the soiling occurred during the night. At school some of the children did not like to go to the school toilet, sometimes were harassed by other children, and on occasions some teachers had not permitted them to leave the class, so sitting in their own faeces was very uncomfortable, apart from the smell and embarrassment it created. One boy said he had been allowed out to the toilet but was unable to perform and about 15 minutes later had the urge to go again but would not ask the teacher.

An issue that was highlighted to me recently by one of the youngsters was the child having to tell lies to their school friends. When he had to take time off school to visit the consultant or had to go to the hospital for treatment, he was too embarrassed to say what was wrong and so would say he had a finger infection or give some other excuse. He said he did not like having to tell lies but was so ashamed at what was happening to him. Another source of embarrassment was when a child's mother was called to the school to 'clean her daughter up'.

Another area of concern for parents was the time taken time off work to take the child to the hospital. One or two parents informed me they sometimes had over two hours to wait as the consultant had been delayed, which meant they were away from work for at least three hours or more. Their employers were none too happy and this all added to the tension in the household and sometimes the frustration was taken out on the child. Several of these children and/or their parents had attended a psychologist as well as a dietician. Pain and discomfort with distension of the abdomen often caused problems with children having to attend A&E for suppositories or an enema.

One day I asked three of the parents at different times if they would like to speak to another mother whose child I was treating. They all agreed to meet one afternoon and felt this was so revealing for them, being able to understand they were not alone, that small things could be done to improve the situation and that help was available. Treating these children has been such a joy and to see the improvement has been truly amazing.

Since commencing Bowen on the ten-year-old girl, I have now treated at least 17 children with chronic constipation. On looking at all these children, I have noted that several of them had had problems within a few weeks of birth and others when the child was about two years old.

All of these children had attended their GP and 50 per cent had been seen by a specialist. All were on medication, some for as long as 5–10 years, and often several doses a day. I have tried to identify similarities in the cause of the constipation but to date have been unable to do so. All the parents fed the children well, tried to give them water and had no major family issues or obviously traumatic births.

Treatment

The number of sessions the children required varied; 3–5 for the very young children (under one year), older children required anything from 6 to 15 sessions. One of the young boys came along monthly for almost one year just to make sure 'he was alright'. I met him a few days ago (which was more than one year later) and he has had no problems at all and is understandably delighted. He said, 'I now have a life!' Twelve children had their medication gradually reduced within about three to four weeks of treatment. I always advised them to do this under medical supervision.

In the majority of children, their bowels opened normally within 24 hours of having Bowen, some children just a few hours after treatment. There was not one child who did not enjoy having Bowen treatment. Even the young ones would run upstairs and jump on to the couch waiting for me to begin. The sessions usually last no more than 30 minutes with the parents present throughout. Generally, they attend weekly for the first three sessions, then every other week until they have regular bowel movements.

Conclusion

Bowen therapy appears to work extremely well on young children with bowel problems. It is non-invasive, is very gentle and children appear to love the treatment. Results in having normal bowel motions within a few weeks have been noticed in most of the children treated. Hospital visits decreased and medication was greatly reduced or not required at all. I have received some lovely hand-made cards from the children and comments of how much Bowen has helped them. The ten-year-old girl had attended on her tenth birthday and her comment was 'It's the best birthday present I could ever have received!'

If only we could get Bowen Therapy into the health service for these young children, a lot of anguish for parents and children could be removed and the family situation would certainly improve. It would also cut down the large amounts of medication required and time spent in hospital waiting rooms, and give the children and their parents a much better quality of life.

ॐ

Bowen Children's Clinics

ॐ *Jo Wortley*

Tom Bowen opened up his busy clinic to disabled and special needs children on a Saturday morning, where he and two of his students provided free treatments. Many Bowen practitioners the world over are now following in his footsteps by setting up similar clinics treating children, either free of charge, for a donation or a nominal fee.

In the UK, Cardiff-based practitioner Howard Plummer was the first therapist to set up a clinic specifically for children, in the hope that it would inspire other therapists to do the same. At the time of publication, there are around 40 BTPA registered clinics in and around the UK. Howard began his Bowen career whilst lecturing in anatomy and physiology for ITEC (International Therapy Examination Council) in 1992. During this time, he began to realize that fascia was actually a far more an important structure than was first believed. His understanding was that, during the development of the embryo, the ectoderm becomes both the neurological system and the skin, both of which are sensory organs responsible for sending signals to the brain. This led him to develop a very different way of administering the Bowen moves, which has now become widely known as 'Fascia Bowen'. Howard teaches his students moves over the superficial fascia, thus affecting the underlying dense fascia, which in turn affects the structure of the fascia and organs within the entire body. Howard gave his first lecture on his approach in Manchester 2002, during which he demonstrated these moves. His teaching of Fascia Bowen took off over the following few years and is now widely used in the treatment of both adults and children alongside regular Bowen.

The Bowen Technique is an ideal therapy for babies and young children, as the moves are gentle, pleasant to receive and can be administered through clothing whilst the child is lying, sitting or standing. The parent or guardian and the therapist remain in the room at all times, even during the breaks, and parents are encouraged to become actively involved in the treatment itself. As a therapist, administering Bowen to this age group can be an extremely rewarding experience. Some children respond very quickly to the moves applied, with improvements being identified during their session. This is likely to be due to an efficient nerve impulse speed, but is also thought to be related to children not having preconceived ideas about what the therapist is doing or the results that might be expected, and so they are more open to change. A child's Bowen session can last anywhere between 10 and 30 minutes, depending on their age, presenting condition and willingness to comply. In general a baby will require far fewer moves than an older child, and 'break' times between moves are often able to be reduced – providing the conduction of nerve impulses is not compromised by a presenting condition. The flexibility of these break times can be particularly helpful when a client is presenting with a condition such as hyperactivity, ADHD or severe autism. Typically, a child would receive one to three Bowen sessions, a week apart, although long-term conditions may benefit from treatments over an extended period of time.

In comparing information received from the children's clinics across the UK, it can be seen that children with certain symptoms of dyspraxia or developmental coordination disorder (DCD) have a tendency to respond in much the same way. As with any other condition, the symptoms of dyspraxia vary between each individual, but commonly a dyspraxic child can present with poor coordination, low concentration, sensitivity to the texture of certain foods, possibly resulting in a monotonous diet. The child can often look small for their age and skin pallor may be evident. It is also common for a child to require frequent trips to the doctor due to illness or infection. In an older child, self-confidence may be a concern. Following a series of Bowen sessions it is often noted that the child appears calmer and is more able to concentrate, coordination may improve in varying degrees, but also the child's sensitivity to food textures can significantly reduce, resulting in a wider, more varied diet. Furthermore, it appears that the child is able to derive more of the nutrients ingested and appears to thrive, with improvements in both growth and pallor. Less frequent and/or severe periods of illness are often noted, suggesting an improvement within the immune system. In response to this discovery, Bowen practitioner Melanie Morgan Jones is at the time of publication conducting a doctoral research programme, via the University of Bath's Health Department, into Fascia Bowen as an intervention for children with DCD. This research is a first in this area of specialization. Melanie already has a qualification in scientific research methods to ensure the design of this study conforms to the highest standards required by the scientific community. This research paper will be available for peer group review and publication in due course.

More and more clinics are opening every year in the UK, treating children who present with conditions such as asthma, bedwetting, colic, cerebral palsy, autism, ADHD, Asperger's, dyspraxia, sleep disorders, growing pains and glue ear. Research carried out on the effects of Bowen on children with autism, as well as case studies and testimonials, and information about clinics, can be found on the Children's Clinics page of the Bowen Therapy Professional Association (BTPA; www.bowentherapy. org.uk) website.

౪

Bedwetting in Children
౪ *Charlotte Meerman*

Bedwetting (also referred to as nocturnal enuresis) is an embarrassing, frustrating and distressing problem that can have a significant impact on a child's self-esteem. There are many different theories on the cause of bedwetting which include physical, developmental and emotional issues, but most likely there are several combined factors that cause a child to wet at night. Every child will have a different combination of these issues and bedwetting needs to be approached with this in mind. Only a small percentage (less than 1%) is caused by a medical condition, such as urinary tract infections, diabetes, seizure disorder, abnormal nerves to the bladder, birth defects, etc.

There are three different types of bedwetting: *primary enuresis* (the child is wet every night), *intermittent enuresis* (the child has occasional dry nights) and *secondary enuresis* (the child has been dry for months or even years and then starts to wet again, which can be a sign of an underlying medical or emotional problem).

Immaturity of the nervous system is a very common cause of primary enuresis, as the sleep arousal centres of the brain have not yet learnt to recognize signals from the full bladder. Bedwetting is also frequently seen in children with sleep disorders such as sleep apnoea. This condition can be very disruptive to sleep patterns and is usually caused by enlarged adenoids and tonsils. Some children have a relatively small bladder which needs be emptied frequently and cannot hold all the urine produced at night.

In some cases, bedwetting can be a response to stressful events. Divorce, new siblings, moving house, death of a loved one and other traumatic childhood experiences (including abuse) may make bedwetting more likely (especially secondary enuresis). It is important, however, not to label every child who is a bedwetter as having an emotional or psychological issue or to label the parents as bad parents. Plenty of children who wet the bed at night live in a loving and stable family. However, parents often find that even small changes to normal routines can make the bedwetting worse.

Parents who wet the bed as children are more likely to have children with the same problem. Genetics, physical traits, personalities and lifestyles are important factors to consider when explaining why bedwetting is more common in certain families.

Children with constipation, urinary frequency and/or urgency are more likely to also suffer from nocturnal enuresis. As many as 20 per cent of children with nocturnal enuresis also suffer from diurnal enuresis (involuntary urination during the day). Some children hold on to their urine until the bladder is extremely full or wait until it's too late. The brain will learn to ignore the bladder's signal when it is full, irrespective of whether it's day or night-time. The pelvic floor muscles, bladder and bowel sphincters become very tight holding on to the full bladder and bowel, which can create a 'trigger happy bladder', and therefore even daytime accidents can occur by the urgency problem. When a child is sleeping, they are not able to consciously wiggle, squat or run to the toilet when the bladder is very full.

ADH (also known as arginine vasopressin, AVP) is a hormone secreted from the posterior pituitary gland which regulates the balance of water in the body and causes the kidneys to produce less urine. Some children with nocturnal enuresis do not produce enough ADH at night and produce too much urine while they are asleep, therefore becoming more likely to wet the bed.

Some children with nocturnal enuresis have nitric oxide (NO) levels more than 11 times greater than normal and twice the average prostaglandin levels. A high concentration of NO (a naturally occurring gas in the body) decreases ADH production and as a result nocturnal urine production is increased. Prostaglandin is a hormone-like substance which has a variety of physiological functions, such as metabolism and nerve transmission. It also acts on mesangial cells in the glomerulus of the kidney to increase the flow rate of filtered fluid through the kidney (increased urine production).

An adequate dietary intake of omega 3 fatty acids is essential in children who wet at night as they play a critical role in the development and function of the central nervous system (Logan and Lesperance 2005). They may address a possible root cause of some cases of nocturnal enuresis, namely the delayed development of inhibitory brain pathways which control micturition. They also have the potential to influence bedwetting by inhibition of prostaglandin and renal nitric oxide production.

A retained spinal Galant reflex is found in a high percentage of children over the age of five years with nocturnal enuresis. In newborns this reflex can be demonstrated by stroking along one side of the spine. The newborn will laterally flex towards the stimulated side and the reflex may also instigate emptying of the bladder (Blythe 2005). Interestingly, if both sides of the spine are stroked simultaneously, the Pulgar Marx reflex is elicited. This leads to lordosis of the spine, elevation of the pelvis, flexion of the arms, lifting of the head, voidance of bowel and bladder, apnoea and cyanosis, followed by a few seconds of rigidity (hypertonia).

The spinal Galant reflex emerges at 20 weeks in utero, is actively present at birth and should be integrated by the time the baby is 6 to 12 months of age. This reflex helps the baby during the birthing process when the mother's contractions stimulate this reflex, causing movements of the baby's hips to enable the baby to work its way down the birth canal. It also allows the foetus to hear and feel the sound vibrations in the womb and is important in the development of hearing and auditory processing, as well as helping to achieve balance when the child is creeping and crawling.

If the spinal Galant reflex is not integrated within the first year of life, it can be elicited by light pressure in the lumbar region. A Bowen practitioner will notice that these children have very reactive lumbar paraspinal muscles which can be observed with the bottom stoppers and moves up the spine over the erector spinae. These children often do not like wearing belts, elastic waistbands or labels inside the waistband as the friction activates the reflex. They may also dislike having their backs rubbed or an arm around their waist. The possible long-term effects of a retained Spinal Galant reflex include bedwetting, bowel control issues, difficulty sitting still ('ants in the pants'), speech development problems, fatigue, attention and concentration problems, poor coordination, extreme ticklishness (especially around the back), poor short-term memory, hip rotation to one side when walking, poor posture and scoliosis.

Unintegrated, active primitive reflexes may be caused by stress of the mother and/ or baby during pregnancy or complications at birth that prevented the baby using this reflex to manoeuvre itself through the birth canal (e.g. breech birth, premature birth, induced birth, caesarean birth, forceps or vacuum assisted delivery). Lack of enough proper movement in infancy may also be a factor as this restricts critical movements required for brain development - for example, being left for long periods of time in baby walkers, baby capsules or bouncers. In some cases, reflexes that are completely integrated can become reactive at a later stage because of illness, trauma, injury, chronic stress, environmental toxins, complications with vaccinations, dietary imbalances or sensitivities.

Children with auditory processing disorders and neuro-developmental disorders such as autism, Asperger's syndrome or ADD/ADHD often have a retained Spinal Galant reflex (as well as other retained primitive reflexes such as the Moro reflex and asymmetrical tonic neck reflex). About 25 per cent of these children wet the bed at night, which is higher than the general child population.

Primitive reflexes are essential for survival in the first few months of life. These automatic, stereotyped movements are directed from the brain stem and provide the training platform for many aspects of later functioning. The brain stem is the most primitive part of the brain which controls life-supporting autonomic functions of the peripheral nervous system. The primitive reflexes transition into more complex, voluntary-based movement patterns when they are inhibited by the higher centres of the brain within the cerebral cortex. This process allows for the development of more sophisticated neural structures which then allow an infant control of intentional response.

The voluntary control of micturition (urination) usually develops by the age of 3–5 years but, if primitive reflexes remain active, the neural structures of the higher brain centres which inhibit micturition cannot fully develop. If the autonomic nervous system is dominant over the somatic nervous system, we are not able to easily access our prefrontal cortex, the higher centre of the brain where we can process and analyze information. Instead, we remain in survival and stress mode. As a child grows up, the unintegrated reflexes trigger the fight/flight response even when there is no logical reason for the stress, so over time this becomes a common pattern of responding, even into adulthood.

Bowen moves activate proprioceptors at multiple tissue levels and create a dynamic rearrangement of the central and peripheral nervous systems, regulating the autonomic nervous system and therefore facilitating the neural pathway to the prefrontal cortex which will allow development of more complex and refined reflexes, especially procedures that involve areas such as the TMJ, respiratory, kidney and coccyx.

Bowen Therapy is a wonderful holistic technique to help children overcome bedwetting as it promotes physical and emotional balance and healing. Parents also play an important role because patience, commitment and a positive approach are essential. It is not helpful for them to get angry or use punishment when the child has an accident at night. Children need support and reassurance and should never be made to feel embarrassed, ashamed or responsible for the bedwetting.

The bedwetting procedure is the most commonly used Bowen procedure for nocturnal enuresis. It may assist in integration of the spinal Galant reflex because of the combination of the two extra holding points on the erector spinae superior to the iliac crests whilst performing the move over the coccyx. The third holding point (which is also used in the coccyx procedure) is immediately inferior to the inferolateral angle of the sacrum, which corresponds with acupoints also used in other modalities to treat urinary dysfunctions and bedwetting. The move over the coccyx stimulates nerve pathways and ganglia of both the sympathetic and parasympathetic nervous systems that control the bladder, lower bowel and reproductive systems.

Tom Bowen used to say that the second move of the bedwetting procedure on the rectus abdominis fascia 'locked in' the first move. This 'boomerang' shape move is done midway between the umbilicus and the mid-point of the inguinal crease which is innervated by T10–T12. The sympathetic nerves which innervate the bladder and internal sphincter originate from T10–L2; therefore, these areas originate from the same level in the spine. They also correspond with an internal kidney meridian trajectory.

At the first session the basic relaxation work and procedures such as the kidney and respiratory procedures balance and relax the child's body and prepare them for the bedwetting treatments which then follow in the subsequent weeks. The kidney procedure is essential when treating any kidney/bladder issues. It stimulates the kidneys and brings energy into the bladder area as well as the nerves which innervate these structures. Kidneys can be associated with fear so the kidney procedure is very useful when children have emotional issues. The respiratory procedure is also very important as it addresses stress or anxiety.

The subsequent weekly sessions usually consist of the bottom stoppers and the bedwetting procedure, alternating between the left and right side every week. If the child hasn't responded after several treatments or only minimal changes have been achieved, other procedures may be indicated by that stage, such as specialized Bowen procedures coccyx oblique or gracilis which stimulate nerves that innervate the bladder. These moves also correspond with kidney and bladder meridians. Other procedures to consider (not all in the same session): gallbladder procedure – essential when treating children for nocturnal enuresis who also suffer from bowel problems because these conditions can be related. This procedure is also effective for emotional issues and in such cases the shoulder procedure may be added. The knee and ankle procedures coincide with bladder and kidney meridians so can be effective in treating bedwetting as well. The upper respiratory/TMJ and additional TMJ procedures, which stimulate the vagus nerve, may be useful in some children with nocturnal enuresis who haven't responded to the bedwetting procedure. There is also an important Bowen procedure that addresses the vagus nerve directly. Vagus nerve branches represent most of the cranial component of the parasympathetic division of the autonomic nervous system. If the sympathetic nervous system dominates, it can cause an excessive activation of the vagus nerve (especially due to physical or emotional stress). In fact, research has shown that children with nocturnal enuresis demonstrated parasympathetic hyperactivity (Yakinci *et al.* 1997). This parasympathetic overcompensation can affect bladder control. The Bowen Technique calms the sympathetic nervous system so the parasympathetic system will no longer need to compensate and therefore bladder agitation is reduced. The mechanism for this 'vagal brake' is described in detail by Stephen Porges (Porges 2001).

Dietary and Emotional Factors

Tom Bowen advised children who suffer from bedwetting to avoid dairy products, apples and apple juice and anything containing malic acid, which is a natural diuretic. A balanced 80/20 diet is also recommended (80% alkaline-forming foods and 20% acid-forming foods). Soft drinks should be avoided (due to their high sugar content and the fact that some (such as cola) contain caffeine which can irritate the bladder) and other sugary and/or highly processed foods. It is highly recommended that the child drinks filtered alkaline mineralized water (alkaline water filtration systems are available in health food stores and online).

If bedwetting treatments with Bowen therapy do not result in a reduction of the bedwetting frequency or any change in the bedwetting pattern, there may be an underlying medical or emotional issue that needs to be investigated by an appropriate professional. In those cases, referral for further investigation by a paediatrician and/or counsellor would be recommended. Referral to neuro-developmental therapists who use remediation techniques with special exercises to integrate retained primitive reflexes should also be considered.

CASE STUDY

Ten children participated in my bedwetting research project (six girls and four boys) ranging in age from 6 to 14 years. They had weekly Bowen treatments in the first 1–2 months, and some continued to see me for a couple of follow-up treatments. Nine of the ten participants had an improvement in the number of dry nights. Four became 100 per cent dry, two were dry almost every night and two others were dry on average five nights a week. One female participant has had some improvement but her sister still had the same average wet nights per week as before. These two sisters have not been able to have regular weekly treatments and also suffer from coeliac disease, which may be a factor in their results. They have been referred back to their doctor.

The Bowen Therapy treatments also had a profound effect in other ways. Five of the ten children settled down to sleep much earlier than they used to. Others started to wake up and go to the toilet themselves during the night, which they had never done before. This is a sign the brain is starting to respond to the bladder's cues when it is full. Anxiety and moodiness also reduced in several children. Some parents observed emotional releases, improved concentration and calmer behaviour in their children. The children have become more confident and a lot more positive since they started to become dry at night.

∽

Afterthoughts on the Ramifications of Bowen in Childhood

During rare idle moments I sometimes ponder an intriguing question: Given the potential of Bowen to instigate long-lasting resolution of physical and psychological trauma, would the history of the world be substantially different today if Henry VIII had had a Bowen treatment when he was young? This might seem a stupid question, but it is well documented that Henry VIII had a bad accident as a young man when he failed to lower his visor during a jousting tournament and was hit just above his right eye. As Lucy Worsley, chief curator of Britain's Historic Royal Palaces, says:

> We posit that his jousting accident of 1536 provides the explanation for his personality change from sporty, promising, generous young prince, to cruel, paranoid and vicious tyrant. From that date the turnover of the wives really speeds up, and people begin to talk about him in quite a new and negative way. After the accident he was unconscious for two hours; even five minutes of unconsciousness is considered to be a major trauma today. (McCarthy 2009)

The reason I ask this question has an element of seriousness to it, because a therapist never actually knows who is going to come into their clinic on a given day. It could be the future CEO of a big company or even a future prime minister. And we never know how the psychological, emotional, physical wellbeing of that person, who might later be in a position of power, will influence the lives of the people that are affected by their everyday decisions. This can be seen all too clearly in characters such as George Bush and Tony Blair whose decisions have had devastating consequences for millions of people. Some commentators have revealed that their early psychological experiences had a profound and detrimental effect on their ability to make sound judgements. The celebrated child psychologist Sue Gerhardt (author of the must-read *Why Love Matters*) devotes a large section of her more recent book *The Selfish Society* (2010, pp.231–251) to this very subject. The British politician and neurologist David Owen points out in his book *The Hubris Syndrome* (2012) the rather shocking prevalence of severe personality disorders in both US presidents and UK prime ministers during the last 100 years.

So the question is, what would have happened if people such as this had had treatment early in life? And, more importantly, how does treatment early in life affect the quality of life not just for the person who is being treated but for their family, friends and colleagues who come into contact with them?

The good news is that there are a lot of therapeutic interventions available such as Bowen, craniosacral therapy and other body-based psychotherapeutic approaches like somatic experiencing and neuro-developmental therapy that can help to address issues arising from pregnancy and birth, as well as many organizations that help address the long-term consequences of how we are born (see web resources below). The bad news is that, despite the large body of evidence and some vocal campaigners, little has been done over the last 30 years to improve the potentially negative impact of the birthing experience on both mums and babies.

References

Blythe, S. (2005) *Reflexes, Learning and Behaviour: A Window into a Child's Mind.* Oregon: Fern Ridge Press.

Campbell-McBride, N. (2010) *Gut and Psychology Syndrome: a Natural Treatment for Autism, ADD/ ADHD, Dyslexia, Dyspraxia, Depression, Schizophrenia.* Soham: Medinform Publishing.

Cuccia, A. and Caradonna, C. (2009) The relationship between the stomatognathic system and body posture. *Clinics* 64 (1), 77–78.

Damasio, A. (2000) *The Feeling of What Happens – Body, Emotion, and the Making of Consciousness.* London: Vintage.

Flanagan, M. (2010) *The Downside of Upright Posture.* Minneapolis, MN: Two Harbors Press.

Gerhardt, S. (2010) *The Selfish Society. How We All Forgot to Love One Another and Made Money Instead.* New York: Simon and Schuster.

Hameroff, S., Rasmussen, S. and Mansson, B. (1988) Molecular Automata in Microtubules: Basic Computational Logic of the Living State? In C. Langton (ed.) *Artificial Life, SFI Studies in the Sciences of Complexity*, vol. VI. Redwood City, CA: Addison-Wesley.

Juhl, J. (2004) Prevalence of frontal plane pelvic postural asymmetry. *Journal of the American Osteopathic Association* 104 (10), 411–421.

Levinkind, M. (2008) Consideration of whole body posture in relation to dental development. *Oral Health Report, British Dental Journal Supplement* 1, 1–7.

Logan, A. and Lesperance, F. (2005) Primary nocturnal enuresis: omega-3 fatty acids may be of therapeutic value. *Medical Hypotheses* 64 (6), 1188–1191.

McCarthy, M. (2009) The jousting accident that turned Henry VIII into a tyrant. *Independent*, Saturday 18 April.

McCarty, W.A. (2012) *Welcoming Consciousness: Supporting Babies' Wholeness from the Beginning of Life – An Integrated Model of Early Development.* Santa Barbara, CA: Wondrous Beginnings Publishing.

NICE (2010) *Constipation in Children and Young People.* Guideline CG99. London: NICE.

O'Dell, N. and Cook, P. (2004) *Stopping ADHD.* New York: Penguin.

Oschman, J. and Oschman, N. (1995) Somatic recall part 1 – soft tissue memory. *Massage Therapy Journal* 34 (3), 36–45, 66–67, 101–167.

Owen, D. (2012) *The Hubris Syndrome. Bush, Blair and the Intoxication of Power.* York: Methuen.

Porges, S. (2001) The polyvagal theory: phylogenetic substrates of a social nervous system. *International Journal of Psychophysiology* 42, 123–146.

Sakaguchi, K. *et al.* (2007) Examination of the relationship between mandibular position and body posture. *Cranio: The Journal of Craniomandibular Practice* 25 (4), 237–249.

Yakinci, C. *et al.* (1997) Autonomic nervous system functions in children with nocturnal enuresis *Brain and Development* 19 (7), 485–487.

Resources

Websites

Birth International
https://www.birthinternational.com

Birth Psychology
birthpsychology.com

Birthworks International
www.birthworks.org/site/primal-health-research.html

Building and Enhancing Bonding and Attachment
www.beba.org

Conscious Embodiment Trainings
www.conscious-embodiment.co.uk

CYMA
www.cyma.org.uk

Fathers to Be
www.fatherstobe.org

The Origins of Peace and Violence
www.violence.de

Womb Ecology
www.wombecology.com

Wonderful Birth
www.wonderfulbirth.com

Further Reading

Blasco, T.M. (2003) *How to Make a Difference for Your Baby if Birth Was Traumatic.* Santa Barbara, CA: Building and Enhancing Bonding and Attachment.

Chamberlain, D. (1998) *The Mind of Your Newborn Child.* Berkeley, CA: North Atlantic Books.

Gerhardt, S. (2004) *Why Love Matters: How Affection Shapes a Baby's Brain.* London: Taylor and Francis (Routledge).

Levine, P.A. (1997) *Waking the Tiger: Healing Trauma – The Innate Capacity to Transform Overwhelming Experiences.* Berkeley, CA: North Atlantic Books.

Schore, A.N. (2003) *Affect Dysregulation and Disorders of the Self.* New York: W.W. Norton.

Siegal, D.J. and Hartzell, M. (eds) (2013) *Parenting from the Inside Out.* London: Penguin.

14

A Sporting Approach to Bowen Therapy

Michael Quinlivan

Despite the widespread clinical use of Bowen Therapy in many countries around the world, the amount of scientific research, in randomized, controlled studies into the efficacy of this technique, is very limited. In my experience, using the Bowen Technique in the sporting environment has achieved very positive outcomes and above average results in comparison to other techniques. My training in soft-tissue therapy is not limited to Bowen but I am also a myotherapist, which, in Australia, is an Advanced Diploma of Remedial Massage. Because of these qualifications I am able to apply a wide variety of philosophical applications to the use of Bowen therapy when treating a variety of athletes who are involved in sporting activities. It is important, however, to understand that when applying the Bowen Technique I believe I have an advantage in that I am able to draw on theoretical knowledge learned in other training and this gives me a greater insight into how to apply the technique in different situations. Because of this, when treating sporting people, the methodology I use enhances the initial Bowen Therapy training, which I originally undertook through the Bowtech system in 1994.

The Nature of Sport

Just the mere mention of the word 'sport' often raises a wide and diverse range of emotions, probably matched only by events at a dinner party when discussions on religion and politics are introduced. There are those who love their sport so much they will drive to distraction any person with whom they are having a conversation and any others who may be within hearing range. There are those who are so passionate about their favourite sport or sporting team that they are almost unable to have a conversation without some mention of these. On the other end of the spectrum are those who simply love to hate sport. In spite of these contradictory feelings, there are literally millions of people on this planet who are involved in some level of sporting activity. These levels range from passive activities that don't require much in the way of an active training regime yet may demand a high degree of mental concentration, such as darts and billiards, to the other end of the range, the extreme sports requiring a huge amount of physical training, mental concentration and possession of a high level of specific skills that are related to these activities, for example, mountain bike riding and triathlons.

Sport can be undertaken just for fun or to attain a desired level of fitness and, in some cases, weight control. Others are involved in competition either in team sports or as an individual. Each individual has their own reason for being involved in their chosen sport. Whatever the sport, whether the level be novice through to elite or casual to serious, it is almost inevitable that those involved will ultimately receive an injury, ranging from simple soreness (often referred to as general soreness) through to very severe soft-tissue ruptures and fractures. The athlete's primary concern is always to get rid of the pain and then return to sport as soon as possible, which is often something that is not necessarily realistically achievable.

Traditionally, treatment of sporting injuries has been undertaken by medical practitioners, physiotherapists, chiropractors, osteopaths and massage therapists and, in many situations, trainers at sporting clubs. In some cases the club trainers have no formal training. In my experience their knowledge seems to have been acquired mainly from trainers who have preceded them and I have experienced some unfortunate adverse reactions as a result of very ordinary practices. Today, with an emphasis on higher standards of training requirements, the incidence of poor-quality practices is diminishing.

This chapter is not so much about specific treatment protocols using Bowen Therapy, but more about the athlete and the background to what makes them 'tick'. I also wish to give an insight into various situations where I have found Bowen Therapy to have been beneficial and how I use the technique differently today from how I learned the procedures in my initial training.

Tom Bowen, the originator of the technique, treated many sporting injuries, both in his clinics and at sporting clubs around Geelong, Australia, where he resided. Ossie Rentsch, who learnt from Tom Bowen and created an instruction programme which instigated the initial training of many thousands of people learning the fundamentals of the Bowen Technique, told me that people would travel vast distances to Geelong to see Bowen for treatment of sporting and other injuries.

With such a variety of treatment protocols already in existence, what does Bowen Therapy have to offer that can match, or improve on, these other methods? The traditional thought process used by an injured athlete is usually to seek treatment from a physiotherapist. Even if any of the other modalities is sought, lack of widespread knowledge and popularity, for an athlete to regard Bowen therapy as the first source of treatment, is a continual problem for a Bowen practitioner. Basically, the fact that Bowen therapy is relatively new, only having been taught to the general populace since 1987 (Rentsch 1987), and lack of general awareness of the technique means it is very low in the pecking order of preferred options for the injured athlete.

To change the status of this situation, all Bowen practitioners must lift their level of professionalism, their profile and that of the technique. This requires all Bowen Therapy training to equate with other soft-tissue modalities so that a Bowen practitioner has a high level of underpinning knowledge of anatomy and physiology, skills of assessment and an understanding and application of the requirements of rehabilitation. I believe any trained Bowen practitioner can easily take their knowledge of the application of learned procedures and adapt them to use in a sporting environment. Within a club environment is where I Iearnt to adapt my clinical training into the sporting world. Basically, I had three tables set up in the changing rooms and gave treatments of no longer than ten minutes to each athlete. By moving from one table to the next I had to minimize the length of treatment time and be very specific about the selection of procedures and the use of prerequisites. Such an experience was very valuable for my learning and I would recommend it to any new or experienced Bowen practitioner.

Depending on what you read about the history of massage, there are claims that it has been in existence for thousands of years. Bowen Therapy training commenced as a four-day training schedule in 1986 but has now progressed into a very professional system of modular units spread over at least a year. The initial level of Bowen Therapy training today is documented in three manuals written by O. and E. Rentsch and produced by the Bowen Therapy Academy of Australia (Rentsch and Rentsch 2005) The Bowtech system is controlled and supervised through a programme of registration and is available in many countries around the world.

Before we look at what Bowen Therapy can do for the injured or, for that matter, the uninjured athlete, we must first turn our attention to what makes an athlete the person that they are. I will refer to any person who is involved in any sporting endeavour as an athlete. I do realize that there may be some conjecture in the mind of some individuals who believe what is and what isn't sport. For example, there are those who will say that unless a sport is included in the Olympic games it can't be considered to be a sport. By my own definition, involvement in a sport allows for the inclusion of any activity that requires some physical exertion and mental concentration with the aim of competition or simply the improvement of one's physical or mental wellbeing.

Physical, Mental and Emotional Aspects of Sport

Whilst I am using a broad definition of what can be considered a sport, I will begin with what I consider is required to be part of sporting endeavour and what a person experiences in participating in a sporting activity. I believe that there are three areas that a person utilizes within their inner self. These are the involvement of *physical* as well as *mental* and *emotional* aspects of human nature so as to achieve an individual's own level of *personal wellbeing*.

The *physical* doesn't need much explaining as it is simply using the body to undertake actions and ranges of movement in a pre-prepared format to achieve goals and standards in line with the actions of their chosen sport. *The mental* aspect requires the participant to concentrate or focus on specified tasks so as to achieve desired outcomes. It is my experience that the mind gives in before the body, so the mind and the body need to be trained to acclimatize to the demands of a specific sport. The *emotional* aspect is an entirely different situation: control of nervousness, self-belief, fear of the unknown and the thoughts associated with the perception of the degree of pain involved in the particular sporting activity. If these three aspects are functioning at less than desirable levels, tension is the end result. This can be tension both physical and mental. To test this for yourself, throw a ball at a target and see how close you can get to hitting the target. The distance from the target is unimportant. Then tense the muscles in your arm and shoulder and throw again and you most likely will miss the target by a greater distance than the first throw. If you managed to hit the target with both throws, congratulations, you are a talented athlete. The positive desire to achieve benefits from sporting participation is usually the driving force behind an individual's involvement and an outcome of *personal wellbeing*. This aspect is achieved by sport being fun, relaxed and tension-free.

Where does a Bowen practitioner fit into this picture? From my experience and observation as a long-time Bowen practitioner, I have seen that Bowen therapy has the capacity to provide relaxation to the somatic tissue of the body, relax the mind and calm the emotions so that the individual can perform the desired tasks in a relaxed and competent manner. As an athlete myself, I have felt body tension to be the destroyer of good body action and performance. For example, while reading this chapter, clench the fist of one hand and hold for a few minutes. I anticipate the entire arm will tire and if you wish to make a quick movement you will have a less than desired reaction. Your mind will react adversely and tell you to stop squeezing the fist. You may feel, emotionally, this is a silly thing to be doing and not beneficial to your body's wellbeing. Imagine then what it would feel like if you whole body was tensed. Perhaps you'd better not.

The point is, if an athlete were to experience overall tension, a Bowen treatment of the three procedures known as the Bowen Relaxation Moves (BRMs) (Rentsch and Rentsch 2005, vol. 1, 1.4–1.14) gives the body, mind and emotions an opportunity to relax. This will have the added benefit of decreasing the likelihood of soft-tissue injuries that are generally in the muscles, tendons, ligaments and fascia, known as somatic tissue. It is interesting that Sebastian Coe would routinely sleep just before an Olympic event in order to feel completely relaxed before the race.

Before we get too excited about relaxing the athlete, we should look at where they are in their training regime. At the start of a sporting season the athlete should prepare for the competition. Well before competition commences the ideal training programme should begin with a pre-season plan of acclimatizing the body's muscle and connective tissue to a state of preparedness for competition.

Complete physical function is critical to successful sporting endeavour. The same applies to everyday life. To achieve any level of physical attainment, a fit and healthy body must have 'strength, balance, power, speed, agility, coordination, endurance and mobility' (Chaitow 2006, p.314). These aspects of human physicality can be present in the natural talent bank of the individual but for the most part they need to be practised and developed through training. For most activities a level of aerobic fitness is essential. *Mosby's Medical, Nursing and Allied Health Dictionary* describes 'aerobic exercise, any physical exercise that requires additional effort by the heart and lungs to meet the skeletal muscles' increased demand for oxygen' (Anderson 2002, p.50). Training for any sport educates the body into improved performance and when done gradually provides a developmental gradient to achieve competitive results. The question then asked is how can Bowen Therapy assist?

The answer is that we really don't have any documented, validated evidence to tell us. But I will relate to you an occurrence that happened by accident. (Some of the greatest discoveries in the history of the world have happened by accident.) A reasonably talented athlete attended my clinic with his wife for help with fertility problems. A treatment requires the use of the coccyx procedure (Rentsch and Rentsch 2005, vol. 3, 5.2–5.4). From our clinical experience, we have learned that this procedure has many benefits, among which is general body relaxation and body balance, but it is generally suggested that after such a treatment no physical exertion be undertaken. That evening I was controlling a training programme, in which this individual was involved, and the plan was that the whole training group was required to run as far as possible in 15 minutes. This exercise was undertaken regularly (usually every three weeks) and on a measured running track. The purpose was to assess the rate of improvement on a measurable scale. On this particular evening, the athlete in question, after receiving a coccyx treatment, ran a personal best distance by more than 100 metres. After the run, he commented that he felt really relaxed and balanced throughout the run. I recognize that one isolated run by one individual is not sound scientific evidence. Three weeks later he ran the trial again and he covered 50 metres less than the previous run and had not received a coccyx treatment on the day. As a trainer of athletes, I would have expected him to at least match his previous distance, especially as he had participated in another three weeks of training. For the remainder of that season, each time he received the coccyx treatment prior to the run he was able to match or slightly improve on his personal best distance.

The point is that here is an instance where a Bowen procedure may have assisted with an improved athletic performance and the application of the procedure may be contrary to the methodology of the originally taught instruction. My suggestion to any Bowen Therapy practitioner is to experiment with different procedures to assess whether or not measured results can be improved upon. In this particular instance I do suggest that the coccyx procedure should only be done during the 'in training' phase of a programme. I further suggest that you don't experiment with an athlete on the day of a very important event as the result may be contrary to the desired outcome and the athlete may not be very happy if their performance is less than satisfactory. This is particularly true if they have never had Bowen before, as treatments can result in a change in proprioceptive awareness – something that needs time for the body to integrate.

The Nature of Sporting Injuries

Bowen Therapy, in my experience, when used in a sporting environment has achieved some amazing results with injured athletes. An injury, in general terms, is a condition where damage has been caused that usually results in pain and restricts activity or may even cause disability to the extent that the athlete is not able to participate in training or competition in their chosen sport (Prentice 2011, p.61).

The injuries that I now wish to discuss are related to somatic tissue such as muscle, tendon, ligament and fascia and are graded in accordance with the severity of the damage caused to the tissue by various forms of mechanical or chemical stimuli. The *Churchill Livingstone Dictionary of Sport and Exercise Science and Medicine* defines injury as 'any process causing damage'. When injuries are presented to me at a sporting contest or in my clinic, I wish to know the cause because my treatment protocol can vary according to the type of injury it is. There are three different types. First, a direct injury is damage to tissue, (tendon, ligament, bone or fascia) that has been caused by direct contact, usually with an opponent (e.g. a knee striking the lateral thigh region) or sporting equipment (e.g. being struck by a hockey stick or crashing into the post of a volleyball net). Second, an indirect injury results from an external source such as 'rolling' an ankle when running and landing on the raised edge of a running track, or tearing a hamstring or a pectoralis major muscle in the course of tackling an opponent during a game of rugby. The third type is an overuse injury, which is usually in a chronic state before an athlete seeks treatment. In my experience, distance runners present with Achilles pain resulting from continual training and competing that result in the bursa surrounding the soleus tendon becoming inflamed and hence restricted in its ability to slide satisfactorily through the sheath. Other causes include wearing in appropriately fitting shoes, continual use of the same range of movement (e.g. serving in tennis) or bad biomechanics.

Whatever the cause or type of injury, pain results and is reported through receptor cells known as nociceptors. The initial stage of injury causes an inflammatory response which creates a chemical reaction that is reported to the brain via afferent fibres. Bogduk tells us that 'The process of nociception involves several components: the detection of tissue damage (referred to as transduction); the transmission of nociceptive information along peripheral nerves; its transmission in the spinal cord; and its modulation. Furthermore it is important to recognize that not all nociception involves peripheral tissue damage.' (Bogduk 1993, pp.49–50). Bogduk goes on to explain that the mechanism to initiate nociceptive message has two known causes, *chemical nociception*, which only occurs in the presence of actual tissue damage, and *mechanical nociception*, which occurs when tissues are being excessively strained (Bogduk 1993, pp.50–51). In certain situations the two processes may also operate in parallel (Bogduk 1993, p.53). I suggest knowledge of the nociceptive process is important for any Bowen practitioner to understand in the treatment of pain management.

Muscle and connective tissue that is forcibly lengthened beyond its normal range of motion is classified by the severity of damage. When a practitioner is presented with an ankle injury it is very likely to be a *sprain*. 'A *sprain* is an injury to a ligament or capsular structure' (Schultz, Houglum and Perrin 2000, p.4). Various authors describe the grading of injuries slightly differently; however, in general terms the descriptions are similar. In regard to sprains, Schultz grades damage as follows:

- *First Degree.* A first-degree sprain is characterized by mild overstretching and does not cause any visual disruption in the tissue.

- *Second Degree.* With a second-degree injury, further stretching and partial disruption or macrotearing of the ligament occur.

- *Third Degree.* A third-degree sprain is characterized by a complete disruption (rupture) or loss of ligament integrity.

(Schultz *et al.* 2000, pp.4–5)

When ligaments have been sprained they have a propensity not to return to their original length, which allows for laxity (looseness) in the joint. Exercises to strengthen the muscles, and their tendons, that cross that joint are necessary to assist in stabilizing the affected joint.

The same text describes injuries to muscles and tendons known as strains and are also described in gradings as follows:

- *First Degree.* A first-degree strain is characterized by overstretching and microtearing of the muscle or tendon, but there is no gross fiber disruption. [A first degree strain may not cause the athlete to stop competing.]

- *Second Degree.* Second-degree strains involve further stretching and partial tearing of muscle or tendon fibers.

- *Third Degree.* In third-degree strains, a muscle or tendon is completely ruptured.

(Schultz *et al.* 2000, p.5)

The information contained here is a brief overview of aspects of the body's physiological reaction to injury, but is by no means extensive. As a Bowen practitioner researching this type of knowledge is invaluable in assisting with treating not only sporting athletes but also any presenting pathology. What is relevant is that the Bowen practitioner will be confronted with a request from the athlete as to when they can return, first, to training, and, second, competition. The practitioner's knowledge must be of an extent that any advice given is as accurate as is possible based on information obtained from observation, assessment and informed knowledge. This knowledge can be acquired in any educational environment which forms the base for learning from formal courses, clinical experience, reading, undertaking further qualifications, continuing education workshops and informal discussions with other professionals and even patients. Personally, I have acquired a huge amount of knowledge from my peers by asking relevant questions about specific needs when looking for answers when treating athletes and other patients.

Using Bowen with Sporting Injuries

Another learning experience is treating patients, particularly in the sporting environment. I am continually surprised at the results the Bowen Technique has given to athletes over the years. Just one example of this was an athlete whom I was training, who was about to participate in a milestone event on a particular Saturday. On the preceding Thursday he limped into the room where I was treating fellow athletes. I did not assess his injury, other than ask him where he was experiencing the pain and how did he damage his right adductors. My initial expectation was that he would not be fit enough to be involved in sport in two days' time. In this situation, I have a ten-minute time frame for each athlete, so the treatment protocol was brief and specific. I did BRM 1 and the pelvic procedure. To my amazement, he not only competed on the Saturday but also on the Sunday without discomfort and did not require a follow-up treatment, even though I suggested he should have one.

Any muscular and somatic dysfunctional conditions should be assessed and treated specifically. It is not good enough to have a patient present in your clinic with a shoulder injury and have a Bowen practitioner think that all they need to do is perform the shoulder procedure (Rentsch and Rentsch 2005, vol. 1, 2.5–2.9). For example, is the injury acute or chronic and what was the cause? Has the dysfunction occurred gradually as in the case of an overuse injury? What is the classification of the injury and is there a state of inflammation (e.g. tendonitis) or has it progressed to a non-inflamed yet painful stage and a likely thickening of the tendon (e.g. tendonosis)? Or is it referred to as a tendonopathy? Tendonopathy is a term often seen on radiographic reports used to describe conditions in a tendon. Brukner and Khan (2009, pp.21–23) describe in great detail the pathology of these conditions which gives a real insight into the physical state of a dysfunctioning tendon. As professional practitioners, Bowen practitioners have a legal obligation to determine a patient's presenting condition as well as a need to achieve desired outcomes for the patient. The patient's answers to the questions asked by the practitioner will give a history upon which the Bowen practitioner will base the plans of treatment and rehabilitation specifically for each patient. I have formulated a series of questions based on the text by Nicola Petty, which as a general process is known as subjective examination (Petty 2011, pp.4–36). This information is very comprehensive; however, any practitioner can formulate their own series of questions, which can be found in many texts published on clinical assessment.

As stated previously, physical function is critical for success of any athlete. Chaitow tells us that 'Strength, balance, power, speed, agility, coordination, endurance and mobility are important elements in most sports' and 'The presence of musculoskeletal dysfunction will most certainly reduce physical function' (2006, p.314). This brings me to the importance of knowing exactly what it is that I am treating. The Bowen practitioner must make good clinical notes from questioning the athlete on all relevant aspects of the history of an injury and observe for any physical abnormalities and postural asymmetry. Palpation of the injured site can often give an insight into the nature of an injury. It is as important for the practitioner to detect if any of the necessary elements are missing (e.g. strength), to detect specific dysfunction (e.g. pain in a hamstring).

To obtain the correct information I have devised an assessment protocol which has its origin in a Muscle Energy Technique (MET) postural-structural model. The assessment begins with the Pelvic Girdle described by Philip E. Greenman (2003, pp.337–363). These assessment techniques are osteopathic in their origin, but by assessing the structural integrity the practitioner can quickly become aware of which tissues are hypertonic (over-toned) or hypotonic (under-toned) and causing osteo-structures to be misaligned. Where uneven stresses are present in tissue, postural stresses are present and neural tension inequality can also exist, resulting in differences in muscle firing capacity in musculature. By being aware of which tissue requires treatment and the specific treatment needed, the Bowen practitioner treats only what is relevant to eliminate causative factors.

Following the pelvic area assessment, I then assess lumbar spine, followed by thoracic spine and finally cervical spine using MET assessment protocols. These assessment tasks are not easily learned but with appropriate teaching and lots of practice the Bowen practitioner will gain great professional skills. Whatever assessment tools are utilized, it is important for each Bowen practitioner to have and use their own assessment protocols.

When a joint or specific musculature is dysfunctional I conduct physical functional tests that are taught in diploma-level soft-tissue courses. The following activities are known as objective examination and are used to obtain factual information. These involve assessing range of movement (ROM) activities with the intention of reproducing normally expected ROMs of various regions of the body.

The tests involve *active movement*. If there is pain on *actives* then the practitioner makes a *passive movement*. If pain presents on *passive movement*, it is expected that the dysfunction is related to the joint structure or ligaments of the joint. The Bowen practitioner should consider a referral to a medical practitioner. For the benefit of the patient, however, I would give a Bowen treatment to assist with decreasing the inflammation. This suggestion is as a result of my own experience. If there isn't any pain on *passive movement,* then it is safe to assume that the dysfunction is muscular. The practitioner then validates the assessment by doing *resisted movements* to confirm the specific dysfunctional muscle. At this point, and to further confirm a positive finding, the practitioner can undertake a *special test* or what is commonly known as an *orthopaedic test.* There are numerous texts containing a wide array of such tests, but there are two that I mostly use. These are Hattam and Smeatham (2010), which is totally devoted to special tests, and Jurch (2009), where special tests are included within the general text. One other book that I use is Hoppenfeld (1976); even though it has been in publication for a very long time, I find its simplicity of explanations easily understood and easy to use. An example of when to use a special test would be when an athlete presents with an aching pain in the unilateral gluteal region with pain referring distally through the hamstring to the posterior knee. The practitioner may suspect sciatica and a special test may be used to ascertain if the cause of pain is disc involvement, facet joint pathology or nerve entrapment. Some special test suggestions would be *slump test* (Jurch 2009, p.180), *Lasegue's (straight leg raise) test* (Jurch 2009, p.179) for lumbar spine dysfunction or *Gillet's (sacral fixation) test* (Jurch 2009, p.199). When the cause is establisheds a management plan can be initiated. It must always be remembered, however, that the Bowen practitioner must refer a patient for medical diagnosis and treatment when necessary.

If the Bowen practitioner has a particular Bowen procedure to employ for the specific problem, then carry it out. If there isn't a known applicable procedure for an identifiable muscle, make a medial Bowen move over the proximal musculotendinous junction (MTJ) followed by a medial move over the distal MTJ. Wait two minutes and make a medial move over the belly of the muscle. Make sure that none of the moves is made on a tear or on a trauma site. The aim is to assist the repair of the dysfunction, not make it worse.

A very common injury sustained by an athlete is hamstring dysfunction. It has been my experience that the general perception of pain in the hamstring experienced by an athlete is that it must be a strain. Indeed, Prentice (2011, p.612) states that:

> Hamstring strains are the most common injuries to the thigh. The exact cause of hamstring strain is not known. One theory is that the short head of the Biceps Femoris muscle is subject to the highest incidence of hamstring strain because, as a result of an idiosyncracy of innervation, it contracts at the same time that the quadriceps muscle does. Another speculation is that a quick change of the

hamstring muscle from the role of knee stabilization to hip extension when running is a major cause of strain.

Prentice goes on to discuss the physiology of the hamstring group and its relationship to its antagonist, the quadriceps.

On many occasions I have had athletes present with hamstring soreness and treated the condition using the Bowen hamstring procedure (Rentsch and Rentsch 2005, vol. 1, 2.10–2.13) and the condition did not resolve. In a discussion with a local physiotherapist, I was introduced to the work of Sandy Fritz in relation to *muscle firing patterns* (Fritz 2004, pp.404–407). My experience has been that there is a need to investigate the relevant muscle firing pattern when the hamstring soreness is chronic and is usually related to a previous injury in the hamstring muscles, quadriceps muscles and gluteal muscles. In one case, quadriceps tightness and hamstring soreness was detected as a result of a hernia operation that turned off the muscle firing of the transverse abdominis muscle and the internal and external oblique muscles. 'Muscles contract, or fire, in a neurological sequence to produce coordinated movement. If the firing pattern is disrupted and muscles fire out of sequence or do not contract when they are supposed to, labored movement and postural strain occurs' (Fritz 2004, p.403). In her text, Fritz describes the firing patterns in a number of body actions; for example, she lists the normal firing pattern of hip extension. It is within this text that Fritz describes one of the symptoms of non-normal firing pattern in hip extension as recurrent strain (2004, p.405). In my experience I have found that, whilst repetition of strains does occur from this problem, chronic pain is also present, and when addressed through rehabilitation exercises the chronic condition generally resolves. The natural inclination of a practitioner is to give the athlete strengthening exercises. I believe that the firing pattern must be restored prior to strengthening the non-firing muscle. The key to restoring a firing pattern is to have the athlete repeatedly go through the 'complaining' action using a small amount of load and continue the repetitions on a daily basis until they feel the specific muscle firing again.

Another example of 'thinking outside the box' is of a footballer (Australian Rules Football) who received an opponent's knee in the lumbar region prior to half-time during a game. His hamstrings in his left leg tightened and after half-time he tore the biceps femoris muscle at the proximal MTJ. The game was on a Saturday and he visited a practitioner of another modality on the Sunday morning. He was diagnosed with a severe grade II tear and told he wouldn't return to competition for eight weeks. He visited me on the next day and, on assessment, I agreed with the grading of the tear; however, I assessed he had a rotation of one lumbar vertebra at L4. This is typical of a presenting trauma and, in my experience, causes the psoas muscle to go into spasm. As stated earlier, a hypertonic muscle can misalign osteo-structures; however, I believe in this situation the vertebra was forcibly rotated by the opponent's knee which in turn causes the psoas to spasm. The misaligned vertebra then alters the symmetry of the sciatic nerve and subsequently the tibial nerve, resulting in tension on the hamstring group. Ultimately, the biceps femoris is over-lengthened when running and consequently tears. My treatment protocol for the first visit was to use BRM 1, BRM 2, hamstring procedure and the psoas procedure (with prerequisites). I was very careful not to make moves over the trauma site. For the next seven days I repeated only BRM 1 (Moves 1 and 2 only) and hamstring after I had assessed that the rotation at L4 had corrected and held. Seven days later I repeated the treatment of the first day and then repeated the second day to day six treatments, every five days for the next two weeks. He returned to competition in four weeks from the date of the injury. His rehabilitation exercise was to use the Bowen hamstring exercise within pain threshold, gentle passive stretching, with gradual lengthening over time and ultimately supine bridging for strengthening. Throughout the treatment time he used rubber bands to actively move the leg to mobilize and strengthen the affected muscle. I wanted to ensure that the muscle did not lose its firing ability.

A Bowen practitioner has the perfect tool to assist the athlete's rehabilitation. This is because Bowen therapy addresses the appropriate nerve pathways to assist the body to correct the dysfunctioning pathology. Having used the Bowen Technique to treat numerous different types of injuries over many years, I am pleased with the results I have achieved with this modality. In particular, in treating chronic-type injuries and looking for causative factors by using investigative assessment, I have often found dysfunctional muscle firing patterns require rehabilitation exercises to rectify this problem. By giving appropriate exercises to refire an affected muscle or muscle group, I can incorporate this into the treatment protocol after a Bowen treatment. I am very confident that using rectifying techniques along with the Bowen Technique gives positive results for a chronically injured athlete.

Bowen practitioners have a remarkable technique at their disposal. However, I believe the use of this modality has far more potential than we are making use of at the moment. I am confident the technique can be used in a wider variety of presenting pathologies in the future, especially if we follow protocols of assessment, treatment and rehabilitation, and we are able to discover evidence-based information as to how Bowen therapy really works on the body's pathology; hence we can extend the varieties of treatment protocols. I am confident that the variation that I apply to the treatment of sporting situations is only one example of where this marvellous technique can be used in the future.

References

Anderson, D.M. (ed.) (2002) *Mosby's Medical, Nursing and Allied Health Dictionary* (6th edition). London: Mosby.

Bogduk, N. (1993) The anatomy and physiology of nociception. In J. Crosbie and J. McConnell (eds) *Key Issues in Musculoskeletal Physiotherapy.* Oxford: Butterworth-Heinemann.

Brukner, P. and Khan, K. (2009) *Clinical Sports Medicine* (3rd edition). Sydney: McGraw-Hill.

Chaitow, L. (2006) *Muscle Energy Techniques*, 3rd edn. Edinburgh: Elsevier.

Fritz, S. (2004) *Mosby's Fundamentals of Therapeutic Massage* (3rd edition). London: Elsevier.

Greenman, P. (2003) *Principles of Manual Medicine* (3rd edition). Philadelphia: Lippincott Williams and Wilkins.

Hattam, P. and Smeatham, A. (2010) *Special Tests in Musculoskeletal Examination. An Evidence-Based Guide for Clinicians*. Edinburgh: Elsevier.

Hoppenfeld, S. (1976) *Physical Examination of the Spine and Extremities*. Upper Saddle River, NJ: Prentice Hall.

Jennett, S. (2008) *Churchill Livingstone's Dictionary of Sport and Exercise Science and Medicine*. Edinburgh: Elsevier.

Jurch, S.E. (2009) *Clinical Massage Therapy. Assessment and Treatment of Orthopedic Conditions*. Boston, MA: McGraw-Hill.

Petty, N. (2011) *Neuromusculoskeletal Examination and Assessment. A Handbook for Therapists* (4th edition). Edinburgh: Elsevier.

Prentice, W.E. (2011) *Principles of Athletic Training: A Complimentary-Based Approach* (14th edition). New York: McGraw-Hill.

Rentsch, O. (1987) *The Bowen Technique. An Interpretation by Oswald Rentsch*. Byaduk: Bowtech.

Rentsch, O. and Rentsch, E. (2005) *Bowtech the Original Bowen Technique. The Bowen Technique Training and Instruction Manual*, 3 vols. Hamilton: Bowen Therapy Academy of Australia.

Schultz, S.J., Houglum, P.A. and Perrin, D.H. (2000) *Assessment of Athletic Injuries*. Champaign, IL: Human Kinetics.

15
Dance, Stretching and Hypermobility

Evidence suggests that dancers suffer a very high rate of injury. Wyon (cited in Wise 2008) reports that 'Dancers have a huge injury occurrence: 80 per cent of dancers incur at least one injury a year that affects their ability to perform.' The incidence of injury in dance is substantially higher than the 20 per cent injury rates sustained by football and rugby players. Typical injury sites for all dancers are:

- lower back 31 per cent
- ankles 24 per cent
- knees 23 per cent
- feet 16 per cent
- lower legs 15 per cent
- groin 14 per cent
- neck 14 per cent
- thighs 14 per cent
- shoulders 12 per cent
- hip 10 per cent.

The perceived causes of injury are:

- overwork
- recurrence of old injury
- fatigue
- repetitive movements
- ignoring early warning signs
- incorrect technique

- insufficient warm-up
- new/difficult choreography
- unsuitable floor
- cold environment
- costume/shoes
- partnering work
- rehearsal schedule
- different repertory
- inadequate diet
- set/props.

(Laws 2005, p.19)

Lateral Rotation of the Hips

Most dance injuries affect the lower back and lower limbs, as reflected in the case studies later in the chapter. These types of injuries often relate to faulty technique, especially in the case of classical ballet dancers who have to dance with their legs in lateral rotation, known within the dance world as 'turnout'. If they do not possess sufficient lateral rotation from the hips, which is dependent upon the shape of the hip socket, and the angle at which the femur is positioned within the acetabulum, they are apt to what is known as 'screwing' their 'turnout' (lateral rotation) from the knees and ankles. If dancers do consistently 'screw' their turnout this can lead to knee and foot/ankle injuries (Clippinger 2007; Khan *et al.* 1995). Most 'serious' or professional dancers require an ideal (but extremely rare!) 180 (certainly over 140) degrees of turnout from the hip, determined from birth and dependent on the angle of the femur and depth of the hip socket. By about age 11, the angle of the femur (however rotated or otherwise) is more or less determined, and those with a more limited range of lateral rotation are unlikely to be selected for serious ballet training or are likely to find classical ballet much more difficult owing to a limiting range of movement from the hip. Of course, as well as the bony articulation of the femur in the acetabulum, the dancer must also use the deep gluteal and hip muscles required to sustain and safely hold the leg at the desired angle of lateral rotation (Clippinger 2007; Daniels 2007).

Daniels writes that:

Turnout involves external rotation of the femur along its long axis in relation to a stable pelvis. In an extended position of the hip with a stable pelvis, external rotation will bring the greater trochanters of the femur closer to the pelvic ischial tuberosities (sit bones). While many muscle groups contribute to hip external rotation, the six deep external rotator muscles (piriformis, gemellus superior and inferior, obturator internus and externus and quadratus femoris) are particularly effective because they lack undesired secondary actions. (2007, p.91)

If these muscles are not correctly engaged it can lead to lower limb injuries (knee/ ankle/foot) (Khan *et al.* 2007).

Types of Injuries

The types of injuries most commonly sustained by dancers might typically include lateral ankle sprains, medial sprains if the dancer lands from a jump with a pronated foot, stress fractures, patellafemoral joint syndrome, iliotibial band friction, back pain (from lordosis or lack of deep core muscles or insufficient use of deep gluteals) and problems with the feet such as bunions, bony spurs and, again, stress fractures (Daniels 2007; Khan *et al.* 2007; Laws 2005). Kennedy *et al.* (2007, p.163) suggest that:

> It is estimated that up to 95% of dancers employed for more than one year will suffer a significant injury. Most of these physical injuries occur to the foot and ankle in female ballet dancers. Many of these injuries are as a result of dancing on the point of the toe.

Although a dancer might sustain a sudden and acute traumatic injury such as tearing an Achilles tendon, for example (Kennedy *et al.* 2007), more injuries appear to be slower and cumulative over time, mostly owing to overwork/rehearsal, fatigue and then poor teaching and technique (Khan *et al.* 2007; Laws 2005; Murgia 2013). Most vocational dance schools and dance companies will have immediate access to physiotherapy, or to the appropriate medical advisor, so it is highly unlikely that a Bowen practitioner will encounter an acute injury; instead they might see dancers who have had the same types of injuries for a long period of time, in other words, injuries that are chronic or older than three months and have not resolved through physiotherapy or other 'more commonly known' treatment modalities.

Dance Treatment and Psychology

In the UK there are now two major specialist dance injury clinics in London and Birmingham (see Dance UK, www.danceuk.org), but dancers do not, in general, have anywhere near the same level of help and support as athletes (Murgia 2013). Additionally, the psychological impact of injury in dancers is often woefully ignored and the stigma attached to injury means that many dancers do not report slow, insidious injuries early on, when early intervention would be advantageous, possibly for fear of losing their role in a performance (Caldwell 2001; Laws 2005; Murgia 2013). Since it appears that Bowen work might address psychological (e.g. anxiety/

stress) issues, as well as physical bodily trauma (Wilks 2007) it makes it an ideal adjunct therapy in addition to what is already offered (i.e. mainly physiotherapy, Pilates or body conditioning work) (Sabo 2013). Although diagnosis is essential, particularly in cases where surgical intervention is required, or for problems such as stress fractures, with this in mind Bowen practitioners can offer invaluable holistic input, including, where appropriate, nutritional advice, particularly as dancers can often present with disordered eating, potentially leading to malnutrition (Laws 2005).

Dancers love to stretch, and although flexibility is highly desirable, especially in classical and contemporary dance, ways of achieving this are not always understood, as Joanne Avison explains.

Stretching Our Ideas About Stretching

&ꝰ Joanne Avison

Recently there has been a great deal of research about stretching, which questions the value of exercise modalities such as yoga and dance and warm-up styles for a range of movement programmes in sport and athletics. It seems that there is stretching and there is stretching. Pulling on the tissues, or actively loading them, or doing what an animal does when it yawns and stretches after rest (Figure 15.1), all appear to have different effects on the tissues of the body.

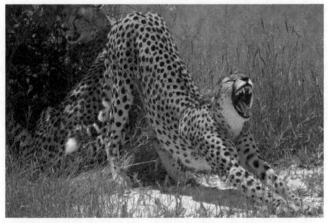

Figure 15.1 Stretching is something animals do instinctively; however, they do it after rest, rather than in preparation for action. Can they teach us something about the fascia?
Source: image taken in the wild and reproduced from McDermott n.d. with kind permission from Shane McDermott ©

Yawning Stretches

Bertolucci has asked if yawning stretches are 'Nature's way of maintaining the functional integrity of the myofascial system'. Bertolucci's research suggests that this kind of stretching, called pandiculation, might be 'to maintain the animal's ability to express coordinated and integrated movement by regularly restoring and resetting the structural and functional equilibrium of the myofascial system' (Bertolucci 2011).

Interesting research in British Columbia revealed that hibernating bears in fact have what we might call a 'daily yawning stretch routine'. A team on Grouse Mountain in Vancouver built a reserve for two orphaned grizzly bears and placed a camera in their hibernation lair. Daily, at around midday, they wake up and do 10 to 20 minutes of padding around, stretching and yawning as if to reset their systems before returning to sleep.

Passive or Active Stretching?

Stretching after sleep or rest is not news, in the sense that we see our domestic cats and dogs do 'Face Up Dog' pose and 'Face Down Dog' pose beautifully, like expert yogis, whenever they uncurl from their favourite chair. However, these are yawning stretches and they have a particular quality. The movements are more like 'lengthening contractions' in that there is an element of both stretching and contracting (or squeezing) as the long myofascial chains are engaged. As shown in Figure 15.2, the whole body participates. Such yawning stretches might be a valuable asset to anyone spending hours sitting in cars or at desks, travelling and working for long periods of relative immobility. A yawning stretch might also reintegrate our fascial tissues; it certainly feels better.

While these movements are recapitulated in yoga and warm-up exercises, they are not necessarily done in this way. Actively loaded stretches have quite distinct effects through the myofascial tissues (Müller and Schleip 2011).

In an 'actively loaded stretch' the muscle is both active and also loaded at the long end of its range; it includes long myofascial chains. Most of the fascial components are being stretched and stimulated in that loading pattern (after Müller and Schleip 2011).

Often, stretching exercises focus more on length for the sake of it (see Classic Stretching (C) in Figure 15.2), using more passive styles of stretching. Research (Nelson 2005) suggests that passive muscle stretching can be detrimental immediately before sprint performance, for example. There is practical evidence (Kelsick, personal correspondence, 2013) to suggest that modern elite athletes benefit from preparation for sprinting with small, spring-loaded jumps to 'elasticate' the tissues ready for a race, as if to 'wind them up' in order to deploy their elastic recoil capacity. Rather than passive stretching, performance shows marked improvement at that stage in the athlete's programme, if the body is warmed up with small, spring-like bounces off the ground.

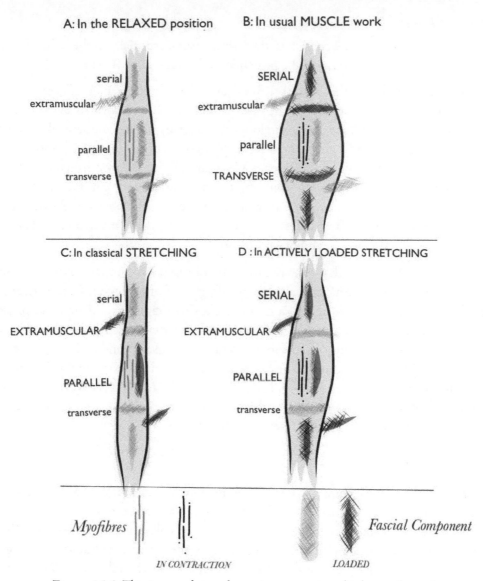

Figure 15.2 This image shows the various ways in which muscle and fascial components are activated by different types of use
Source: reproduced with kind permission from Art of Contemporary Yoga Ltd (image modified after Robert Schleip)

Kangaroos 'warm up' to their long bounds by leaping in smaller ones. It would be unusual to find footage of an animal stretching its tissues before peak performance, such as hunting. If anything, they appear to tighten their form, globally tensioning the body to adopt a stalking stance and raising their fur to animate their 'intention' by literally putting the tissues 'in tension'.

Fascial Recoil

This all makes sense in the context of the fascial tissues, especially in the light of their innate architecture based upon the principles of biotensegrity (Levin 2013).

> it has been shown that fascial stiffness and elasticity play a significant role in many ballistic movements of the human body... First discovered by studies of the calf tissues of kangaroos, antelopes and later by horses, modern ultrasound studies have revealed that fascial recoil plays in fact a similarly impressive role in many of our human movements. How far you can throw a stone, how high you can jump, how long you can run, depends not only the contraction of your muscle fibres; it also depends to a large degree on how well the elastic recoil properties of your fascial network are supporting these movements. (Robert Schleip, cited in Stecco and Stecco 2009)

Fascial stiffness is a term that gives rise to some confusion, given that 'stiffness' carries connotations in bodywork and movement of discomfort and pain. It is, at least in general language, something that a client or class participant wants to avoid or get rid of. Indeed, it may be part of the description for the ailment that led them to seek treatment. The feeling of stiffness is in fact more usually indicative of *shortness* (Richards 2012). In terms of stiffness, fascial elasticity relies upon the elastic storage capacity of the fascia. That is not just a property of the material, it is also innate to its biotensegrity architecture. This is the foundation of our elasticity. It is a balance essentially described between stiffness and stretchiness.

The Fabric

The fibre of the fascial connective tissues in the body are made up of collagen, elastin and reticulin (which is immature collagen). There is a common misconception that the elastin fibre makes the tissue elasticated and the collagen fibre stiffens it. (Thus the notion that if these elements are in balance, then we have sufficient 'spring'.) However, the elasticity of the fascial matrix relies upon the relative *stiffness* of the collagen. Elastin is a component of the suite of tissues used by the body in wound healing (Zorn 2012). In order to see why suitable stiffness is so important, the engineering terms for elasticity can be explored briefly.

Elasticity is the measure of deformation and reformation in a material. It goes together with stiffness like the back and front of your hand. They are relative terms that can be applied to any material.

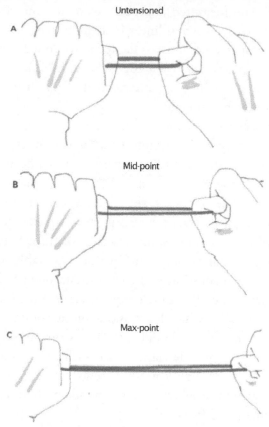

Figure 15.3 This image shows the band at rest, at the
mid-point of stretch and fully stretched
Source: reproduced with kind permission from Art of Contemporary Yoga Ltd

The action (in Figure 15.3) demonstrates the material's *resistance to deformation* (i.e. its stiffness). We can sense it *stiffening* as it becomes more resistant. When the last position is released, the band's ability to restore to the first position, after deformation, is a measure of its capacity to return (elasticity). All materials can be measured for their elastic capacity.

Thus, if you pull on an elastic band, you are measuring its stiffness – that is, its *resistance to deformation.* As you release it, the speed of its elastic return (*its capacity for reformation*) is the elasticity. If it doesn't reform (i.e. goes beyond its elastic limit), it enters a stage of plasticity. This means it deforms, but doesn't reform; in other words, the 'spring back' doesn't happen. A metal slinky toy has low stiffness and elasticity, whereas a car spring has very high stiffness and elasticity. It offers support as well as strength and resilience. It has to be regulated, however, and the actual material cannot be too brittle (or it will break) or too soft (or it will bend and be unsupportive). On this basis, steel has higher elastic storage capacity than rubber. 'The collagen fibril is stronger in tensile strength than steel wire – it requires a load ten thousand times its own weight to stretch it (Vezar)' (Juhan 1987).

Many materials are measured for their elasticity on stress–strain graphs. However, the human body is a non-linear biologic system, so our tissues, besides having visco-elastic properties that act as dampers (to slow down the rate of elastic return), exhibit a J-shaped stress–strain curve (Levin 1980). It never reaches zero, because we never reach the point of an untensioned band. The shape reflects the way the body moderates stretch gradually.

When you zip up a neoprene wetsuit, so that it is stretched, it stays semi-tensioned or semi-stiffened, wrapping snugly around you. Your limbs act as the compression struts. When you take the suit off, it lies untensioned in a heap of fabric. We don't 'untension' or deflate in that way. We remain an open, animated form, as a tension-compression structure. The bones are the 'floating compression' (Snelson 1989) elements that it is thought may act as struts in the tensional 'guy wires' and fabric of the various fascial forms (tendons, myofascia, aponeurotic sheets and so on). If they were very *elasticated*, they would not function as suitably organized structures for their role of force transmission and support. Although it is not an enclosed tensegrity architecture as such (because it requires an external frame for support), it helps to imagine a trampoline which is a tension-compression structure. If the fabric isn't strong enough or appropriately tightened to its surrounding frame with steel springs, then it would not provide elastic recoil such as it is designed for. It must have appropriate stiffness. Elasticity means 'energy storage capacity', so this is an innate feature of our structure, allowing us to bound and bounce, if it is sufficiently tensioned, or has 'suitable stiffness'.

On this basis, there are questions to be asked about the value of stretching as if stretching is the common denominator of useful exercises (i.e. we should all do it). In fact, if someone is hypermobile and their tissues already exhibit high flexibility, they may benefit from the stiffening of their tissues. In their case, resistance exercise may prove more beneficial to the fostering of a spring in the step than stretching. A very strong body builder, however, erring towards a description such as 'muscle bound', may find stretching and animating the glide between the tissue layers highly beneficial.

If we go back to the elastic band (Figure 15.3) measuring stiffness and elasticity, we rest in the semi-tensioned state, the mid-point. The lungs 'rest' there, semi-tensioned and half-filled. It is the basis of our architecture; we can expand globally (stretch) by inhaling and contract globally (squeeze) by exhaling – think of a puffer fish!

ELASTIC BREATH CYCLE

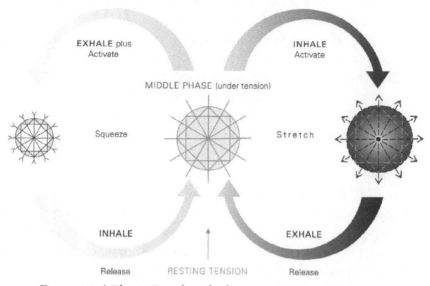

Figure 15.4 Elastic Breath cycle shows our Resting Tension, or semi-stiffened state when the body is relaxed between the inhale and exhale
Source: reproduced with kind permission from Art of Contemporary Yoga Ltd

Elastic Integrity (soft graph)

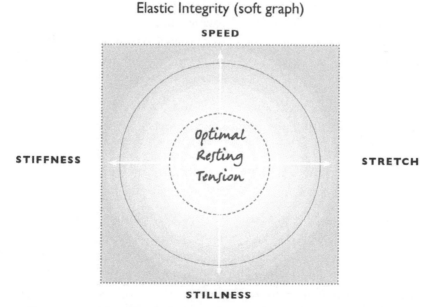

Figure 15.5 We seek a balance, in terms of yoga practice and types of practices (relative to Fascial Body Types) between these possibilities
Source: reproduced with kind permission from Art of Contemporary Yoga Ltd

This is the basis of our elasticity: the body's ability to rest in suitable *tensional integrity* so it doesn't collapse or over-stiffen. It is also the most economical basis of energy storage in motion. Elastically tuned movements are metabolically less expensive to the body in terms of effort. To preserve that elastic 'mid-point', the stiffer structure may indeed benefit from stretching, but the stretchy one might benefit from stiffening to find the balance nature tends to prefer.

In both cases, the common denominator is in fact the preservation and promotion of elasticity as energy storage capacity. The body, then, benefits from a balance between appropriate stretch and appropriate stiffness. In the movement field, these can be expressed on a graph, albeit a 'soft' one (Figure 15.5). In terms of yoga, for example, the X-axis can represent a range from stiffness to stretch. It is beyond the scope of this chapter, but a summary of a particular aspect of yoga can be proposed as the Y-axis. For the purpose of illumination, these can be summarized as a balance between speed and stillness. (In yoga practice, this would encompass the faster, flowing practices to the stillness of meditation.) This soft graph becomes a very useful metaphor for the practice of a technique such as Bowen – that is, if scale and time frames can be suitably adjusted.

Bowen Technique and Stretching

The above description is used in a very general sense in a movement assessment context, to encourage an individual to find overall balance in the type of practice most appropriate to bring them towards balance. In Bowen, a single move or series of moves offers all of these possibilities in a very immediate time frame. It is a different scale, but nonetheless in a single Bowen move there is a remarkable combination of these assets:

1. A 'squeeze–stretch' technique on the body, where it could be said a single intervention incorporates both these aspects in very rapid succession or simultaneously.

2. A 'speed–stillness' balance between the rate of the move, relative to the time the tissue is left to rest and assimilate immediately afterwards.

The idea that all four of these aspects are deployed within a Bowen session, albeit on a very subtle level, would in fact bring it in line with yoga in many ways. The localized intervention may 'reboot' the tissue and allow it to find its own ability to reset or find suitable balance regionally. It points to the benefit of both the subtlety of approach and the invitation to self-regulation in the body, within the smaller time frame of the Bowen session. In a movement class, or series of classes, the participant is invited to work with their whole body. Is it possible that the Bowen Technique assists the proprioceptive enquiry, with small reminders that invite the tissues to join the dots?

In Summary

In a movement context, then, we could say that stretching is useful and welcome under certain circumstances. However, we might suggest in the context of fascial matrix that it is one of at least four different aspects of understanding the tissues that can be considered. Appreciating all these aspects may bring balance on the larger scale (of a movement practice) to the smaller time frame of a manual session, particularly in a therapy such as Bowen. Both may contribute to a sense of balance and comfort in the body and the individual ability to self-regulate, moment to moment and movement to movement.

Yawning stretches (as a natural way of pressing the 'reboot' button) may have quite distinct values to the tissues, after a period of rest, for everyone. However, stretching for the sake of stretching might depend more on the individual and which particular type of stretching is being undertaken and for what particular pupose.

ex/

What Is Joint Hypermobility?

Hypermobility is very common within the dance and performing arts population, and from a performance point of view is highly desirable, providing that it is asymptomatic (Knight 2011). A hypermobile joint is one with a greater than average range of movement (ROM) and a joint that is passively hyper-extended in excess of 10 degrees when measured by eye or more accurately with a goniometer, as shown in Figure 15.6 (Knight, McCormack and Bird 2012).

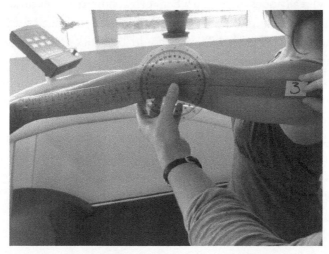

Figure 15.6 A hypermobile elbow joint being measured with a goniometer

Grahame describes hypermobility as 'the result of ligamentous laxity, which is inherent in a person's make-up and determined by their fibrous protein genes' (Grahame 2003, p.2). Hypermobility is a heritable condition, which is predominant in females (Raff and Byers 1996; Simpson 2006) and more common within African and Asian populations than the Caucasian population (Grahame 2003; Russek 1999; Simpson 2006). Hypermobility is also prevalent within the dance sector, up to 70 per cent, particularly within the ballet and contemporary dance community, compared with 10–30 per cent within the non-dance population (Desfor 2003; McCormack *et al.* 2004; Ruemper and Watkins 2012).

Hypermobility could be described as a useful asset to dancers and performing artists because it often means that a person has improved flexibility and can achieve varied and interesting body postures (Simmonds and Keer 2007). Indeed, one of the key components of dance is flexibility and the ability to produce aesthetically pleasing postures, often at the end range of normal joint movement (Clippinger 2007; Deighan 2005; Desfor 2003; Liederbach 2000). Joint hypermobility has been documented as advantageous during the selection process for a career in dance (Desfor 2003; Grahame and Jenkins 1972; McCormack *et al.* 2004), with some dancers acquiring hypermobility by virtue of their training in order to produce the beautiful extensions that many choreographers require (Bird 2007; Klemp, Stevens and Isaacs 1984; Knight 2011; Knight, McCormack and Bird 2012).

Measuring and Assessing Dancers

One problem in assessing dancers for hypermobility is in determining how much of their hypermobility is acquired through training (Bird 2007; Desfor 2003; Keer and Simmonds 2007; Klemp, Stevens and Isaacs 1984). Ruemper and Watkins (2012) suggest that it is still not clear whether the forward flexion test from the Beighton Score (see below) really does distinguish between acquired and natural hypermobility. Dancers who are warmed up before the test might easily manage the forward flexion assessment (shown in Figure 15.7), but would be unlikely to manage a modified (more challenging) forward flexion (Figure 15.8) by virtue of hypermobility acquired through training (Bird 2007; Desfor 2003; Keer and Simmonds 2007; Klemp, Stevens and Isaacs 1984). Bird suggests that 'acquired hypermobility' when measuring elite gymnasts shows an appreciable loss within 15–20 minutes at the end of training when the body is cool again (Bird, Walker and Newton 1988). Bird and colleagues are therefore perhaps suggesting that the acquired hypermobility is temporary, and that true hypermobile dancers can therefore manage the modified forward flexion test at any time (Bird, Walker and Newton 1988; Ruemper and Watkins 2012).

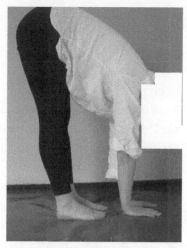

Figure 15.7 Dancer in forward flexion
Source: Knight 2011

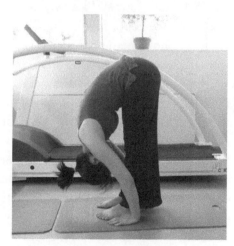

Figure 15.8 Dancer in modified forward flexion

What Is the Difference between General Joint Hypermobility (GJH) and Ehlers-Danlos Syndrome (Hypermobility-Type) (EDS-HT)?

General joint hypermobility (GJH) is hypermobility that is asymptomatic and not causing pain (Grahame and Hakim 2008; Simpson 2006). Research has shown that dancers with GJH could have a successful career with no increased risk of injury compared to the non-hypermobile dancer (Desfor 2003; Grahame and Jenkins 1971; Ruemper and Watkins 2012). Some dancers, however, have a heritable connective tissue disorder that naturally gives them extensions, but there might be a price to pay for their disordered joint laxity (Grahame 2003, p.2; Liederbach 2000; Ruemper and Watkins 2012). The price of disordered joint laxity is joint hypermobility syndrome, which has now become known as Ehlers-Danlos Syndrome (Hypermobility-Type) (EDS-HT). It is the symptomatic (e.g. pain) element that distinguishes dancers who have EDS-HT from GJH (Desfor 2003, Grahame and Jenkins 1971; Ruemper and Watkins 2012).

Ehlers-Danlos Syndome (Hypermobility-Type) is a heritable, genetic connective tissue disorder systemically affecting collagen fibres and fibrous protein genes (Grahame 2003, p.2; Russek 1999). The term 'hypermobility syndrome' was first developed by Kirk, Ansell and Bywaters in 1967, in response to what Grahame describes as the occurrence of musculoskeletal symptoms in otherwise healthy individuals (Grahame 2003, p.4). Research has shown that it is often easy for medical professionals to misdiagnose HMS/EDS-HT, and patient's symptoms are often dismissed, with only 1 in 20 correctly diagnosed, on the sole basis of how the patient looks – for example, healthy and well, and apparently without obvious illness (Grahame 2009, p.4). Amending the term HMS to Ehlers-Danlos Syndrome, a group of several different types of connective tissue disorders, was only recently done, and so HMS is now formally known as Ehlers-Danlos Syndrome (Hypermobility-Type) (Castori et al. 2012; Hakim in Knight 2015).

The overriding complaint that is made by these healthy individuals is pain, resulting from ligamentous laxity at the joints that are often working within an extra range of movement and thus placing an additional strain on the surrounding soft-tissue (Grahame 2003; Keer 2003). There are rarely signs of inflammation, but hypermobile dancers often suffer from soft-tissue conditions such as tendonitis, bursitis and overuse (Simpson 2006). Dancers, despite their increased range of movement, also report feeling stiff and experience clicking and popping sensations in their joints. They are also prone to subluxations and dislocations (Simmonds and Keer 2007) which can make them feel vulnerable. Partly, perhaps, because of their continued experience of extra movement and regularly being in pain, people with EDS-HT are more likely to experience fatigue and flu-like symptoms (Keer and Simmonds 2007). Furthermore, because their symptoms are often dismissed, EDS-HT dancers (and patients) do not always receive adequate support from the medical profession, which can lead to feelings of anger and mistrust (Grahame 2009; Harding 2003; Knight 2013; Simmonds 2003).

Continual movement into an extra range of joint movement and joint instability, owing to collagen laxity, can make patients with EDS-HT more prone to injury (Keer 2003; Knight 2011; Ruemper and Watkins 2012). One possible theory for an increased risk of injury is because patients with EDS-HT have a poor sense of joint proprioception (Knight et al. 2012). Proprioception is determined by the spatial awareness of one's joints. In patients (and dancers) with EDS-HT, their joint proprioception, particularly at the end range of movement into their hyperextension, can be impaired (Ferrell 2009; Hall et al. 1995).

A poor sense of proprioception could perhaps explain why dancers with EDS-HT become injured, because of the lack of sensation in the joint at end of range (Batson 1992; McCormack *et al.* 2004). Furthermore, dancers and others with EDS-HT often have poor muscular tone and joint stability, increasing further the likelihood of injury (Keer 2003; Ruemper and Watkins 2012). Keer also suggests that because females have less muscle bulk and manage an increased ROM, it might explain why they suffer greater instability than males (Keer 2003). Additionally, there are further implications for women, in that symptoms can increase prior to menstruation, caused by an increase in the hormone progesterone, which further relaxes collagen (Bird 2004). In female adolescents, both growth spurts and the onset of menstruation can make symptoms (e.g. pain and joint instability) worse, and therefore increase the overall risk of injury (Bird 2004; McCormack *et al.* 2004). Research has confirmed that once a dancer with EDS-HT or 'Hypermobility Syndrome' becomes injured, the chances of further injury are very likely (McCormack *et al.* 2004; Ruemper and Watkins 2012).

How Do You Assess Hypermobility?

The Beighton Score

Historically, the diagnosis of hypermobility has not been without controversy, and it remains a topic of contentious debate amongst clinicians. Hypermobility was originally diagnosed using the Carter Wilkinson Scale (Carter and Wilkinson 1964; Russek 1999) which included some of the movements described in Figure 15.9. However, the assessment of forward flexion was absent, and instead excessive dorsiflexion and eversion of the foot was present (Carter and Wilkinson 1964; Russek 1999). The Beighton Score superseded the Carter Wilkinson Scale, and is still considered the bench-mark in the measure of hypermobility (Carter and Wilkinson 1964; Russek 1999). The Beighton Score is a simple, nine-point clinical method of assessing hypermobility in some joints (Grahame 2003; Russek 1999; Simpson 2006). A positive score for each joint indicates hypermobility (see Figure 15.9).

One of the problems with the Beighton Score is that it does not assess the foot and ankle joint. This is a disadvantage when working with dancers because ankle stability would be considered an important component in injury prevention (Deighan 2005; Liederbach 2000; McCormack *et al.* 2004; Ruemper and Watkins 2012). Another problem with the Beighton Score is that it looks at a small range of joints only, and it cannot quantify hypermobility and joint laxity, neither does it look at other major joints such as the hips and shoulders, which would certainly be useful in working with dancers (Bird 2007). Research has also shown that the number of joints affected does not necessarily correlate with the amount of symptoms experienced in the affected individual (Grahame 2007, 2009; Russek 1999). There is therefore a need for a further measure in extinguishing GJH (asymptomatic hypermobility, which is desirable in some dance styles) from assessing the symptomatic condition EDS-HT, which is the underlying reason for the Brighton Criteria (Grahame 2003).

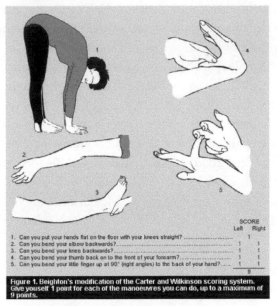

Figure 1. Beighton's modification of the Carter and Wilkinson scoring system. Give youself 1 point for each of the manoeuvres you can do, up to a maximum of 9 points.

Figure 15.9 The Beighton Score

Source: reproduced with kind permission from the Hypermobility Syndromes Association

The Brighton Criteria

It is the Brighton Criteria (see Box 15.1) that provide the important distinction in separating hypermobile dancers from those who have Hypermobility Syndrome (HMS) or EDS-HT (Simpson 2006). One of the problems with EDS-HT is that it is difficult to diagnose because patients with EDS-HT frequently appear healthy (Grahame 2009). However, the Brighton Criteria are crucial to the diagnosis of EDS-HT because it is a multi-systemic condition (Grahame 2009) and so there are questions in the Brighton Criteria relating to joints, skin and blood vessels, as all these can be affected in patients with EDS-HT and are ultimately related to faulty collagen fibre structures, systemically (Russek 1999; Simpson 2006). In addition to widespread pain, there are a range of conditions that are linked to EDS-HT because of the known tissue laxity and resultant faulty collagen fibres. Some examples are asthma (Bird 2007; Simmonds 2003), varicose veins (Russek 1999), rectal or uterine prolapse (Simpson 2006), digestive problems and autonomic dysfunction – symptoms of dizziness, palpitations and light-headedness (Grahame 2003). Furthermore, there is an overlap in diagnosis between EDS-HT and two other connective tissue disorders: Marfan and other types of Ehlers-Danlos syndromes (EDS), particularly in relation to assessment of stretchy and thin skin with EDS and overly long fingers and thumbs in Marfan syndrome (Bird 2007; Grahame 2007; Raff and Byers 1996; Russek 1999; Simpson 2006).

Box 15.1 Brighton Criteria: Revised Diagnostic Criteria for Hypermobility Syndromes

Major Criteria

- A Beighton score of 4/9 or greater (either currently or historically).

- Arthralgia for longer than 3 months in 4 or more joints.

Minor Criteria

- A Beighton score of 1, 2 or 3/9 (0, 1, 2 or 3 if aged 50+).

- Arthralgia (> 3 months) in one to three joints or back pain (> 3 months), spondylosis, spondylolysis/spondylolisthesis.

- Dislocation/subluxation in more than one joint, or in one joint on more than one occasion.

- Soft-tissue rheumatism. > 3 lesions (e.g. epicondylitis, tenosynovitis, bursitis).

- Marfanoid habitus (tall, slim, span/height ratio >1.03, upper: lower segment ratio less than 0.89, arachnodactily [positive Steinberg/wrist signs]).

- Abnormal skin: striae, hyperextensibility, thin skin, papyraceous scarring.

- Eye signs: drooping eyelids or myopia or antimongoloid slant.

- Varicose veins or hernia or uterine/rectal prolapse.

HMS is diagnosed in the presence two major criteria, or one major and two minor criteria, or four minor criteria. Two minor criteria will suffice where there is an unequivocally affected first-degree relative.

Source: reproduced with kind permission from the Hypermobility Syndromes Association

A crucial aspect of the Brighton Criteria is that an element of joint pain or soft-tissue rheumatism forms part of both the major and minor criteria, so injury could therefore be a determining factor in fulfilling the criteria for many EDS-HT dancers (Keer 2003; Knight 2011; Ruemper and Watkins 2012; Sharp 2008). The evidence suggests that a major factor in predicting injury is in previous injury (Gamboa *et al.* 2008; Hiller *et al.* 2008; Wiesler *et al.* 1996). For instance, Hiller and colleagues conducted a study into predictors of lateral ankle sprain in adolescent dancers. The conclusion was that previous ankle sprain is a predictor of future ankle sprain (Hiller *et al.* 2008). Hiller and colleagues' study interestingly suggests that further research is needed to explain why some people re-sprain ankles whilst others recover completely. In a similar manner, it is well known that once dancers (and patients) with EDS-HT become injured, they are highly likely to injure again (Deighan 2005; Liederbach 2000; McCormack *et al.* 2004, Ruemper and Watkins 2012); however, to date, no one has yet attempted to explain how and why some patients and dancers with generalized joint hypermobility (GJH) manage to avoid injury, and what tactics they might be using to avoid injury (Ruemper and Watkins 2012).

Characteristics of People with Hypermobility

It seems possible that people with hypermobility might exhibit certain characteristics. Physiotherapist Harding describes the patients she sees at the INPUT Pain Management Centre as having a quality of 'grace and drape' (Harding 2003, p.149), which she also observes in the family of the hypermobile patients, which would certainly relate to EDS-HT being a genetic condition (Raff and Byers 1996; Simpson 2006). Harding describes how the EDS-HT patients behave in stretch class. She writes that 'Most patients look rather unhappy with the stretches; however, those with joint hypermobility seem to love it and are practically purring afterwards!' (Harding 2003, p.155). The relief that Harding describes EDS-HT patients (and dancers, too) gaining from stretching might be linked to relief of feelings of muscle stiffness which is related to the condition (Keer 2003, p.79), and stretching might relieve growing pains in adolescents (Middleditch 2003). However, it might be that EDS-HT dancers enjoy stretch class simply because they are good at it!

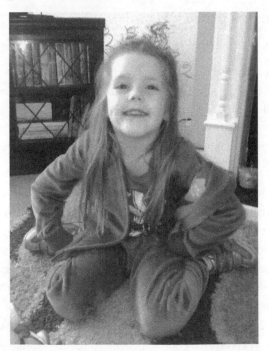

Figure 15.10 Hypermobile pose – sitting in the 'W' posture
Source: Knight 2011

Physiotherapists Keer and Simmonds report observing their patients behaving in a variety of ways (see Figure 15.10) including 'fidgeting' and describe them as 'slouching...adopting end range of postures, such as entwining their legs' (Simmonds and Keer 2007, p.302). Keer additionally describes hypermobile patients habitually standing on one leg (Keer 2003, p.79), and 'resting on the lateral border of their feet in standing or sitting, producing a sustained stretch to the lateral ankle' (Keer, Edwards-Fowler and Mansi 2003, p.96). These behaviours are also common in dancers (Knight 2011). Children who may have EDS can even be labelled as inattentive or hyperactive because of fidgeting in class (Middleditch 2003).

Characteristics of Dancers with Hypermobility

Anecdotal evidence suggests that it might also be possible to recognize hypermobile dancers by virtue of their behaviour. Batson, for example, writes how she observes dancers with hypermobile spines hanging in forward flexion (see Figure 15.11) and going into prolonged stretches (Batson 1992, p.42). A Laban classical ballet teacher with more than 30 years of experience, T. Kelsey, in an informal discussion about hypermobile dancers, made the following observations: 'that their sense of spatial awareness appears under-developed, that they have a tendency to lack proprioception, that they have difficulty in sensing their dynamic alignment and that their concentration can be inconsistent and their focus dispersed' (personal communication, 9 June 2009, in Knight 2011).

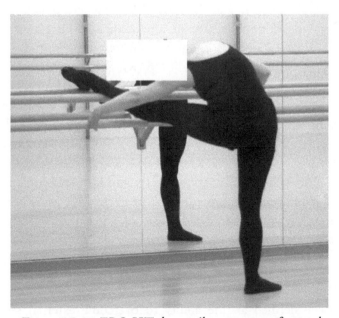

Figure 15.11 EDS-HT dancer 'hanging into forward flexion' and 'into her joints' at the barre
Source: Knight 2011

Rationale behind Physiological Behaviour Exhibited by EDS-HT Patients and Dancers

The characteristics of dancers and patients with GJH and EDS-HT could be related to their physiology. Keer writes that 'patterns of movements that patients adopt during assessment give clues to muscle imbalances' (2003, p.79). Part of the problem for both GJH and EDS-HT patients (and dancers) is that they appear to de-condition and lose muscle tone more quickly (Harding 2003; Simmonds 2003; Simmonds and Keer 2007) and often stop exercising either due to injury or because of resultant pain. It may be that patients (and dancers) with both GJH and EDS-HT de-condition and lose muscle tone quickly, partly because of time loss from injury (Knight *et al.* 2012) and because it is physiologically harder for them to strengthen their weaker collagenous tissues (Harding 2003, p.152). Research has also shown that muscle tissues had atrophied greatly in the first 5–7 days during inactivity, particularly the endurance slow-twitch muscle fibres (Keer 2003, Simmonds 2003). Additionally, and interestingly, muscles also atrophy in response to pain and fear, which might be a problem for some patients (and dancers) with hypermobility (Simmonds 2003). Simmonds observes that hypermobile people often display considerable joint instability, reduced muscle strength, endurance and poor proprioception and vulnerability to injury (Simmonds 2003, p.111).

Research has also shown that patients and dancers who are hypermobile do not tolerate overuse or repetition well, partly as a result of a lack of muscular endurance, which can lead to further injury (Knight *et al.* 2012; McCormack *et al.* 2004; Roussel *et al.* 2009; Ruemper and Watkins 2012). Hypermobile dancers might be less able to tolerate repetition because the muscles are working harder to control an extra range of movement, which might explain why their muscles fatigue sooner than in non-hypermobiles, and they feel tired (Knight *et al.* 2012).

Potential theories to explain patients' and hypermobile dancers' behaviour might be that their poor muscle tone makes it difficult for them to sustain postures. In particular patients with hypermobility seem to exhibit poor muscular endurance, which might explain their inability to sustain positions, hence the 'fidgeting' and potential relationship to attention deficit disorders (Middleditch 2003; Simmonds 2003). Nevertheless, it is crucial that both GJH and EDS-HT patients and dancers develop muscular endurance to provide support to their lax joints (Bird 2007; Keer *et al.* 2003) and to improve posture and therefore reduce injury (Knight *et al.* 2012; Maillard and Murray 2003; Phillips 2005; Simmonds 2003).

Dancers and Strength

Strength has been defined as 'the ability to overcome external resistance, or to counter external forces by using muscle' (Koutedakis, Owolabi and Apostolos 2008, p.87; Koutedakis *et al.* 2007; Phillips 1999). Research has shown that dancers have poorer and weaker strength compared with athletes (Wyon 2007). Research has also shown that lower levels of strength amongst dancers have been linked to increased injury rates (Koutedakis *et al.* 2008). Additionally, Koutedakis and colleagues write that 'poor posture increases the stress on supporting structures and therefore the risk of developing injury' (2008, p.86).

Research has shown that there is a correlation between injury and EDS-HT, and part of the outcome of the Brighton Criteria is dependent on joint arthralgia and soft-tissue rheumatism (Grahame 2003; Ruemper and Watkins 2012). Desfor recommended research into the relationship between strength and EDS-HT in terms of injury management, and to date no one has explored that link (Desfor 2003). Sharp worked with dance students in holding knee-strengthening classes for those with hypermobile knees, showing an improvement and fewer injuries if the hypermobility was better managed (Poggini, Lossasso and Iannone 1999; Ruemper and Watkins 2012; Sharp 2008).

Although being GJH might be highly desirable compared with symptomatic EDS-HT, where a dancer is to get to the top of their career ladder (principal dancer) (McCormack *et al.* 2004), the management in terms of the musculoskeletal system remains very similar for both groups, with strengthening work, physiotherapy exercises and Pilates work to strengthen the increased ROM, and perhaps the use of adjuncts such as kinesiotaping (Knight 2011; Knight *et al.* 2012; Sabo 2013). Bowen work can help with hypermobile people in terms of fascial re-patterning, and improving joint proprioception (Knight 2011, 2013), as well as encompassing the other holistic aspects of Bowen as a valid treatment modality of dancers. For more detail about hypermobility and dancers, readers might find Knight (2011) helpful and, for medical professionals, Knight (2013) for detailed information about working with people who have EDS-HT and other related complex and chronic conditions.

Bowen for Dancers and the Hypermobile

Given that Bowen is a 'holistic' therapy, it has been shown to provide a range of other health benefits, including better sleep quality, improved energy levels, a feeling of relaxation and other known benefits (Baker 2001; Wilks 2007). Additionally, Bowen work is very economic, with most patients requiring a few treatments only (Baker 2001; Wilks 2007). One reason for the beneficial effect of Bowen on people with hypermobility syndromes may be because the treatment simultaneously affects muscles, joints and fascia, as well as having a powerful effect on the autonomic nervous system. Because Bowen affects the connective tissue directly, it is important to understand the physiological changes involved in hypermobility so that treatment can be tailored specifically. This is primarily concerned with increasing tonus in the core muscles and contractile strength within the fascia, as well as initiating a lowering of sympathetic tone in the autonomic nervous system.

In hypermobility there are a number of observations that have been made concerning the effect of this condition on connective tissues, in particular the superficial and deep fascia. Soft-tissue techniques such as the Bowen Technique rely on effecting structural change by directly influencing the biotensegrity aspect of the fascia, which is why it can be so effective in the management of hypermobility. Gentle therapeutic approaches that directly affect the myofascial system would appear to be the most obvious choice. Some therapies such as Rolfing and myofascial release involve direct manipulation of fascia but many clients experience these techniques as too strong and painful due to their inherent tissue sensitivity.

As stated earlier, tissue laxity and fragility is determined by the action and composition of collagen fibres, particularly the ratio of type I to type III, as well as the density and action of myofibroblasts in the fascia. From the point of view of hypermobility, an increase in myofibroblast contractile quality would seem logically to be beneficial in encouraging joint and tissue stability, which is something that can be encouraged through Bowen work.

The Bowen Technique is not yet well known amongst the dance population, but it would be highly advantageous to consider Bowen alongside other rehabilitation models (e.g. physiotherapy), and the following case studies might show why. At this stage further research needs to be conducted within the dance population with case studies and larger studies to show how Bowen Technique might be an invaluable treatment modality when working with dancers who suffer both acute and accumulative injuries.

The following are a series of case studies involving the use of Bowen work to support the rehabilitation of dancers who dance in a variety of dance styles.

CASE STUDY

Jim (pseudonym) was a dancer in his early 50s who was an ex-professional ballet dancer. He had come for Bowen to help his back pain, but also for very tight hamstrings.

Although Jim had tried physiotherapy, osteopathy and chiropractic, he had also tried Bowen a long time ago and thought it was going to be 'the next new thing' for the future in terms of treatments. Bowen was yet unknown in the dance world and dancers are very traditional and rather limited in what they choose (if they do anything at all about their injuries).

Treatment

I gave Jim a minimal session including the lower body relaxation procedure and upper stoppers. He returned reporting an improvement to his lower back. During the second treatment I repeated the work from the first treatment and added in the pelvis and hamstring work. He returned the following week and said that his hamstrings felt looser and, as with all dancers, who love lots of external hip rotation as befits the dance style (known as turnout), felt this was also looser.

Conclusion

Although Jim still had some remaining problems with his hamstrings, he still strongly maintained that the Bowen was helpful to him and improved his back pain, and he still felt it would be the next 'new thing' in the future, when people got to find out more about it!

CASE STUDY

Amy (pseudonym) was a student contemporary dancer in her early 20s. She attended for Bowen for restricted lateral rotation of the hips and also for back pain. In addition, Amy was very hypermobile with a diagnosis of EDS-HT.

Treatment

Amy was given BRM 1 (lower body Relaxation Procedure), BRM 2 (1–4) and pelvic procedure. She then had to rush off for a ballet class and came back to tell me that she felt that her hips had felt much more 'open' and less restricted during the class. I asked her if her teacher had noticed, and she said that she hadn't, but that she felt it was great she had improved range of movement in lateral rotation and even better that she was able to sustain it.

Conclusion

Amy came for Bowen on an occasional basis and maintained that Bowen certainly helped maintain her turnout.

CASE STUDY

Ella (pseudonym), a recreational dancer, came for Bowen to help with poor hip alignment, leg-length differences and a tight inflamed Achilles tendon and a hamstring injury.

Treatment

The first treatment consisted of a whole body rebalance (full body relaxation procedures) and pelvis. Ella reported that she felt good after the session and that, although her Achilles tendons and hamstrings still felt tight, two days post-treatment during her class she felt that her turn out or lateral rotation really opened up. A follow-up treatment included hamstring, knee and ankle work, and Ella remained fine and able to continue dancing.

CASE STUDY

Karen (pseudonym) was an ex-professional contemporary dancer. She was incredibly hypermobile and was attending for back pain (she had disc calcification and slipped discs at L4/5) and shoulder pain. It was my professional opinion that some of her pain was related to her hypermobility and a lack of core stability. Karen said that she was now dancing much less and therefore had de-conditioned.

Treatment and Conclusion

Karen attended for many Bowen treatments over a long period of time and felt that Bowen really helped with her back pain. Her shoulders, however, remained more of a problem owing to her ligamentous laxity and instability. She realized that she would need to do the necessary strengthening work to support her vast range of movement in order to sustain the muscular tone needed to support her shoulders and hips. It has been said to me before that Bowen puts the body back together, but that physiotherapy keeps it there. I think this is an excellent description. Another dancer wrote:

> I feel that Bowen has given me more space around muscles and joints, has settled my body better, and given it some balance. It has opened up around my lungs and given them more space to expand after some of the tightness around my ribs has been relieved. There has been quite a significant reduction of pain in my knees and I hardly have stabbing pains at present. They are better placed and I have been able to address what I need to do keep my alignment. I feel calmer and my IBS and sleep have also improved after these sessions. All of it has encouraged me to move again, which is something I have felt quite reluctant to do for a while because of the pain. (A.B., from Isobel Knight's website, www. bowenworks.org)

CASE STUDY

One professional dancer and dance lecturer thought that the short breaks throughout Bowen sessions were so fascinating that she decided to employ these during her teaching. She writes:

> After my Bowen treatment I was relaxed beyond the level of relaxation you get simply from lying down, which often makes me feel sleepy and heavy, and I felt a softness and clarity not only in my thoughts but in my movement work that day. After the treatment it was very interesting to observe shifting landscape of symptoms and sensations that rippled through the week and they seemed to shift to, often and too distinctly to be simple coincidence. My back pain and general tightness is definitely less despite a heavier workload. I also felt that it had a profound effect on my teaching practice. By taking the idea of stepping out of

someone's territory, putting them at the centre of the situation and allowing them the space to connect with their intuitive understanding I had a great result with my students who became more centred, engaged and awake. The idea of providing someone with information and then leaving them alone can seem quite radical. In practice I found it liberating and effective and also a relief that with Bowen I might not need to continue with a high maintenance programmeme of repetitive and expensive expert manipulation treatments that my body can't integrate or maintain. (Dance Lecturer, from Isobel Knight's website, www.bowenworks.org)

CASE STUDY

Lily (pseudonym) was a semi-professional Latin/ballroom dancer who presented with hip and back pain and had been born with hip dysplasia. Lily had a number of hypermobile joints – notably in her knees and hips.

Treatment

Treatment involved work to support her back and hip pain – including the pelvic procedures, sacral and knee and ankle. Lily said that her pain had reduced and that her hips felt better. After a second treatment she said that she was now 'a lot better', that dancing had become a lot easier, and that it was easier to stand upright. She attended six Pilates sessions upon my recommendation and found that this supported the Bowen work in strengthening the vast range of movement related to her hypermobility. Over time, treatment also included work to support and open out her thoracic spine with some very specific procedures to help her contain and manage her 'frame' and keep her 'out of her hips' and lifted upwards – something very important for this dance style.

Conclusion

Lily continues to do very well with her dancing and Bowen supports her perhaps through re-addressing her fascia combined with the appropriate strengthening work to manage her hypermobility.

Lily says:

I have had several Bowen treatments and they have helped to get rid of my hip pain completely. I am hypermobile in my hips and due to incorrect Latin dance teaching technique, I suffered from severe hip pain and stiffness. I found after a few sessions of Bowen, I had a greater range of movement in my joints and muscles. I have stretched and lengthened my spine by two inches. I also have more freedom of movement in my arms and legs. Bowen has helped me to become a high level dancer with more flexibility and grace in my movements.

CASE STUDY

Alastair McLoughlin, Bowen practitioner, Skipton, North Yorkshire, England (www.mobiletherapyservice.com)

Jessica, 18 years old, writes:

After 12 years of travelling the length and breadth of the country attending freestyle dance competitions and festivals, it was heart-breaking to have to retire due to my ongoing hip problems that had developed over the last two years of my life as a dancer. The pain was becoming unbearable even after just small amounts of exercise. Physiotherapists were perplexed, and no amount of deep heat and painkillers would touch it. Eventually I was referred to a surgeon in the northwest of England where I underwent further physiotherapy and steroid injections to no avail. Finally, I was placed on the waiting list to have surgery to release my iliotibial band one side at a time.

By now I had missed several weeks of college as my muscles kept going into spasm which meant guaranteed trips to the hospital via ambulance where I was pumped full of painkillers and muscle relaxers until I was sick! Work was also becoming an issue: as a sales assistant I spent long periods of time on my feet which left me crippled with pain. I couldn't arrange to do anything with friends if it involved walking, and even my favourite high heel shoes had to be thrown in the back of the wardrobe!

I had surgery on my left hip in March 2013 which seemed successful. I then returned to the hospital to have physiotherapy in order to re-strengthen my muscles and ligaments. After just three sessions I was told that they could no longer help me as I needed to go to a gym to build up my core muscles. I was subsequently discharged from being under the care of my surgeon.

Depression eventually set in and I was extremely unhappy. My mum then told me about the Bowen Technique. I had no idea what Bowen involved, and if I'm honest I didn't believe it would do any good, but I was willing to try anything.

Bowen practitioner Alastair McLoughlin chatted with me about my past history and then carried out an assessment. At first it was painful to even have my hip area touched let alone anything else. After the first session I didn't feel all that different, but I did have fewer aches and pains. The following week Alastair returned and spent a full hour working on various areas. The main areas being my hips, back and neck. I had not felt that good in years!

By the fourth session I could stand on my tip toes, even on one leg, without falling and I could bring my knees up to my chest area, all of which I had not been able to do because of the restriction in movement and the severe pain. The treatment has given me a normal life again and I have since treated myself to a full day's shopping in Manchester city centre, been out for walks and also nights out. I walk to and from the bus stop every day and now only have the odd twinge.

Within the space of just one month my life has completely changed with very few painkillers and thankfully no trips to hospital. I now also have a full-time job alongside studying for my NVQ. I will now go on to practise yoga or Pilates to continue to strengthen my core muscles and hope to return to some form of dancing very soon.

Postscript by Alastair: On 4 January 2014 Jessica had her fifth appointment. During the intervening month between session four and five she hadn't taken any analgesia and is now fully mobile.

Conclusion

Dancers have a very high injury rate, approximately 80 per cent (Wyon, cited in Wise 2008) and are often slow to report injury for fear of losing their roles to others (Murgia 2013). It is well known that fatigue is a major reason for injury (Laws 2005; Murgia 2013, Sabo 2013), so Bowen might be excellent to help dancers to rest and to aid tissue healing, preferably in advance of injury. The case studies in this chapter help to show how Bowen has helped various dancers who have presented with different injuries, predominately back, pelvis, hamstring and lower limb injuries, as might be expected from the list of common injury sites (Laws 2005). It now remains for Bowen to be more widely introduced to the dance community, starting with presentations to local dance schools and more academically at conferences such as the International Association of Dance Medicine, so that both dancers and the medical profession at large can be made aware of Bowen work. It is hoped that this chapter provides a useful introduction, focusing on stretching (because flexibility is highly desirable for most dance forms) and hypermobility, owing to a high prevalence within the dance world (Bird 2007; Knight *et al.* 2012; Desfor 2003; Ruemper and Watkins 2012).

References

Baker, J. (2001) *The Bowen Technique.* Chichester: Corpus Publishing.

Batson, G. (1992) Spinal hypermobility in the dancer: implications for conditioning. *Journal of Kinesiology and Medicine for Dance* 14 (2), 39–57.

Bird, H. (2004) Rheumatological aspects of dance. *Rheumatology* 31 (1), 12–13.

Bird. H. (2007) Joint hypermobility. *Musculoskeletal Care* 5 (1), 4–19.

Bird, H., Walker, A. and Newton, J. (1988) A controlled study of joint laxity and injury in gymnasts. *Journal of Orthopaedic Rheumatology* 1, 139–145.

Bertolucci, L.F. (2011) Pandiculation: nature's way of maintaining the functional integrity of the myofascial system? *Journal of Bodywork and Movement Therapies* 15, 268–280.

Caldwell, C. (2001) *Dance and Dancers' Injuries.* Chichester: Corpus Publishing.

Carter, C. and Wilkinson, J. (1964) Persistent joint laxity and congenital dislocation of the hip. *Journal of Bone and Joint Surgery* 46 (1), 40–45.

Castori, M., Morlino, S., Celletti, C., Celli, M. *et al.* (2012) Management of pain and fatigue in the joint hypermobility syndrome (a.k.a. Ehlers-Danlos syndrome, hypermobility type): principles and proposals for a multidisciplinary approach. *American Journal of Genetics, Part A* (158A), 2055–2070.

Clippinger, K. (2007) *Dance Anatomy and Kinesiology*. Champaign, IL: Human Kinetics.

Daniels, K. (2007) Teaching sound turn-out. *Journal of Dance Education* 7 (3), 91–4.

Deighan, M. (2005) Flexibility in dance. *Journal of Dance, Science and Medicine* 9 (1), 13–17.

Desfor, F. (2003) Assessing hypermobility in dancers. *Journal of Dance Science and Medicine* 7 (1), 17–22.

Ferrell, W. (2009) The sixth sense and joint hypermobility syndrome. *Hypermobility Syndrome Association Newsletter*, Spring, 10.

Gamboa, J., Roberts, L., Maring, J. and Fregus, A. (2008) Injury patterns in elite preprofessional ballet dancers and the utility of screening programs to identify risk characteristics. *Journal* of *Orthopaedic Sports Physical Therapy* 38 (3), 126–136.

Grahame, R. (2007) The need to take a fresh look at criteria for hypermobility. *Journal of Rheumatology* 34 (4), 664–665.

Grahame, R. (2009) Hypermobility: an important but often neglected area within rheumatology. *Hypermobility Syndrome Association News*, Spring, 4–5.

Grahame, R. and Hakim, A. (2008) Hypermobility. *Current Opinion in Rheumatology* 20, 106–110.

Grahame, R. and Jenkins, J. (1972) Joint hypermobility – asset or liability. *Annals of the Rheumatic Diseases* 31, 109–111.

Grahame, R. (2003) Hypermobility and Hypermobility Syndrome. In R. Keer and G. Grahame (eds) *Hypermobility Syndrome – Recognition and Management for Physiotherapists*. Philadelphia, PA: Elsevier.

Hall, M., Ferrell, W., Sturrock, R., Hamblen, D. and Baxendale, R. (1995) 'The effect of the hypermobility syndrome on knee joint proprioception.' *Rheumatology* 34 (2), 121–125.

Harding, V. (2003) Joint Hypermobility and Chronic Pain: Possible Linking Mechanisms and Management Highlighted by a Cognitive-Behavioural Approach. In R. Keer and G. Grahame (eds) *Hypermobility Syndrome – Recognition and Management for Physiotherapists*. Philadelphia: Elsevier.

Hiller, C., Refshauge, K., Herbert, R. and Kilbreath, S. (2008) Intrinsic predictors of lateral ankle sprain in adolescent dancers. A prospective cohort study. *Clinical Journal of Sports Medicine* 18, 44–48.

Juhan, D. (1987) *Job's Body*. Barrytown, NY: Station Hill Press.

Keer, R. (2003) Physiotherapy Assessment of the Hypermobile Adult. In R. Keer and G. Grahame (eds) *Hypermobility Syndrome – Recognition and Management for Physiotherapists*. Philadelphia: Elsevier.

Keer, R., Edwards-Fowler, A. and Mansi, E. (2003) Management of the Hypermobile Adult. In R. Keer and G. Grahame (eds) *Hypermobility Syndrome – Recognition and Management for Physiotherapists*. Philadelphia: Elsevier.

Kennedy, J., Hodgkins, C., Colombier, J., Guyette, S. and Hamilton, W. (2007) Foot and ankle injuries in dancers. *International SportMed Journal* 8 (3), 141–165.

Khan, K., Brown, J., Way, S., Vass, N. *et al.* (2007) Overuse injuries in classical ballet. *Sports Medicine* 19 (5), 241–357.

Kirk, K., Ansell, B. and Bywaters, E. (1967) The hypermobility syndrome – musculoskeletal complaints associated with generalized joint hypermobility. *Annals of the Rheumatic Diseases* 26, 419–425.

Knight, I. (2011) *A Guide to Living with Joint Hypermobility Syndrome: Bending without Breaking*. London: Singing Dragon.

Knight, I. (2013) *A Multidisciplinary Approach to Managing Ehlers-Danlos (Type III) Hypermobility Syndrome, and Other Chronic Complex Conditions*. London: Singing Dragon.

Knight, I., McCormack, M. and Bird, H. (2012) *Managing Joint Hypermobility for Dance Teachers. Foundations for Excellence, Sheet 7*. London: South West Music Schools (Dance UK).

Koutedakis, Y., Owolabi, E. and Apostolos, M. (2008) Dance biomechanics – a tool for controlling health, fitness and training. *Journal of Dance Medicine and Science* 12 (3), 83–89.

Koutedakis, Y., Hukam, H., Metsios, G., Nevill, A. *et al.* (2007) The effects of three months of aerobic and strength training on selected performance and fitness-related parameters in modern dance students. *Journal of Strength and Conditioning Research* 21 (3), 808–812.

Laws, H. (2005) *Fit to Dance 2: Report of the Second National Inquiry into Dancers' Health and Injury in the UK*. London: Dance UK.

Levin, S. (1980) Continuous tension, discontinuous compression: a model for biomechanical support of the body. Address to the North American Academy of Manipulative Medicine.

Levin, S. (2013) Lecture at the University of Leuven, Belgium. Available at www.biotensegrity.com.

Liederbach, M. (2000) General considerations for guiding dance injury rehabilitation. *Journal of Dance Medicine and Science* 4 (2), 54–65.

Maillard, S. and Murray, K. (2003) Hypermobility Syndrome in Children. In R. Keer and R. Grahame (eds) *Hypermobility Syndrome: Recognition and Management for Physiotherapists*. Philadelphia, PA: Elsevier.

McCormack, M., Briggs, J., Hakim, A. and Grahame, R. (2004) Joint laxity and the benign joint hypermobility syndrome in student and professional ballet dancers. *Journal of Rheumatology* 31 (1), 173–178.

McDermott, S. (n.d.) *Wild Earth Illuminations*. Available at www.shanemcdermottphotography.com, accessed on 16 May 2014.

Middleditch, A. (2003) Management of the Hypermobile Adolescent. In R. Keer and G. Grahame (eds) *Hypermobility Syndrome – Recognition and Management for Physiotherapists*. Philadelphia: Elsevier.

Müller, D.G. and Schleip, R. (2011) Fascial fitness: fascia oriented training for bodywork and movement therapies. *Terra Rosa e-magazine* 7. Available at www.somatics.de/FascialFitnessTerraRosa.pdf, accessed on 16 May 2014.

Murgia, C. (2013) Overuse, fatigue and injury – neurological, psychological, physiological and clinical aspects. *Journal of Dance, Medicine and Science* 17 (2), 51–52.

Nelson, A.G., Driscoll, N.M., Landin, D.K., Young, M.A. and Schexnayder, I.C. (2005) Acute effects of passive muscle stretching on sprint performance. *Journal of Sports Sciences* 23 (5), 449–454.

Phillips, C. (2005) Stability in dance training. *Journal of Dance, Medicine and Science* 9 (1), 24–28.

Poggini, L., Losasso, S. and Iannone, S. (1999) Injuries during the dancer's growth spurt. *Journal of Dance Medicine and Science* 3 (2), 73–79.

Raff, M. and Byers, P. (1996) Joint hypermobility syndromes. *Current Opinion in Rheumatology* 8, 459–466.

Roussel, N., Nijs, J., Mottram, S., Van Moorsel, A., Truijen, S. and Stassijns, G. (2009) Altered lumopelvic movement control but not generalized joint hypermobility is associated with increased injury in dancers: a prospective study. *Journal of Manual Therapy* 14 (6), 630–635.

Ruemper, A. and Watkins, K. (2012) Correlations between general joint hypermobility and joint hypermobility syndrome and injury in contemporary dance students. *Journal of Dance, Medicine and Science* 16 (4), 161–166.

Russek, L. (1999) Hypermobility syndrome. *Physical Therapy* 79 (6), 591–599.

Sabo, M. (2013) Physical therapy rehabilitation of dancers – a qualitative study. *Journal of Dance, Medicine and Science* 17 (1), 11–17.

Sharp, E. (2008) The bee's knees. Does hypermobility of the knee predispose students of musical theatre to knee injuries? *Dance UK News* 68, 24–25.

Simmonds, J. (2003) Rehabilitation, Fitness, Sport and Performance for Individuals with Joint Hypermobility. In R. Keer and G. Grahame (eds) *Hypermobility Syndrome – Recognition and Management for Physiotherapists*. Philadelphia: Elsevier.

Simmonds, J. and Keer, R. (2007) Hypermobility and the hypermobility syndrome. *Manual Therapy* 12 (4), 298–309.

Simpson, M. (2006) Benign joint hypermobility syndrome: evaluation, diagnosis and management. *Journal of American Osteopathic Association* 106 (9), 531–536.

Snelson, K. (1989) Exhibition: The Nature of Structure. The New York Academy of Sciences, January–April. Available at www.kennethsnelson.net/articles/joelle_burrows_piece_intro.htm, accessed on 16 May 2014.

Stecco, L. and Stecco, C. (2009) *Fascial Manipulation – Practical Part*. Padova: Piccin Nuova Libraria.

Wiesler, E.R., Hunter, M., Martin, D.M., Curl, W.W. and Hoen, H. (1996) Ankle flexibility and injury patterns in dancers. *American Journal of Sports Medicine* 24 (6), 754–757.

Wilks, J. (2007) *The Bowen Technique*. Sherborne: CYMA.

Wipff, P.-J. *et al.* (2007) *Myofibroblast Contraction Activates Latent TGF-B1 from the Extracellular Matrix*. Laboratory of Cell Biophysics, Ecole Polytechnique Fédérale de Lausanne, CH-1015 Lausanne, Switzerland.

Wise, J. (2008) Project seeks to improve dancers' health. *British Medical Journal* 337, a721.

Wyon, M. (2007) Testing an Aesthetic Athlete: Contemporary Dance and Classical Ballet Dancers. In E. Winter, A. Jones, R. Davidson, P. Bromley and T. Mercer (eds) Sport and Physiology Testing Guidelines. Abingdon: Routledge.

Zorn, A. (2012) Walk with Elastic Fascia. In E. Dalton (ed.) *Dynamic Body; Exploring Form, Exploring Function*. Oklahoma City: Freedom from Pain Institute.

Resources

Dance UK
www.danceuk.org
Dance UK is the national voice for dance – provides information sheets, resources on dance and health.

Hypermobility Syndromes Association (HMSA)
www.hypermobility.org
Provides help and support for those affected by hypermobility syndromes.

International Association for Dance Medicine and Science (IADMS)
www.iadms.org
IADMS enhances the health, wellbeing, training, and performance of dancers by cultivating educational, medical, and scientific excellence.

The Rudolf Nureyev Foundation Medical Website
www.nureyev-medical.org
A useful website packed with different articles on dancer health/injury.

16

Parkinson's, Multiple Sclerosis and Diabetes

John Coleman

Parkinson's disease is a diagnosis accompanied by dire predictions of continuing degeneration, discomfort, distress and hopelessness. For most, a picture is painted of a future filled with distressing and embarrassing symptoms that, inevitably, get worse; drugs that give some relief for a relatively short time; surgery that may or may not be effective and, if helpful, only temporarily. This is a medical prognosis based on the Western medical view of what Parkinson's disease is, how it can be defined and how it develops.

Conservative View

Parkinson's disease affects six to seven million people around the world. The severity of the disease varies from mild, untreated symptoms (stages 0 to I) to debilitating symptoms necessitating full-time care (stage V). Idiopathic Parkinson's disease is thought to be primarily a problem associated with advancing age; however, there are significant numbers of early-onset Parkinson's disease sufferers, some as young as their 20s. Non-idiopathic, or secondary Parkinson's disease, has no age barriers but is a much less common condition.

Parkinson's disease (also known as Parkinson's syndrome, Parkinsonism, paralysis agitans and Shaking Palsy) is a chronic, progressive disorder of the central nervous system (CNS) characterized by slowness and poverty of purposeful movement, muscular rigidity and tremor. Parkinsonism is essentially a set of symptoms rather than a disease, as pathological changes can only be surveyed post-mortem.

Variants, or extensions, of Parkinsonism ('Parkinson's Plus') are Multi-System Atrophy (MSA), idiopathic orthostatic hypotension, Shy-Drager syndrome and Progressive Supranuclear Palsy.

Parkinson's disease was first described in detail by James Parkinson in 1817 in his essay on the Shaking Palsy; however, some researchers believe it to be a condition as old as man in that it is thought to be essentially a condition of cell death during the ageing process. This view is not necessarily universal as there is a developing body of thought linking Parkinson's disease with pollution and heavy metal toxicity. An even more recent (and more credible) view is that the degenerative process leading to Parkinson's disease symptoms is created by long-term repression of the fight/flight/freeze response which leads to cell starvation and damage (Goldstein 2008). Free radical damage is also postulated as a possible cause, again linked to our polluted, nutritionally poor lifestyle.

The classical manifestations of Parkinson's disease are resting tremor, muscle rigidity and an impairment of voluntary movement (akinesia). These symptoms may develop alone or in combination but, as the disease progresses, most will be present to some degree. The symptoms usually develop asymmetrically but eventually become truly bilateral, although there may still be asymmetry about the severity of some symptoms. Postural abnormalities, autonomic-neuroendocrine symptoms and, sometimes, dementia are also part of the syndrome. The pathophysiology of Parkinson's disease post-mortem shows both a progressive reduction in the number and activity of nigrostriatal dopamine neurons that are responsible for transmitting dopamine from one region of the brain to another, and also a massive reduction in the striatal dopamine content. However, in most cases, the cause of these changes is still a matter for conjecture.

Idiopathic Parkinson's Disease

The disease does not show any hereditary pattern or strong familial tendency, nor any particular population patterns. Epidemiological studies have suggested vascular, viral and metabolic factors as possible causes but there is, as yet, no consensus on any one or combination of these factors as a definitive cause. One hypothesis is that age predisposes the nigrostriatal pathway to damage by viruses or toxins. However, this begs the question of why only 1 per cent of the ageing population develops this disease when rationality would suggest that all those who age with exposure to the same viruses or toxins would display some or all Parkinsonian symptoms before death. Again, more recent epidemiological studies indicate that continuous hyper-production of cortisol (during fight/flight/freeze response) can, itself, become a trigger for production of cortisol after only a few weeks (McEwen 1998). This mechanism can lead to cell damage and death at a speed determined by other lifestyle choices.

While there is a significant amount of research into methods of controlling Parkinsonian symptoms, and into trying to understand the processes involved during the development of Parkinson's disease, little is yet known by Western medicine about likely causes and the developmental pathway. Many millions of dollars are being poured into research projects looking at the minutiae of chemical imbalances, genes and protein expressions, but the studies ignore non-medical research demonstrating the likely aetiology and pathogenesis of Idiopathic Parkinson's and similar disorders.

Stages of Parkinson's Disease

The stages of Parkinson's disease are often assessed on the Hoehn and Yahr Scale:

- STAGE 0 = no clinically discernible syndrome
- STAGE I = syndrome is unilateral
- STAGE II = bilateral syndrome without balance impairment
- STAGE III = syndrome impairs balance or walking
- STAGE IV = syndrome markedly impairs balance or walking
- STAGE V = syndrome results in complete immobility.

While this scale is extremely limited in the scope of symptoms it references, it is useful in enabling a uniform classification of disease severity where required. A more complete assessment of the progress of Parkinson's disease can be obtained using the Unified Parkinson's Disease Rating Scale (UPDRS). The UPDRS scores an extensive range of symptoms and lifestyle deficits across a wide range of functions and activities for a more thorough judgement of illness progression. For instance, when my Parkinson's symptoms were at their peak, I was assessed at stage IV on the H&R scale, but 127/199 on the UPDRS.

A Naturopathic View

Since my recovery in 1998 I have treated over 2000 people around the world diagnosed with Parkinson's disease, multiple sclerosis and a variety of neurodegenerative and autoimmune disorders. It has become obvious to me that these are not separate diseases, but sets of symptoms arising from a common degenerative process. Just as each person manifests acute disorders such as influenza or hay fever slightly differently, each person will manifest long-term degeneration with slightly different sets of symptoms. Western medicine has conveniently grouped these sets of symptoms into 'diseases' that can be treated with sets of medications or put aside as 'incurable'.

Finding a pattern of unresolved stress or trauma in the lives of all those diagnosed with Parkinson's disease who came to my clinic set me off on a search for answers. Could unresolved stress prepare our bodies for the expression of Parkinson's disease symptoms? I began to study the chemical processes that occur in trauma and stress, and the long-term effects of those chemicals when they remain at an abnormal level over long periods.

The Physiology of Stress

There is excellent research into genetic factors and the physiological processes that take place during the development of Parkinson's disease. It seems to me, however, that most research looks at factors too close in time to diagnosis. While family history is considered and either held as a risk factor or discounted as such, the full life and health history of the patient is rarely taken or considered important.

One factor stands out as a common denominator among all my patients with Parkinson's disease: each person has experienced high stress or trauma at some stage during their first 15 years of life. Most had this experience during their first ten years. Many of the traumas are obvious – abuse of various types, loss of a parent or sibling, life-threatening disease or accident. Some are not so obvious. For instance, a woman who was implicitly blamed by her father for her mother's miscarriage; a woman adopted into a loving family after nine months of bonding to her birth mother; a man whose father was a workaholic and was not around for any of his son's activities, or to develop a relationship.

Stress can be good for us, as it motivates us to activity and provides the physiological resources for that activity. Without some level of stress, we would not get out of bed in the morning.

Trauma need not be physically damaging if it is treated and resolved healthily and holistically. But this is rare in the sorts of trauma mentioned above. Prolonged stress and unresolved trauma trigger our body into continuous stress reactions that, over a long time, become damaging.

The initial physiological reaction to any type of significant stress or trauma is the 'flight/fight/freeze' response. Simply put, the process is this:

- The adrenal glands have two major parts, the medulla and the cortex.

- Excretion of adrenal medullary hormones is directly triggered by stress and trauma.

- Stress and trauma stimulate the hypothalamus to release corticotropin-releasing hormone (CRH).

- CRH stimulates the release of adrenocorticotropic hormone (ACTH) from the pituitary gland.

- ACTH regulates excretions from the adrenal cortex.

Hormones released by the adrenals are:

- Medulla (amino acid derivative): adrenaline (plus small amounts of noradrenaline).

- Cortex (steroids): mineralocorticoids (aldosterone), glucocorticoids (cortisol), adrenal androgens (testosterone).

Effects of Adrenal Hormones

Adrenaline:

- increases blood glucose by activating cyclic AMP

- increases glycogen breakdown (decreases reserves)

- increases intracellular metabolism of glucose in skeletal muscles (ready for action)

- increases breakdown of fats in adipose (fatty) tissue

- increases heart rate

- increases force of heart contraction

- constricts blood vessels in skin, kidneys, gastrointestinal tract and other organs not needed for fight/flight

- dilates blood vessels in skeletal and cardiac muscle.

Aldosterone:

- increases rate of sodium reabsorption in kidneys leading to

  - increased plasma sodium

  - increased water reabsorption (that can lead to oedema)

  - increased blood volume (that can lead to hypertension)

- increases potassium excretion (lower plasma potassium)

- increases hydrogen ion excretion (leading to acidic urine, increased metabolic pH – alkalosis)

- causes changes in sodium/potassium balance that can affect cellular hydration, cell membrane function and transport to and from cells.

Cortisol:

- increases catabolism of fats

- decreases glucose and amino acid uptake in skeletal muscles

- increases glucose synthesis from amino acids in the liver leading to increased blood glucose

- increases protein degradation (leading to muscle weakness/atrophy, osteoporosis)

- decreases inflammatory response by decreasing number of white cells and the expression of inflammatory chemicals (leading to a depressed immune system).

Testosterone (indirect and mainly in women):

- increases pubic and axillary hair

- increases sexual drive (but may reduce potency).

Short-term stress is a normal part of life. We need it for motivation, and we need the physiological responses to stress in order to survive. Our forebears faced immediate dangers and stimuli every day in living; for instance, they needed to chase down prey, or run away from predators, or fight enemies to protect their territory or families. In all these cases, the stress was resolved quite quickly – they won or lost, caught the prey or waited until the next day, got away or got eaten.

We have negative feedback systems to adjust levels of adrenal hormones so they do not become damaging. However, stress can override these negative feedback systems so that we go on over-producing these chemicals. Professor Bruce McEwen has found that, in the dentate gyrus of the hippocampus, chronic stress reduces neuron number and contributes to cognitive impairment. In the hippocampus, chronic stress causes neurons to undergo remodelling of dendrites. Excitatory amino acids – in particular, NMDA receptors – are important regulators of neuronal remodelling, acting in concert with glucocorticoids. The lab has also shown that the stress-induced remodeling is largely reversed once the stress is removed (McEwen 1998). Professor McEwen estimates that continuous hyper-production of cortisol for only a few weeks may lock the body into ongoing fight/flight/freeze response with resultant long-term damage.

Many stresses in this society are not resolved, and many traumas go unrecognized (Victoroff 2002). We live surrounded by noise, pollution, busy-ness and poisons. Child abuse is the world's best-kept secret; family breakdown is seen as traumatic for the partners, but not necessarily for the children; the loss of a sibling or grandparent or friend is often borne in silence by the young in our society.

Prolonged and unresolved stress or trauma can result in:

- increased plasma sodium

- decreased plasma potassium

- cellular dehydration

- reprogramming of the hypothalamus

- chronic heart stress and eventual failure

- alkalosis (often treated with antacids!)

- hypertension

- weak skeletal muscles

- acidic urine

- hyperglycaemia leading to diabetes mellitus

- deficient immune system

- muscle atrophy

- general weakness and debility

- osteoporosis

- weak capillaries

- thin skin that bruises easily

- impaired wound healing

- inappropriate fat distribution (face, neck, abdomen)

- mood swings (euphoria and depression).

In women it can additionally result in:

- hirsutism

- increased sex drive

- diminished breast size

- menstrual irregularities.

People facing prolonged unresolved stress or trauma will respond in different ways, possibly influenced by their genetic inheritance, but primarily by lifestyle choices and environment. Some may develop heart disease, cancer, arthritis, diabetes, skin disorders, depression or other psychological disorders, gastric ulcers or inappropriate behaviours such as substance abuse, addictive gambling or violent behaviour (McEwen 2005).

Some will develop Parkinson's disease. The reprogramming of the hypothalamus and cellular dehydration, as well as many of the other effects shown above, allow some brain cells to become damaged or inactive, or even die, over many years, ultimately resulting in the expression of Parkinson's disease symptoms.

Stress and or trauma is not necessarily the cause of Parkinson's disease, but can begin the slow degeneration that leads to cell fragility and damage. All those I see also have a history of stress triggers throughout life, and a high degree of imposed responsibility for others. This is also a factor in disease development.

Once we recognize that there is a logical development process for Parkinson's disease, we can create strategies to reverse the process and, perhaps, recover.

Bowen for Parkinson's

There are many forms of excellent bodywork available that can bring comfort and assist mobility for those with Parkinson's disease. Many forms of bodywork will bring comfort simply because we are receiving loving touch from a caring practitioner; some will generate chemical reactions (e.g. producing endorphins or natural painkillers) that provide physical comfort; a few modalities will bring positive therapeutic effects to our lives.

During my journey with Parkinson's disease I experimented with a number of bodywork modalities – massage of various types, craniosacral therapy, Feldenkrais, reflexology, osteopathy and Bowen Therapy (Coleman 2012). I found advantages and disadvantages with most and it became clear that *the most important component in delivering the therapy was the practitioner.* If my therapist was of the type who simply 'sells' their therapy or 'processes' their clients, then I rarely gained any benefit and often felt much worse. If, on the other hand, the therapist showed they cared about me and my journey, took time to understand what I, and my body, needed in the way of duration and intensity of treatment, I always gained some benefit.

It became clear, and this has been confirmed by my experience in practice, that people with Parkinson's disease need *very gentle* bodywork, no matter how robust or confident we may appear. This makes sense when we consider that an underlying condition with Parkinson's disease is cell fragility. If our cell membranes are fragile, they need gentle persuasion to resume their 'normal' function and resilience; hard or rough bodywork is likely to have an adverse effect.

After trying many forms of bodywork during my journey with Parkinson's disease, I found that Bowen Therapy, combined with the Aqua Hydration Formulas and self-help activities, brought the greatest benefit (Coleman 2012).

My observations below are borne from personal experience, clinical observation and research with many experienced practitioners.

Bowen Therapy: Pumping Water

There are a number of hypotheses concerning the way Bowen Therapy works. Current research indicates that there are probably two major effects created by the therapist's moves during a Bowen Therapy session. The first is the movement of water through the fascia, and movement of fascia itself (Oysten 2004). Fascia consists of proteins, made up of proteoglycans and glycosaminoglycans, contains collagen and reticulin fibres, and fills all the apparent spaces in our body between organs, muscles, bones, tendons and ligaments and the brain (the dura) – in other words the 'gaps' between the various parts of our body that appear separate in anatomy charts. Fascia carries fluids, immune system cells and other elements vital to our wellbeing. During times of illness, injury, fatigue or stress, fascia can become 'cooked', like an egg white, and firmly attached to the muscle or bone it surrounds, and no longer allow free movement of fluid and nutrients. This can create discomfort, stiffness or pain (often distal to the fascial pressure on a nerve) and inhibit our return to wellness.

The second major effect of a Bowen therapy treatment appears to be movement of electrical energy throughout the body. This can be thought of as electrical current,

Qi, Prana or life-energy depending on the philosophy you're coming from. However we view it, it is vital to have a balanced electrical energy flow throughout our bodies for us to feel well. The moves in a Bowen therapy session serve to remove blockages, correct imbalances and restore free flow of electrical energy over the whole body, even though the moves are made only at specific points. This is similar to the work done in acupuncture or acupressure.

I started treating people with Parkinson's disease using Bowen Therapy and Aqua Hydration Formulas in the second half of 1998. This was very much an experiment because I had used a large number of therapies to obtain my own recovery. However, intuitively and intellectually, I believed that Bowen Therapy and hydration were the major therapies instrumental in my full recovery. In part, this was wrong, as I now know, because at least 80 per cent of recovery depends on thought processes, belief systems and lifestyle choices. Physical therapies and remedies constitute only about 20 per cent of the recovery process. In saying that, however, of that 20 per cent, Bowen is certainly important.

Since 1998 I have treated people displaying the symptoms of Parkinson's disease, multiple sclerosis, Multi-System Atrophy, motor neurone disease/Amyotrophic Lateral Sclerosis/Primary Lateral Sclerosis, spasmodic torticollis, lupus, ankylosing spondylitis and a variety of other degenerative disorders, using the combination of Aqua Hydration Formulas and Bowen Therapy, still with a focus on self-help.

Bowen therapy is very powerful treatment for pain, injury and a number of illnesses. However, I have found, in the treatment of neurological disorders, that it works best in conjunction with the Aqua Hydration Formulas and some accompanying therapies described in other writings (Coleman 2005). While some improvement in Parkinson's disease symptoms can be obtained by using only Bowen therapy, the results are generally slow and unsatisfying. Using the hydration effect of Aqua Hydration Formulas plus the hydrating and balancing effect of Bowen therapy is very powerful medicine indeed. All those who have come to me with Parkinson's disease and persisted with this therapy while adopting necessary lifestyle changes have made great steps forward in returning to health.

Any Bowen practitioner treating a patient with neurological disorders needs to remember that the pain and stiffness displayed by their patient is neurological in origin – not physical. Therefore, the therapy needs to be gentle and balancing, despite the often asymmetrical nature of the symptoms displayed. Treatment that is too firm or asymmetrical in approach can be detrimental to progress, as well as causing unnecessary pain.

The timing of treatments is important also. Many therapists try to see their Parkinson's disease patients frequently in the hope of gaining significant result within a short period. My experience indicates that this is rarely satisfactory. Occasionally, I see patients weekly in order to help them over a difficult patch – for instance, when they are reducing medication or experiencing extra stress in their lives. Generally, however, I find that treatments two weeks apart work well.

Remember, recovering from Parkinson's disease takes at least three years or more. It is very important to establish a supportive, comforting relationship with your patients so you can both enjoy and learn from this exciting, challenging journey.

There are a number of interpretations of Tom Bowen's principles of healing that are now available for study or treatment. Bowtech, Bowen Essentials, Neurostructural Integration Technique, Fascial Kinetics, Smart Bowen and International School of Bowen Therapy courses are available throughout many countries. There are practitioners, colleges and associations around the world.

Is There a Standard Protocol for Treatments?

Neurological disorders are difficult to treat for three reasons:

1. The skeletal and muscular dysfunctions we observe are neurological in origin and do not respond to Bowen in the same way as injuries and skeletal imbalances.

2. The symptoms occur as a result of damage to or destruction of brain cells over a wide area. Therefore, long-term or permanent improvement can only result from repair or regeneration of these brain cells.

3. Repair, and consequent resolution of symptoms, takes a very long time and cannot be hurried.

Each Bowen session serves a number of purposes. Each of these purposes is equally important, and it is vital that we do not concentrate solely on the physical manifestations of the disease.

At each session, a practitioner brings their Parkinson's disease patient the following gifts:

1. Contact with a professional health practitioner who believes they can become well.

2. Contact with a health practitioner who gives them time to speak and listens to what they have to say.

3. The knowledge that they are complete, beautiful human beings, worthy of undivided care and attention.

4. The healing touch of Bowen Therapy.

5. The certainty that they will receive the comfort the practitioner give them on a regular basis.

6. An assessment of their current condition and progress over time.

Even though there are a number of Bowen Therapy schools teaching different interpretations of Tom Bowen's work, all are valid; all can help people with Parkinson's disease move toward health. There are, however, principles of treatment which should be observed closely:

- *If it hurts, it's too hard.* The purpose of Bowen Therapy in treating neurological disorders is to move and hydrate fascia, balance energy and encourage regeneration/reactivation of brain cells. Therefore, the therapy does not need to be hard or deep. In my experience, digging too deeply into muscles that are rigid, locked and painful is counter-productive; it causes the muscles to become even more rigid, creates pain and operates on a physical, rather than a neurological, level.

- *All treatment should be symmetrical, except for the coccyx move, specific neuro balance moves and extraordinary circumstances.* Two of the purposes of using Bowen Therapy are to encourage symmetrical energy within the brain and symmetry of physical movement. Therefore, the therapy needs to be symmetrical. The coccyx move is, of its nature, asymmetrical and serves to promote symmetry of energy along and around the spine. Occasionally, there is a need to treat a specific asymmetrical condition such as a frozen shoulder or asymmetrical back pain. Asymmetrical treatment is appropriate here, but it needs to be understood that this is simply treating the physical symptoms of a neurological condition.

- *Bowen Therapy can't do it alone.* It is tempting to think that persistent use of Bowen Therapy will eventually create a healing pathway without recourse to any other therapy. In my experience, this is not possible with Parkinson's disease. Bowen Therapy is a critical, integral part of a synergistic recovery programme. It helps give mobility and peace as well as the benefits described above, but 80 per cent of recovery depends on the patient's own lifestyle choices and determination.

- *Many people with Parkinson's disease are old, frail and rigid. All are very sensitive.* It is very important to move each muscle group or limb only as much as is comfortable for the patient. The rigidity, pain and slowness of movement shown by our patients is neurological in origin and we must be patient in 're-educating the brain' to allow freedom of movement. It has been my personal experience that attempting to create freedom of movement by challenging rigidity is painful, depressing and inclined to set us back or discourage us from trying to get well.

Bowen Therapy is one way to gain a real appreciation of the progress toward health each person is making.

Following the first one or two treatments, I find it most effective to give my clients a 'complete' treatment at each visit. I do not intend to describe specific moves to use during any one treatment; rather I wish to set down principles of treatment I have found to be effective over the last five years. Because each interpretation of Tom Bowen's work names moves differently, I will give general descriptions only.

Each practitioner should assess his or her client on each visit as you do now. Treatments may need to be varied from a set routine because of particular stresses, accidents or changes in your client's condition.

On the first two visits, I suggest that basic moves only be used covering the back, neck and legs. On the second visit, it may be useful to introduce the TMJ moves if your client is robust enough. This can assist with balance and mobility.

From the third visit, I like to do a 'complete' Bowen treatment each time. This includes the basic back moves (sometimes freeing the erector spinae muscles) and, often, extra hip moves where mobility is a problem, plus sacrum and hamstrings while prone. I often include the pelvic moves including psoas. In the supine position, I use abdominal/respiratory moves, neck, knee, ankle, shoulder, elbow and wrist (carpal tunnel) and, almost invariably, the TMJ. I work slowly and very lightly, with variable pauses, to let each client relax and gain full benefit from the treatment.

I also incorporate a form of Yin Tuina on the feet and a specific cranial move. Information on these moves is available from Return to Stillness (www.returnto stillness.com.au).

If you are skilled in any other form of foot or cranial work, you may wish to incorporate some individual moves into your routine. However, people receiving basic Bowen Therapy from a caring practitioner who uses a *very light* touch make good progress. I cannot emphasize enough how important it is to use *extremely light* touch. Firmness of touch will only result in discomfort and aggravation of symptoms. The maximum weight I suggest for any Bowen move is the pressure you would willingly apply to your closed eye without causing discomfort. This equates to less than five grams of weight.

Remember, you are the practitioner your client sees most often. Therefore, you have a unique opportunity to join them on their great adventure. I encourage you to participate fully and enjoy the experience.

CASE STUDY

A 79-year-old male with stage IV Parkinson's disease. Unable to walk, dress, shower, toilet or eat without assistance. Constant nausea, stiffness, pain and depression. He was taking 11 prescribed drugs with little effect.

Commenced Aqua Hydration Formulas, Bowen Therapy each two weeks from a therapist in his local area (not me), and slowly introduced important food choices. Additional herbal remedies were used for nausea and a variety of peripheral symptoms.

After one year, 11 months and two weeks of treatment with little apparent progress, he was suddenly able to leave his walking frame in the house and walk unassisted outside.

Over the next four years of treatment his drug load was reduced to one low-dose blood pressure tablet and one occasional sleeping tablet. Digestive herbs were continued at low dose while Aqua Hydration Formulas and Bowen were continued as before.

Now in his mid 90s, this gentleman has no symptoms of Parkinson's disease, remains active and involved in his community. He benefited greatly from regular Bowen from a practitioner who spent time in understanding his needs and accompanied him on his journey to recovery.

Multiple Sclerosis

Multiple sclerosis (MS) is usually considered to be an autoimmune disease entirely different from Parkinson's disease. However, are autoimmune diseases actually a sign that our immune system is attacking our body?

While immune-suppressing therapies can mitigate symptoms, nobody actually gets well with these therapies. In fact, those who have fully recovered from MS (i.e., replaced all the missing myelin and live without any symptoms) have, in fact, boosted the performance of their immune system.

Multiple sclerosis is actually the result of exactly the same process as that creating Parkinson's disease, except the damaged cells are supposed to produce myelin (oligodendrocytes) rather than levodopa. Unresolved stress/trauma creates long-term dysfunction of the hypothalamic-pituitary-adrenal (HPA) axis, widespread symptoms of cell dehydration and toxicity, a high degree of systemic inflammation and a reduction in the production of myelin.

As we all turn over myelin cells daily (as we turn over every cell in our body over time), myelin loss may exceed myelin production, thus creating 'gaps' in our myelin sheath – or MS plaque. By improving HPA-axis function and rehydrating oligodendrocytes, myelin production is increased and the process of Multi-System Atrophy (MSA) reversed.

It is not an easy journey, especially as a diagnosis of MS brings enormous pressure to take immune-suppressing drugs that may reduce symptoms temporarily, but exacerbate the degenerative process over the long term. It takes great courage for patients (often young, vulnerable women) to defy family and doctors to embark of a journey to discovery and change.

Critical components of MS recovery are self-love, laughter, meditation; food choices are enormously important and exercise will certainly help. I have found, time and again, that a combination of Aqua Hydration Formulas and appropriately applied Bowen will assist patients in their journey towards wellness.

CASE STUDY

A 42-year-old female diagnosed with MS via MRI and spinal tap. Symptoms included fatigue, tingling and numbness in right arm, poor mobility and fine motor skills in right arm, neck pain and headaches. The MRI showed significant MS plaque over a wide area. She was prescribed tegretol (carbamazepine) twice daily.

She made all critical food choice changes, commenced meditation, self-love activities, reduced her workload and began Aqua Hydration Formulas with gentle fortnightly Bowen.

A second MRI after ten months showed a 60 per cent reduction in myelin plaque (that is a 60% replacement of myelin). Over the next three years her symptoms disappeared, and all myelin was replaced as shown by subsequent MRI. She remains well to this day.

Chronic Lyme Disease and Co-infections

Lyme disease and co-infections, perhaps more properly called multiple systemic infection disease syndrome (MSIDS), a name coined by Dr Richard Horowitz, has reached epidemic proportions worldwide (Horowitz 2013).

This is not the place for a treatise on treating this debilitating scourge, but we need all be aware of its rise and prepared to look beyond traditional diagnosis if our patients' symptom patterns seem beyond the ordinary.

MSIDS can, and does, mimic nearly every degenerative, inflammatory and autoimmune disease and can lead to years of frustration and inappropriate treatment for patients. An excellent reference is Dr Horowitz's book *Why Can't I Get Better?* (2013) as this will give a deep insight into symptoms, diagnosis and treatment options.

Diabetes (Types 1 and 2)

This scourge is largely the result of unrecognized and unresolved stress, very poor food choices common in Western society, an almost total lack of good health education in schools and clinics, and medical focus on insulin.

There is no doubt that insulin production is guided by the level of stress we experience consciously or subconsciously. If we are constantly under stress, we will automatically reduce insulin production to enable immediate use of glucose for energy production (for running or fighting). Insulin facilitates the utilization and storage of glucose (sugar) released into the blood stream. This is a very complex process, of course, but the simple view is that, if we are constantly preparing ourselves for action, even when we don't need to or can't act, the reduction in insulin production becomes damaging and, over time, can be diagnosed as diabetes (types 1 or 2).

While it is important to monitor and manage blood sugar levels and insulin receptor sensitivity, treating the source of dysfunction will always reap better results and more permanency in health status.

Reversing the dysfunction in the HPA axis via methodologies already described for Parkinson's disease (Coleman 2005), and utilizing homeopathic support for the pancreas, we can often reverse the process of diabetes and achieve good health.

Bowen can be a most useful and effective treatment for symptoms management and prophylaxis. Peripheral neuropathy (especially in the lower limbs) is very common among diabetics, and often badly managed. Gentle Bowen on a weekly or fortnightly basis, with particular focus on overall balance plus circulation to the lower limbs can play a large part in relieving, reversing and preventing peripheral neuropathy.

CASE STUDY

| *Maureen Pettigrew, Ardrossan, Ayrshire, Scotland*

This lady, born 1960, first came to me in 2007 having been diagnosed with MS 12 years earlier. Her main areas of concern are her feet, legs and hips where she has altered sensations and loss of muscular control and strength. At that point she walked with one stick but gradually she has deteriorated and now uses a rollator. Also she has IBS and other bowel and bladder issues, and sleeps very poorly.

At her first appointment I remember her telling me her feet felt like she had rubber boots with 6-inch thick soles and the day after that first treatment the soles felt only 2 inches thick. She was impressed. She often describes spongy feet, lead legs and pulling sensations on top of feet and ankles.

She continues to report positive effects from her treatments, sometimes subtle and sometimes quite impressive. Some last and some are temporary but she is delighted with either. Examples are feeling each individual toe, which she hadn't for years, reduced tightness, more warmth in feet and surprisingly being delighted to feel some pain in her foot where her sock had been wrinkled. Previously she wouldn't have felt it. For some considerable time her right leg had been outward rotated from the hip with the foot falling out in an uncontrollable fashion when getting up and on walking. Nothing I did was helping this till I did Alastair McLoughlin's 'Art of Bowen' course and I used his opening up moves down the front of thigh and release of IT band. Instant response which has held ever since. Leg now lies straight and foot stays straight as she walks!

I have been able to 'experiment' with this very positive-minded lady as she has continued to have regular treatments – monthly and more recently every three weeks. I have tried the less-is-more approach and, once I knew she was reacting positively, I tried putting in lots of work. Things that work one day may not on another – it is a learning journey. She has never had a bad reaction to Bowen and says there was only once she didn't get any positive changes. She reports fairly quick changes after treatment with reduction in the bothersome sensations. I tend to focus on whatever is troubling her most on the day, which might be her legs or general stress and tension or, more recently, neck and shoulder tightness. I try to be aware of where there is obvious tension and use lateral moves which often release things there and then.

I know Bowen is not performing miracles and it will never be job done. She rarely presents with the same body and generally things are deteriorating slowly. There are areas which have not responded, such as her insomnia and I have made little impression on her bladder and bowel problems but I have so many times seen improvement to skeletal muscle and nerve sensation issues which she appreciates even when they are temporary. Her family and carers also comment and know when she has just had Bowen. She is a lovely lady with a great sense of humor and it is a pleasure to work with her.

Joyce writes:

I have had Bowen now for just over six years. I have multiple sclerosis, being diagnosed in 1995. My main symptoms are numbness in my feet, legs and hands. Both legs feel like lead weights. I feel as if a scarf is being pulled very tightly round my feet and legs. This feeling never lets up. My feet feel very spongy and my balance is not so great. I also have a foot-drop.

After my very first treatment back in 2007 my left foot felt less tight the next day. I have continued with Bowen because after every treatment, apart from one, in all the years I have had a good response. After a Bowen session I feel upbeat. I feel the benefit the second I get off the bed. I want to skip up and down the living room but instead make do with walking up and down with my three-wheeler walker or sometimes just my walking stick. I often put on a CD, hold on to my walker and dance, as I call it, as I sing or rather 'roar' along.

My immediate reaction after each session is of tingling down my legs and a loose feeling inside both legs and my feet feeling less tight. Some treatments that I have been overwhelmed by include:

- The day I just so happened to say that my teeth were sensitive and I was dreading my scale and polish at the dentist. My therapist had just finished working on my jaw. My next visit to the dentist was pain-free!

- Whilst pushing my feet against the bottom of the bath (in the days I was able to get in and out a bath) one night, having had Bowen that morning, I was amazed that my feet felt like 'real' feet again. For the first time in ages I could feel my feet through my usual numbness!

- Just recently my therapist worked on my legs. My right leg now is back to its normal position when standing and walking. It is not pointing out to the side like it has been for years!

I would definitely recommend Bowen to others.

CASE STUDY

| *Ozana Pope-Gajić, Osijek, Croatia (www.ergovita.hr)*

Z.M. is a physician, born 1971, who diagnosed with MS ten years ago. When she came for a Bowen treatment (first time in 2008) Z.M. presented with symptoms of vertigo, instability while walking, tiredness and paresthesia on her both feet. Patient was taking corticosteroid injections every other day.

After her first treatment, which was very gentle, she felt extremely tired, but after that first day she was full of energy and her working days passed easy. After the second visit changes with her symptoms began – vertigo was still present, but lasted for only ten minutes when she lay down, no instability while walking and she felt more energy in her body. There were still no changes with the paresthesia in her feet. However, on the third treatment hamstrings and ankle work were added to address the paresthesia in her feet, and she had great response. Her numbness centralized in one little spot on the metatarsal region on both feet.

It has now been five years that she has been having Bowen sessions with smaller or bigger gaps between treatments. Meanwhile Z.M. has stopped taking any other medication for MS, and her condition has improved. She is able to work full-time as a physician in her medical practice. From time to time when she gets stressed or if she has a cold she can feel a worsening of her symptoms (paresthesia, vertigo, tiredness). If that happens she makes a few consecutive appointments, and her body responds very quickly with improvements in her condition. If she feels well then I treat her every few months as a maintenance programme.

Z.M. writes:

I started with Bowen Therapy in 2008. From the beginning, I saw a positive treatment effect. Easing muscle tension and a sense of relief throughout the body would follow after each session. I would single out the effect of Bowen on the reduction of paresthesia felt in the feet, and of maintaining this condition, for which there is no further spreading which might be expected. My problems with insomnia also have successfully resolved after a few Bowen treatments. For the last three years, Bowen Therapy is my only treatment, despite my diagnosis. I listen to my body, and it tells me, usually after four weeks, when it's a time to regain balance by having another treatment, which I do on a regular basis.

CASE STUDY

| *Joanna Austen, Bodmin and Liskeard, Cornwall, England*
| *(www.bowenincornwall.co.uk)*

This lady came to try Bowen treatment to see if it would help her. MS had affected her ability to walk and she was finding that she was very tired, could not walk far and generally was not getting full enjoyment out of life. She responded really well to Bowen and initially weekly treatments were carried out for six weeks, then fortnightly and then monthly. She felt that monthly was too long and eventually it was decided to carry out short treatments every three weeks. After nine months we have been able to go back to longer gaps between treatments and are now trying six-week gaps with longer treatments being carried out. Her stamina and balance have improved greatly, and she is now able to help take care of her granddaughter. She writes: 'Since seeing Jo my energy has increased and I can walk further – I even managed to climb 130 steps after being all day at a wedding. Would have been impossible before Bowen.'

Another client writes: 'Bowen with Jo helps me keep my job whilst having a chronic condition; by having regular Bowen treatments it helps prevent vertigo, fatigue and muscle pain. I am a different person once I have had a 30 min session of Bowen, it wakes my body up. I find Bowen very relaxing and non-invasive, having Bowen helps me manage my life with MS.'

CASE STUDY

| *Ros Elliott-Özlek, Izmir, Turkey (www.bowen.web.tr)*

I have used Bowen quite successfully in a group setting, with about 15 men and women, aged from mid-teens to around 50, suffering from multiple sclerosis here in Izmir. In Turkey there are many regional support groups for MS patients who meet regularly for activities such as painting, Emotional Freedom Technique (EFT), Reiki and meditation, or Yoga Therapy. A friend recommended that we try the Bowen after this group's weekly yoga session, as I had indicated that it could be done seated, lying down or even standing, so that we should be able to accommodate all conditions of the group if they were willing to try it.

They were. In fact they were willing to try anything, and so I began to understand one aspect of this illness, being that motivation is an issue and group activities are extremely helpful. Some sufferers can get so demoralized that they won't even make the effort to go to the group meetings, and perhaps this is another reason why new 'topics' are needed regularly to encourage the people to keep coming and socializing for an activity, rather than focusing on their disease.

The members who came to the yoga sessions were mainly mobile or walking with the aid of crutches or a stick, rather than wheelchair-bound, and the activities were open to non-MS patients as well, so they would bring their friends along too. I never saw anybody with an official 'helper' or 'carer', but Turkish people are a sociable lot and every new contact is immediately labelled as a 'friend'.

I started a six-week trial, aiming to do some Bowen after the yoga session, which I also joined in with. The set-up was not ideal as it was not possible to create a suitably quiet space to treat in, and also some patients were also receiving Emotional Freedom Technique (EFT) treatments at the same time (it is usually advised not to mix Bowen with other modalities).

Nearly everybody reported some good effects after each of these sessions. Results were mixed due to the issues mentioned above, with the main one being their regularity of attendance. However, the ones who came regularly said that generally they felt:

- able to walk better, and for longer, generally

- had less pain or no pain on standing/walking that week

- had more energy generally/did not get so tired so quickly each day

- had more *joie de vivre*/felt lighter

- were happier/less depressed or angry

- had reduced their problems with incontinence.

One or two who never missed the treatment were a bit more specific about more energy, more leg movement and better walking/less problems in their hip/s on standing or walking.

The director of this particular group, Sema Turkel, has written a brief summary of the benefits she noticed with herself and the group in general. This is a translation:

When I met Ros, she offered to treat our members with the Bowen Technique for a short trial period. The helpful effects I particularly noticed, both personally and with the group, were relief from Restless Leg Syndrome and a deep relaxation of any muscles that were tight, knotted or in spasm.

References

Coleman, J. (2012) *Shaky Past: Return to Stillness*. Lancefield, Victoria, Australia.

Coleman, J. (2005) *Stop Parkin' and Start Livin': Reversing the Symptoms of Parkinson's Disease*. Melbourne: Michelle Anderson Publishing.

Goldstein, D. (2008) Computer models of stress, allostasis and acute and chronic diseases. *Annals of NY Academy of Sciences* 1148, 223–231.

Horowitz, R. (2013) *Why Can't I Get Better?* New York: St Martin's Press.

McEwen, B. (1998) Protective and damaging effects of stress mediators. *New England Journal of Medicine* 338, 171–179.

McEwen, B. (2005) Interview by Dr Norman Swan on ABC Radio National 'The Health Report', 10 January.

Oysten, B. (2004) *A Simple Explanation of the Science of Bowen Therapy*. Unpublished ms.

Victoroff, J. (2002) *Saving Your Brain*. Milsons Point, NSW: Bantam Books (Random House Australia).

Resources

John Coleman has presented a webinar on Parkinson's and other degenerative diseases. The recording is available to view at www.trainings.co.uk.

17

Bowen in Palliative Care

Nickatie diMarco

Complementary Therapies in Hospices

Palliative care is the care that is given to patients with life-limiting illnesses and their families. As defined by the World Health Organization (WHO), it is based on the prevention and relief of suffering through various means such as pain relief and aiding psychosocial, spiritual and physical problems. Palliative care is designed to be holistic and to help not just the patient but also their families to be able to live as well as possible until the person's death. The approach that is used with palliative care is a team approach and that is quite important for the Bowen practitioner as he or she must try to be part of the multidisciplinary team that looks after the patient. If the patient is under either the hospital or hospice palliative care services, then it would be ideal to try to work with these professionals for the patient's good. Although complementary and alternative therapies are not considered to be part of conventional medicine (National Center for Complementary and Alternative Medicine definition) and are often seen as questionable and unproven luxuries (Barnett 2001; Cassileth and Schulman 2001), within the hospice environment they are used extensively.

The majority of evidence lacks a large enough population base, with the uniqueness of the treatments being a possible reason why large randomized control trials have not yet been done (Patterson 2002, cited in Heller *et al.* 2005). However, it is widely documented that an estimated at 64 per cent of cancer patients worldwide resort to some means of complementary therapy (Ott 2002). Most studies show the use of massage, acupuncture, guided imagery, reiki, hypnosis and reflexology, which are the most accepted mainstream therapies.

There are a number of hospices that use Bowen in the UK, and this number is growing. However, hospices often struggle with what they can provide due to restraints in funding and the number of suitable volunteers that can give up their time freely. Most volunteers are asked for two years' post-qualifying experience in order to treat in the hospice environment; they also need to undergo a Disclosure and Barring Service (DBS) check. There are small pockets across the country of NHS and other organizations that offer treatment to palliative patients using Bowen but these numbers are not yet documented.

Bowen within the Hospice Movement

The hospice movement was started in the 1950s by Dame Cecily Saunders with the aim of providing good end of life care for people with terminal illness. Since then, the work of hospices has evolved, dealing with not just the imminently dying, but also with those who have terminal diagnoses that have a longer life expectancy. Hospices, in the main, offer their services for free and rely (in differing degrees) on the support and fundraising of their local communities.

With cancer patients, Bowen can be useful both pre- and post-chemotherapy, but often when sessions can be given is down to logistics more than anything else. Quite a large number of cancer patients will feel tired or fatigued with their illness and treatments, and it is these symptoms are helped most by Bowen. The basic relaxation moves can be given lightly and sometimes not even this much is needed. With cancer patients the maxim 'less is more' needs to be adhered to.

Another common problem with many clients is breathlessness, which often goes hand in hand with fatigue. The top stoppers seem to instantly aid the breathing of the patient and then the respiratory procedure is always excellent for these symptoms. I teach patients how to do the last move of the respiratory procedure themselves, which they find helps. Again, the respiratory procedure is really effective when used with the chest procedure for the breast cancer patients, who will usually have lymphoedema as well. Bowen is excellent for lymphoedema, with clients often noticing a marked reduction in oedema and limb volume.

Often cancer patients will experience pain – when this is the case, then it usually works to use the most appropriate procedure for that pain as a Bowen practitioner would in any situation. However, there are many different types of pain and my experience is that Bowen is particularly successful at treating neuropathic type pain – even when drugs can't help.

Bearing in mind that most chemical treatments and pain-killing drugs can have significant side effects such as sickness, constipation and low mood, Bowen can be a Godsend. I found that simple lateral thinking, such as using the kidney procedure to help with the toxin overload that drugs can bring, respiratory and gall procedures to help with constipation as well as the more advanced gut-based procedures can all be very therapeutic.

If Bowen doesn't work, there may be reasons for this. Sometimes I have found the treatment does not work or does not last long – maybe a few hours or a day or two. I believe that this may have something to do with the particular drugs that a patient is taking; some of the chemotherapy drugs and steroid-based drugs seem to make the treatment less effective or last longer. We also have to consider if the correct procedure was used for the treatment.

One of the other effects of Bowen on these patients is the feeling of improvement of quality of life – the feel good factor. This is measurable on any of the scales such as Measure Yourself Concerns and Wellbeing scale (MYCAW) that are often used by hospices. This is a valuable way of showing medical professionals that the treatment is helping quality of life.

Palliative care requires a different mindset from that of active curative treatment. This can be quite challenging to the therapist who is new to it. We are so used to Bowen being the missing link that solves problems for lots of people. However, we are still solving symptoms and helping to improve quality of life even though we cannot necessarily 'cure' someone. Palliative care is an exceptionally rewarding area to work in, and one that I would recommend wholeheartedly to any practitioner who wants a more rounded practice.

CASE STUDY

Gentleman P: age 68. Diagnosed in spring 1960 with myasthenia gravis and in the mid-1980s with mitochondrial myopathy. Both of these are extremely rare neuromuscular conditions. P's life expectancy when diagnosed in 1960 was a few years at best. When he got married, they expected his wife to be widowed very quickly.

However, he has survived for many years with both conditions. He retired in 1999 on health grounds. In 2010 walking and other activities became very difficult and his sight has virtually gone now in 2013. For about the last five years he has been in the care of the mitochondrial research unit of Newcastle University and Professor Doug Turnbull.

I met P following his wife attending a carers' course that we ran. I spoke to him of the Bowen Technique and that I had had success with helping the symptoms of those with neurological conditions and he agreed to give it a try. P's symptoms tended to be that he was stooped in his posture, needing a stick to walk. He suffered from shortness of breath, muscle cramps and trembles as well as mild ataxic symptoms. He also has pain in both of his quadriceps that does not seem to go away. Muscular pain is made worse by certain types of alcohol but food has limited effect. P takes many pain killers but not many drugs to control the condition as none have been found to have any effect.

The first treatment was basic relaxation moves. P reported feeling relaxed and having enjoyed the treatment. When he returned, he explained that his general feeling of wellbeing had improved, however, the pain in the legs had not.

Over the following weeks treatments were done to work on the leg pain – ease gracilis, quadriceps procedure, etc. as well as using respiratory procedure to work on shortness of breath. Although the leg pain dulled, it did not go away, although his breathing improved. The other major improvement was that posture improved and after the treatment P would walk out standing up straight. These improvements only every lasted for 36 or 48 hours post-treatment though. This led me to think about using psoas work, which had been successful when used with other neurological conditions. Following the psoas treatment P had the best week he had had since starting Bowen. The improvements were quite dramatic – he was more upright, had more stamina and energy and the effects lasted well over a week before they wore off.

P reports the following on his take of Bowen:

Short-term results:

- general feeling of wellbeing for a minimum of 36 hours post-treatment

- walking and posture much improved

- can speak faster and more easily

- stamina improved – after treatment two weeks ago I went shopping at Cribb's Causeway and walked around Marks and Spencer and other stores for about 1½ hours (with rests and walking stick) – I could not have done this until very recently.

Longer-term results:

- generally it's now easier to walk

- breathlessness appears to have reduced

- wife has noticed an improvement in suppleness of my movements.

CASE STUDY

Forty-year-old female with breast cancer re-occurrence, 2010 diagnosis of breast and lumpectomy followed by chemotherapy and radiotherapy. Told surgery was curative. In 2011 re-occurrence of breast cancer plus another new diagnosis of another type of breast cancer (non-hormonal related) in the other breast. Patient had a husband and two children under nine, so huge emotional issues linked within the other issues of pain, lymphoedema and loss of role, etc.

I started treating her when she attended as an in-patient to the hospice. She had already seen externally a person who was studying to be a Bowen practitioner who had done basic work on her. One of her main symptoms was shortness of breath exacerbated, I would imagine, by the anxiety of her situation. The first few treatments were just basic work and respiratory procedure. Not only did this have a positive effect on her respiratory distress, but it also had a big impact on the lymphoedema.

The lymphoedema still progressed though and she began to literally 'fill' with fluid up her torso and into her right arm. Pressure hosiery did little to contain it. However, every time she had a Bowen treatment she felt better, could breath better and her fluid reduced – not massively but enough to make her more comfortable. With these treatments I used either basic work and triceps procedure or the sternal procedure. The client could not be treated lying down due to the fungating and oozing wounds from her skin, its integrity being compromised by the lymphoedema, so we used to manage on a massage chair. This lady died a few weeks later in the hospice but with the lymphoedema bandaging and Bowen we managed to keep her as comfortable as possible during this time.

Hospices Currently Using Bowen Therapy

St Michael's Hospice, Hereford

Dorothy House Hospice, Bath

Great Oaks Hospice, Forest of Dean

Nightingale House Hospice, Wrexham

Weldmar Hospicecare Trust, Dorset

Rowcroft Hospice, South Devon

St Margaret's Hospice, Somerset

Sobell House Hospice, Oxford

St Catherine's Hospice, West Sussex

Phyllis Tuckwell Hospice, Farnham

North Devon Hospice

The Florence Nightingale Hospice, Aylesbury

St Oswald's Hospice, Newcastle-upon-Tyre

Newark Hospice

Marie Curie Hospice, Bradford

St Richard's Hospice, Worcester

St Giles Hospice, Staffordshire

References

Barnett, M. (2001) Complementary Therapies in Palliative Care. In J. Barraclough (ed.) *Integrated Cancer Care: Holistic Complementary and Creative Approaches.* Oxford: Oxford University Press.

Cassileth, B R. and Schulman, G. (1987) Complimentary Therapies in Palliative Medicine. In D. Doyle, G. Hanks, N. Cherny and K. Calmen (eds) *Oxford Textbook of Palliative Medicine.* Oxford: Oxford University Press.

Heller, T., Lee-Treweek, G., Katz, J., Stone, J. and Spurr, S. (eds) (2005) *Perspectives on Complementary and Alternative Medicine*. London: Routledge.

Ott, M. (2002) Complementary and alternative therapies in cancer symptom management. *Cancer Practice* 10 (3),162–166.

18

Bowen in the Workplace

Stress is now the most common reason for workplace absenteeism, something that appears to be predominately related to high workloads (Chartered Institute of Personnel and Development (CIPD) 2012). Conditions that seem to have the highest prevalence of short-term absence from work are:

- colds, flu, stomach upsets, headaches and migraines

- musculoskeletal injuries, back pain and stress.

(CIPD 2012, p.6)

Conditions that are most common causes of longer-term absence include:

- stress

- acute medical conditions (stroke, heart attack, cancer)

- mental health problems

- musculoskeletal problems and back pain.

(CIPD 2012, p.6)

As many employees struggle with the pressure of workloads or face the prospect of redundancy (two-fifths of public sector organizations and a fifth of other sector organizations reported staffing cuts in 2012; see CIPD 2012), there is, more than ever, a pressure to reach workplace targets, and work longer hours in order to achieve demands. This increase in working hours has an impact on both social and family life. In addition, dealing with challenging behaviour from colleagues or managers can be an extra difficulty in the workplace, placing further burden on the employee. It is therefore no surprise that there is an increase in stress-related absenteeism, as well as the more 'standard' long-term chronic medical conditions, such as back pain, and mental health conditions, such as stress, anxiety and depression (CIPD 2012).

Some employees can be reluctant to insist that companies abide by their legal obligation to provide a working environment that is ergonomically conductive to their health, even when it is causing them specific health problems, such as neck or shoulder pain caused by an incorrectly set-up workstation. Such a client can be supported by a Bowen practitioner offering to write to their employer expressing concern that their health problem is being exacerbated by their work environment. Because of companies' legal obligation and the fear of litigation, employees will usually take action quickly.

It should be clear by now that Bowen has the potential to be a useful and cost-saving tool in getting people back to work as well as maintaining both physical and emotional heath in the workplace. Particularly in the area of prolonged stress, physical therapies such as Bowen and massage can be helpful if used in conjunction with counselling or cognitive behavioural therapy (Mackereth *et al.* 2005).

All workplaces have policies relating to sickness and staff absenteeism. Workplaces that are large enough to have Human Resources (HR) managers mean that they will look at ways in which they can help support a staff member to return to work, particularly if absenteeism relates to 'within work' issues such as bullying or stress. HR managers will regularly refer to an occupational health therapist or GP for further assessment with the aim of speeding up a return to work. Many companies already provide access to counselling, gyms, private medical insurance, health screening and even treatments such as physiotherapy (Broadway 2012). However, there is little evidence in the CIPD's report of providing employees access to complementary and alternative medicine, or treatments such as Bowen Therapy. There is, however, anecdotal evidence that Bowen is being used informally in some work environments, especially where repetitive tasks are involved. Despite that fact that Bowen practitioners are seeing work-related injuries every day in their clinics, Bowen's potential to assist in these kind of injuries has not yet been realized by the corporate sector. This is not helped by the fact that employees can be reluctant to report that they are seeing a complementary therapist for a specific health issue to their employer, GP or even occupational therapist.

The remainder of this chapter focuses on the West Scotland project, where Bowen has been successfully used in conjunction with occupational therapy and physiotherapy as a way of supporting staff at work and in returning to work after sick leave.

The West of Scotland Bowen Therapy Team for Supporting Staff Return to Work

∾ Ann Winter, Rosemary MacAllister, Maureen and Gerry Ryan, Jean Hanlin, Ann Tennent and Julia Blake (The West of Scotland Bowen Therapy Team)

In the West of Scotland a scheme was originally set up in 2006 which involved a team of seven Bowen practitioners based in Lanarkshire. These therapists were asked to see clients from various projects within an organization called SALUS – Occupational Health, Safety and Return to Work Services. One of these projects is called Early Access to Support for You (EASY), which was originally set up for staff who were absent from work on sick leave.

Staff were contacted by a member of the EASY team and offered non-judgemental support, and were then sent to the available support services such as occupational health, counselling, physiotherapy, clinical psychology and Bowen therapy. After deciding which service was most suitable for them, if the client then chose Bowen Therapy, they were able to choose from one of nine venues throughout Lanarkshire.

There were anticipated outcomes from the interventions following treatments, and once these targets had been met, the EASY remit was then expanded. Within nine months EASY was offered not only to staff who were off sick but to those who, because of various health issues, were struggling to stay at work. The Bowen team was funded for three treatments for each client, but if at their third treatment the Bowen practitioner considered the client might benefit from a further one or two treatments, then that was offered.

The Bowen practitioners within the project created their own standardized treatment programme for all clients, although this was not set in stone. If something different was required (e.g. a more specialized Bowen procedure), the Bowen practitioner would use their professional judgement to vary the treatment programme.

The programme involved three treatments being given at weekly intervals, three weeks without treatment and then, if necessary, one or two more treatments at weekly intervals as per Bowen protocol. As EASY was extended, it was understandable that the director of the project required an evidence-based report that would help to show that Bowen was effective. In order to do this, a request was made to produce a three-monthly audit report.

The reporting spreadsheet encompassed:

- an ID number for each client in order to protect client confidentiality

- the reason for referral

- the start and finish date of treatment

- job/family circumstances

- work base

- noting whether they were at work or off work during their initial visit

- noting whether they had returned to work upon discharge

- noting the number of Bowen treatments given

- the outcome of treatment (e.g. improved/no change or worse)

- wellbeing score before treatment

- wellbeing score after treatment (0–10 where 0 = feel terrible, 10 = feeling really good)

- pain score pre- and post-treatment

- Canadian Occupational Performance Measure Score (COPM) before and after treatment

- comments and feedback column.

The COPM score looks at five activities at work or everyday life that a client might find difficult. It is scored in a 0–10 basis for performance and satisfaction, where 0 = cannot do the activity and feel unsatisfied, with the score ranging to 10 where there is no problem in carrying out the activity and the client feels really positive about it. In a nine-month period, the team treated 102 clients. Of those 102:

- 40 per cent had been referred for back pain

- 17 per cent for neck problems

- 15 per cent for shoulder problems

- the remaining 28 per cent were referred for a variety of different conditions including joint pain, headaches, fibromyalgia, gastric problems and pregnancy.

Although most had musculoskeletal complaints, many conditions were accompanied by varying degrees of anxiety and depression.

Usually by the time the team saw the clients they had already engaged with an occupational health advisor, who not only gave sound advice but, where necessary, visited the client's workplace and carried out workplace assessments. The Bowen team believes that the advisors play a huge part in providing an essential listening ear for the staff, who may have home and workplace issues to discuss. The advisor can, where they think it would be appropriate, send a client to an Employee Counselling Service (ECS). This is an important part of not only helping the client to start to feel better, but also helping them to remain so. Without this type of support, the client can often end up trapped in a cycle of continuing health/work and home issues.

Almost without exception, our clients believe that Bowen has helped them in many different ways including reducing their pain, helping them to reduce or stop their medication, improving and restoring their musculoskeletal function, increasing their sense of wellbeing and helping them to get back and remain at work.

CASE STUDY

| *Rosemary MacAllister*

GC presented with early onset arthritis in both hips causing pain and reduced mobility. She had seen an orthopaedic surgeon who wanted to operate giving her a bilateral hip replacement. However, at only 37 years old, she wished to prolong this option as long as possible. GC had been diagnosed with arthritis as a young adult. Two years ago she had a rapid and severe onset of pain in both hips. She had constant pain marked with increased degenerative changes and marked loss of mobility. She had great difficulty in walking and getting in and out of the bath. She was not sleeping well because of the pain.

GC was referred for Bowen Therapy initially and was given three sessions at weekly intervals, followed by a treatment gap of three weeks and then offered three more weekly sessions. GC responded 'really well' and was able to continue working. The Bowen practitioner treating GC recommended more Bowen treatment sessions and permission was granted. These were given at monthly intervals for five months.

On commencement of treatment her wellbeing score was 2/10 (0 = awful, 10 = feeling very well). Her pain score at her initial treatment was 8/10 (0 = no pain, 10 = severe) and following treatment was 3/10. GC has subsequently come off all analgesics, her mobility has improved and she was 'delighted' with the outcome. GC said she was 'crippled' when she first attended Bowen. The Bowen sessions allowed her to reduce her pain relief and greatly improved her mobility and now, more than 18 months later, she has still not yet required the bilateral hip operation. GC is now able to walk pain-free with no analgesics and is enjoying life!

CASE STUDY

| *Ann Winter*

This client was a 37-year-old female who had been diagnosed with Eustachian tube dysfunction and had recently fallen and injured her left shoulder. She was initially referred for physiotherapy, but because of a 7–11 week waiting list, she agreed to a Bowen assessment and treatment. She was given pain medication from her GP and, although she was back at work, was struggling with shoulder pain.

On assessment, although she had no pain when she turned her head, she said her neck felt tight on the left side when she turned her head to the right and on bringing her neck into forward flexion. Her right shoulder/arm had a good range of movement and extension (upward), but her left arm was restricted to 80 degrees outstretched. Her hand-grip was good with no pain at the wrist, elbow or shoulder (she was right-handed). She had difficulty in extending her arm forward, and flexing her left arm behind her back. On trying to do this she experienced acute pain near her shoulder tip and down her left arm to her elbow.

Her lower torso was relatively pain-free apart from her right hip which sometimes became sore on 'fast walking'. On the Canadian Occupational Performance Measure (COPM) assessment, she had difficulty reaching for any object, fastening her bra, doing up her dress with a zip at the back or lifting her small son, and her sleeping was poor because of pain on moving in bed. Her COPM score was 1/10 for performance and 0/10 for satisfaction. Her pain score was 8/10, her wellbeing score was 7/10.

Treatment

The basic relaxation and shoulder moves were done. Her latissimus dorsi muscle on the left felt tight as did her posterior and anterior deltoid, on the left. However, her shoulder/arm range of movement improved from 80 to 100 degrees. Shoulder exercises were explained and she was given written exercises to take home. Following the pelvic procedure and the second shoulder move on the second treatment, her arm raise was much improved and she said her muscles felt much less tight. On her third treatment, her shoulder/arm ROM improved to 180 degrees, although she still had some tightness on bending her arm outwards and behind her. Triceps and bicep procedures were carried out. To her surprise her right hip was pain-free and she was now running up the stairs.

On her last (fourth) treatment, she had re-injured her arm. Because she was relatively pain-free by this time, she had thrown her arm above her head whilst in bed! Despite this, her pain-score which had been 8/10 was now 4/10 and her wellbeing score remained at 7/10. She had reduced her pain medication for her left shoulder. Although the zip at the back of her dress was frustratingly still out of reach, she could now lift her two-year-old son from a chair-height position and reach out for objects more easily and could now fasten her bra.

Satisfyingly for her, and her therapist, she remained at work. She was amazed at the results that Bowen had achieved and aimed to tell her work colleagues about Bowen Therapy.

CASE STUDY

| *Ann Winter*

The client was referred from the Occupational Health, Safety and Return to Work Services. She had a history of recurrent left-sided lumbar pain radiating into her left knee. This pain, which had previously resolved itself, was now persistent and impinging on her work and everyday life activities. She had attended her GP, who diagnosed sciatica and prescribed pain relief. She was at work, but struggling with her back pain.

Assessment

On 'top-to-toe' assessment, she was slightly out of alignment. She had no complaints and no obvious pain or stiffness in her head, neck, upper arms or thoracic area. Pain experienced around lumbar discs (L4/5) would radiate down her left buttock and hamstrings to the popliteal space behind her knee. On gentle forward flexion she could flex to approximately 50 degrees. On returning extension she had no problems with lateral movement of her spine. She sometimes experienced pins and needles in her left foot. On the COPM measure she had difficulty with walking, sitting, lifting, doing household duties and sleeping. Her COPM score was 3/10 for performance and satisfaction. Her pain score was 7/10 and her wellbeing score was 6/10.

Treatment

The basic relaxation moves and pelvic procedure were performed. The client was sensitive during the moves over the gracilis and adductor longus, which is not unusual with this type of complaint. Pelvic exercises were shown and given, with written instructions to take home. These gentle exercises are carried out each morning before getting out of bed. She was advised not to go to the gym for a few days.

On her second treatment one week later, she reported that she had been sleeping much better, although she had jumped out of bed the day before and experienced really terrible pain in her back and 'felt bad in herself'. She was experiencing pain in her left buttock and above the centre posterior pelvic girdle. Some basic Bowen moves were followed by the hamstring procedure. On doing the coccyx procedure she had pain at the right side of the symptomatic side of the coccyx (assessment is made of the coccyx by gentle palpation to either side, the more 'sore' or 'tender' side being considered the side to work on). There was no coccyx injury reported and she was advised to continue doing her pelvic exercises.

On the third visit she reported that she had a sore back following the last treatment, but was now much better with little back pain reported. As she still had pins and needles in her feet, the quadriceps procedure was performed, with knee, ankle and hammer-toe procedures (this being to activate the fascia on the sole of the feet to aid the remaining sciatic symptoms).

Her fourth and final treatment was two weeks later and no specific back moves were required as there was no need. However, as she had a terrible cold with nasal congestion, the upper respiratory and TMJ moves were performed.

Evaluation

Her COPM score, which had been 3/10 was now 10/10 for performance and satisfaction. Her pain score which had been 7/10 was now 0/10. Her wellbeing score which was 6/10 was now 10/10. She had no difficulty in walking, sitting, lifting or performing household duties. Her pins and needles had resolved.

Conclusion

A very satisfied client. She felt that Bowen had helped keep her at work and to cope with her home and her job without the stress, strain and pain of struggling with back pain and sciatica.

CASE STUDY

| *Ann Tennent*

Michael is a 56-year-old married man with children and grandchildren. He has a job which involves driving, heavy lifting, pushing and pulling. His main hobby is walking with a marching band. He was referred for Bowen Therapy after a year-long history of lower back pain which resulted in a severe attack of sciatic-type pain for 16 days with radiation down his right thigh to his knee which he described as 'burning' in nature.

He had seen his GP and had an X-ray which did not show anything significant, and he was taking pain killers and muscle relaxants while awaiting physiotherapy. His past medical history included an overactive thyroid which was treated with radioactive iodine, and an appendectomy. His medication included tramadol, diclofenac and a muscle relaxant.

On appearance he was bent over, struggling to walk, was unable to straighten his back and obviously in great pain. His wife brought him to his appointment as he was unable to drive. He was having great difficulty with sitting, walking, standing, bending, dressing, bathing, lying and sleeping. After examination, and satisfied there were no red flags, I began treatment.

Treatment

Cushions were positioned under his ankles to reduce the strain on his back. He was able to lie prone on the treatment table for some of the treatment and supine for the remainder. Moves were done over the lower erector spinae and major gluteal muscles initially, gradually adding moves on the iliotibial band, upper back, trapezius and the neck muscles.

On return the following week, he was considerably improved with much reduced back pain, he was now able to sleep, stating 'it was the first time in weeks', and was sitting with more ease. The burning sensation in his knee was much less intense, and his main complaint now was pain in the lateral aspect of his right knee. Similar moves were employed with addition of a move over the coccyx.

By the third treatment one week later his back and knee pain had resolved, but he now had a numb sensation in his knee and was apprehensive going up and down high kerbstones lest he should he trigger pain. He reported having been to see his GP and had informed him of how he had improved with Bowen Therapy. Treatment this time consisted of basic Bowen moves with addition of kidney and psoas moves.

At the fourth treatment the client reported the past week had been his best so far and he was completely pain-free. The final treatment two weeks later was as the previous session. He had by now made a full recovery and was planning a phased return to work.

Another client wrote:

I'm still pain-free thanks to you. Still talking and referring everybody for Bowen Therapy. Before having Bowen Therapy I was having difficulty walking, getting dressed and managing everyday tasks, plus my work life was really difficult and I was on the verge of having to take sick leave.

However, after having Bowen Therapy, I feel great, I am able to walk long distances without having to stop every few minutes, have no problems at work completing my duties and can manage everyday tasks, for example, putting on my socks, which was difficult before the therapy.

I still do the exercises you gave me and have a bath in Epsom salts three times a week. This is fantastic stuff and most of the staff I work with are having one as well. I can't believe the difference Bowen has made to my life and would recommend it to everyone. I am seriously thinking about becoming a therapist myself! (L.A., 8 June 2013)

⁊

Summary of the Project

The West Scotland Bowen Project is one of the first formal pieces of research work to document the efficacy of Bowen Therapy to help with workplace sickness. The project highlights the potential of Bowen Therapy as a serious contender for a treatment that might support staff to work and also as a preventative measure for staff absenteeism by reducing stress levels. Many Bowen practitioners would be happy to run workshops to explain the benefits of Bowen. They need the opportunity to do so and for companies to consider Bowen as a wellbeing benefit for staff.

The added advantage of Bowen is that it is a short form of treatment, so potentially a cheaper form of therapy, with clients often requiring a few sessions only, compared to some other forms of treatment. Bowen also has the added advantage that it is possible to treat several people at the same time, thereby further reducing cost. This is a highly advantageous consideration, especially during the current economic climate.

References

Chartered Institute of Personnel and Development (CIPD) (2012) Absence Management: Annual Survey Report 2012. Available at www.cipd.co.uk/binaries/5982%20AbMan%20SR%20 (WEB).pdf, accessed on 26 June 2014.

Mackereth, P.A., White, K., Cawthorn, A. and Lynch, B. (2005) Improving stressful working lives: complementary therapies, counselling and clinical supervision for staff. *European Journal of Oncology Nursing* 9 (2), 147–154.

Further Reading

Winter, A. and MacAllister, R. (2011) An Evaluation of Health Improvements for Bowen Therapy Clients. Available at www.therapy-training.com/research/scottish-occupational-healt.html, accessed on 19 May 2014.

19

Research

Introduction

One of the problems for therapies such as Bowen and lesser-known Complementary Alternative Medicine (CAM) modalities is that they lack sufficient evidence-based research that makes them acceptable to the medical profession – in other words, research that has undergone clinical trials with blind and double-blinded trials or randomized controlled trials (RCT) with sufficiently large cohorts.

Within the Bowen profession, there is a strong interest in research being conducted to try to explain both how the therapy works and prove its efficacy. One of the problems encountered is the cost involved in the types and sizes of trials that would make them more acceptable and sufficiently evidence-based for the wider medical profession. Although there has been some research published in peer-reviewed journals, the research data is limited. However, this should not preclude therapists from documenting case studies that follow a standardized protocol as these can be an excellent starting point for larger pieces of work that might follow.

The Bowen Technique Literature Review

∾ Michael Morris

Research into the clinical efficacy of Bowen Therapy clearly shows the modality to be an effective, cost-effective and safe treatment that can be used within hospitals or within private practice to treat a range of conditions including injury as a result of trauma or surgery, as well as those relating to the nervous system, mental health and behavioural disorders.

'While it is evident that further research is needed to systematically test the modality before widespread recommendations can be given' they concluded: 'Bowenwork is a cost-effective, non-invasive treatment modality that can be introduced into diverse health care settings such as acute-care hospitals, outpatient settings, and rural environments' (Hansen and Taylor-Piliae 2011, p.5).

A Tough Act to Follow...?

Tom Bowen's work was first assessed in 1975 in the Report of the Committee of Inquiry into Chiropractic, Osteopathy, Homeopathy, and Naturopathy by the Victorian Government, which found that he saw more than 13,000 clients a year with an 80 per cent success rate in alleviating symptoms for both acute injuries and chronic conditions (Hansen and Taylor-Piliae 2011).

A Systematic Review

Hansen and Taylor-Piliae (2011) conducted a systematic review of available published literature relevant to Bowen Therapy from 1997 to 2009 with the aim of examining the methodologies utilized and summarizing the scientific findings to that time. A systematic review is defined as 'a review of the evidence on a clearly formulated question that uses systematic and explicit methods to identify, select and critically appraise relevant primary research, and to extract and analyse data from the studies that are included in the review' (Centre for Reviews and Dissemination 2012). Systematic reviews with narrowly defined review questions provide specific answers to specific questions, and can be replicated if necessary. The objectives of the systematic review were to assess the literature available on the complementary approach to healing known as Bowenwork (as it is called in the USA) and to examine reported research methods. The literature search included the following search terms: Bowen Technique, Bowen Therapy, Bowtech and Bowenwork.

Of 309 citations included in the Systematic Review, 15 published articles met the inclusion criteria. Studies were included if (1) they referenced the original Bowenwork, (2) provided health-related outcomes and (3) provided quantitative or qualitative data – eight research studies and seven case studies. Individual studies aimed to assess the effectiveness of Bowen Therapy for a number of health-related outcomes, including frozen shoulder, hamstring flexibility, work-related injuries and quality of life. The majority of these studies reported favourable outcomes for pain relief, fewer migraines and improved shoulder mobility. However, not all of the studies reviewed reported improvements in health-related outcomes following treatments using Bowenwork.

To date, only two randomized control trials using Bowenwork have been reported: Marr, Baker, Lambon and Perry's (2011) investigation into the effects of the Bowen Technique on hamstring flexibility over time, and Hipmair and colleagues (2012) into the efficacy of Bowen therapy in post-operative pain management. In Marr's study, the intervention group of 120 subjects receiving a single Bowen Treatment, the study found significant within-subject and between-subject differences for the Bowen group, with continuing increases in flexibility levels observed over one week and reported a statistically significant improvement in hamstring flexibility using an electro-goniometer (independent t test, $p < 0.01$).

Hipmair and colleagues (2012) produced some research funded by the Upper Austrian Medical Society that looked into the Efficacy of Bowen therapy in post-operative pain management – a single blinded (randomized) controlled trial, involving 91 patients. The population was randomly split into three groups: in addition to standard post-operative pain therapy, group A underwent Bowen therapy, group B received a manual sham therapy, and group C constituted the control group without additional treatment. Post-operative pain was assessed with the visual analogue scale (VAS). The results showed a trend of lower VAS scores in the Bowen group within the first two days of treatment (p-values < 0.001 and < 0.008, respectively), indicating that in the early period after knee replacement Bowen therapy may be an effective additional treatment tool for pain reduction.

A total of seven case studies reported between 1999 and 2008 on Bowenwork were reviewed. These case studies are defined as reports in the literature by practitioners who described a client's presentation of symptoms, the course of treatment and an observed health-related outcome. Similar to the research study findings above, the case studies reviewed revealed a common theme of relief of back and neck pain and improvement in other mobility and soft-tissue dysfunction.

Applications of Bowenwork are many, according to the articles reviewed. Over half of these studies (53%) reviewed reported that Bowenwork was effective for pain reduction and 33 per cent reported improved mobility.

Other Documented Studies

The first study to take place in the UK was by Kinnear and Baker (1999), titled the Frozen Shoulder Research Programme. Results from this show that Bowen significantly improves shoulder function through increasing range of motion and reducing pain. The improvement in shoulder function was significantly greater for the treatment group than the placebo group, and placebo patients who had not responded showed considerable improvements once Bowen was administered. One hundred subjects were randomly assigned to either a treatment or placebo group.

A Whitaker, Gilliam and Seba (1997) study found that Bowen clearly had a positive health effect, particularly on fibromyalgia subjects. These results were documented by measuring changes on the autonomic nervous system (ANS) balance by heart rate variability (HRV) and clinical assessment. The data showed the fibromyalgia group showed signs of a decrease in sympathetic nervous system activity, and an increase in parasympathetic nervous system activity.

A study conducted by Pritchard (1993) at the University of Melbourne, Australia, indicated that the Bowen Technique consistently brought about an enhancement of individuals' positive moods, reducing feelings of tension, anxiety, fatigue, anger, depression and confusion. The therapy was also found to be associated with a decrease in heart rate, indicating a suppression of sympathetic activity, and a trend for an extensive decrease in individuals' general muscle tension.

The Hipmair *et al.* (2012) study aimed to evaluate the effect of Bowen Therapy in pain management after total knee replacement. The study of 91 subjects found a decreased pain score in the early post-operative period and concluded that, in the early period after knee replacement, Bowen Therapy may be an effective additional treatment tool for pain reduction.

Winter and MacAllister (2011) have reported on extensive occupational health research in which 778 individuals were allocated Bowen Therapy with a range of presenting conditions. The report showed significant clinical improvement in the clients' occupational abilities, a significant improvement in general health and wellbeing, and high client satisfaction with the treatment. The clients assessed as part of this research report ranged in age from 19 to 67 years and their health limitations were assessed using the Canadian Occupational Performance Measure (COPM) at both entry and discharge.

Duncan *et al.* (2011) undertook a pilot study of 14 subjects involved in a case series format to explore the potential impact of Bowen Therapy in chronic stroke. The authors found, as a result of this pilot study, that Bowen Therapy was associated with improvements in neuromuscular function and recommended further research.

In addition to the research outlined above, the following studies investigating the efficacy of Bowen Therapy have been recently conducted, or are underway.

A feasibility study designed to investigate the use of Bowen Therapy as a treatment for people who live with chronic, non-specific lower back pain (Morris 2012). Thirty-seven participants were randomly allocated to either receive three treatments of Bowen or 'Sham Bowen' (blind to treatment). Pain and functioning levels, psychosocial/somatic changes and general health were measured and 24 'categories' developed. The Bowen group recorded a positive change by the second follow-up in 20 of these categories. By contrast, the control group showed an improvement in only 12 of these categories at the same time point. This research is currently being documented for publication; meanwhile, however, an abstract of the study is available (Morris 2012).

Flinders University, Adelaide, Australia, conducted a randomized controlled trial to evaluate changes to lymphatic flow in the trapezius muscle following Bowen Therapy treatments in patients with damaged fascia due to radiotherapy, surgery or soft tissue injuries. The results of this study will be known late in 2013.

The Bowen Therapy Professional Association (BTPA) of the UK is currently conducting a national study into the treatment of repetitive strain injury with Bowen Therapy (case series) (BTPA 2014).

A US pilot study (quasi-experimental design, PhD dissertation) has been conducted to examine the feasibility of using Bowenwork as a complementary intervention for symptom management of breast cancer treatment-related lymphoedema in 21 female breast cancer survivors. Participants received four sessions of Bowen Therapy, which was 'shown to be an effective management strategy' with statistically significant improvements in mental health, quality of life, daily functional status, reducing arm circumference and increasing range of motion. The researcher, Christine Hansen, has recommended a full-scale study to further explore the findings. The complete PhD is publicly available (Hansen 2012).

A Multidisciplinary Team (MDT) Medical Model, which includes Bowen Therapy, began in late 2011 in the UK under a service level agreement with the National Health Service (NHS). Initiated after two audit reports on Bowen Therapy were prepared for the NHS, results after the first six months showed a high 47 per cent discharge rate among sufferers of chronic pain. The lead service centre, the Northern Integrated Health Practice, works closely with the pain management team at the participating NHS hospital(s). Approximately 40 patients per week have been seen from the NHS as part of Tier 3 secondary care, which involves a stringent monitoring and measurement process. The pilot project is already expanding into other regional NHS trusts. The contact for the project is Paula Esson, Clinic Director, Northern Integrative Health Practice (www.healthnorth.co.uk), which is an approved NHS Centre for pain services (see below for more details of this project and the role for Bowen within the NHS).

ℰℛ

CAM Research

The Cochrane Collaboration for Complementary and Alternative Medicine (CAM) has accepted the following as a definition: 'CAM is diagnosis, treatment and/or prevention which complements mainstream medicine by contributing as a common whole, by satisfying a demand not met by orthodoxy or by diversifying the conceptual framework of medicine' (Ernst, Cohen and Stone 2004, p.156; Ernst 2000). Whilst in Bowen it is against our professional code of conduct to make any medical diagnosis, the rest of the definition would be an acceptable premise for Bowen work.

Various surveys about CAM and data from 2000 suggests that approximately 20 per cent of the UK population (42% in the USA, 48% in Australia) are using CAM (Ernst 2000; Ernst, Cohen and Stone 2004; Frenkel and Borkan 2003; Ong *et al.* 2002). Although this data now seems a little out of date, even if the figure remained similar (i.e. 20% using CAM in the UK), that is still a reasonable percentage of the population, and is likely to have increased (I am basing this anecdotally on the increase in my clinics over the past ten years). It is therefore interesting to explore the reasons why clients both want and like CAM.

Based on the CAM literature, it seems that one reason that people like CAM is because the consultation sessions are frequently longer than allowed for in NHS and Western medicine settings, allowing clients an increased period of time to 'tell their story' and to be listened to (Ernst *et al.* 2004; Frankel and Borkan 2003;

Hyland, Lewith and Westoby 2003). To be listened to may also be linked to people's dissatisfaction with the length of time of other medical encounters which they find 'brief and disempowering' (Hyland *et al.* 2003). Patients may therefore have a preference for a more holistic encounter, frequently completely dismissed within a Western medicine setting. Few medical practitioners take a holistic view of the body, seeing only the injured part (e.g. merely looking a shoulder injury), without taking into account the patient's other injuries or problems, including social and psychological factors. As Hyland *et al.* (2003, p.34) write, most patients express 'a dislike of the reductionist, mechanical model of medicine and the preference for a holistic, integrative model of health'.

Bowen (CAM) practitioners often encounter clients who have chronic and long-term conditions such as cancer, MS, fibroymyalgia or chronic fatigue, all of whom present challenges to the medical profession in different ways. With cancer patients, it can be because it is very difficult to eliminate some of the unpleasant physical and psychological effects of treatment (see Chapter 17). With other conditions, particularly those that affect the autonomic nervous system, there isn't necessarily a 'cure' as such, so CAM is often used to support both these types of patient groups (Frenkel and Borkan 2003; Ong *et al.* 2002). Such clients are some of the most frequent types encountered in the clinic, as they continue to seek help for their myriad of symptoms. Whilst doctors might be aware that their patient is receiving CAM, they seldom enter into dialogue with a CAM practitioner, even if that CAM practitioner is more than willing to do so. However, this depends upon the attitude of the doctor and the time they might have to dialogue with a CAM therapist. This is most likely to happen in a palliative care setting where CAM therapists volunteer or in some larger hospitals where they might be paid to work in this type of setting.

Although as Bowen practitioners we couldn't do without the formalized medical expertise and diagnosis of our doctors and Western/orthodox medicine, it would be more useful if physicians would consider CAM as a way of supporting patients in the true spirit of 'complementary' medicine. Frenkel and Borkan (2003) suggest that, although medical schools are now starting to teach trainee doctors about CAM, this is a neglected area of research, in particular the nature of the dialogue between the medical profession and the CAM practitioner.

I recently had a third-year medical student attend my clinic, who wrote that:

> I was given the opportunity to shadow Isobel. It immediately became apparent that her clients benefited from the holistic approach that she took. At the beginning of every consultation, she would discuss all aspects of the client's life and asked them to give themselves an overall energy score. The clients found this particularly useful as they felt as though the therapist was considering everything that was going on in their lives.
>
> The users had a wide range of health complaints. One client had been treated for back and shoulder pain in March 2010. She returned to the clinic with neck

pain and said that she had not encountered any back or shoulder problems since her first Bowen therapy session last year. She was also 'amazed' at the Bowen practitioner's ability to pinpoint exactly where the pain was in her neck without the client showing it to her. It is evident that she was more than satisfied with the health benefits provided by Bowen therapy. I also learned that the benefits of Bowen therapy can be enjoyed by everyone, from neonates to adults.

On the whole it was clear that clients chose Bowen therapy as it is non-invasive, gentle and allows the body to repair itself using its innate mechanisms. (A. Ragavan, from Isobel Knight's website, www.bowenworks.org)

Although there are many good reasons for patients to seek CAM, not everyone is in a position to do so (unless it is provided within an NHS setting) owing to the costs of seeing CAM therapists, even if they offer discounted treatment sessions. Therefore, CAM clients are more likely to be those with higher incomes since CAM is usually only available privately and is therefore often too expensive for many – something that is clearly unfair. Tom Bowen himself did free clinics for the disabled and for children, and many Bowen practitioners are generous enough to still offer low-cost clinics. My own view is that I would rather someone was able to have access to some treatment, where I know it will benefit them, than deny them recovery owing to financial constraints. However, CAM practitioners also have their own income to earn within altruistic limits.

Many medical practitioners are disparaging of CAM therapists owing to their perceived lack of training (Ernst *et al.* 2004; Vickers 2000). However, this is now improving with the introduction of regulatory bodies such as the Complementary and Natural Healthcare Council (CNHC) that ensure standards of training, professional conduct and continuing professional development. Bowen practitioners are required to have completed an anatomy and physiology course, First Aid, as well as successfully completing all the assessments within their Bowen training course. The length of the core Bowen curriculum training varies a little throughout the world, from nine months to three years in some countries. Additionally, in order to remain a registered practitioner of the Bowen Association UK, it is also a requirement to do a minimum of 16 hours of continuing professional development on an annual basis. CAM therapists are also not permitted by the Advertising Standards Agency to use any such word as 'heal' or 'cure' or list any specific medical condition they may purport to treat. For example, they may say that Bowen might help with elbow problems but not list 'tennis elbow', even if it is something that Bowen might well help with – because 'tennis elbow' is a named medical term. It is to be hoped that there are now fewer charlatans out there, as regulations are more strictly enforced. This greatly improves the chances of CAM practitioners being more respected by the medical profession at large. However, we are still some way off many medical professionals accepting and valuing the work of CAM and Bowen – hence the need for this book!

The largest argument against CAM and Bowen for the purposes of this book is the lack of evidence-based research, which is why doctors continue to be dismissive and disparaging of CAM (Ernst 1995; Ernst *et al.* 2004; Hyland 2003; Mason, Tovey and Long 2002; Vickers 2000). Michael Morris describes some positive and constructive ways forward below.

Challenges in Designing a Bowen Study

ↄ Michael Morris

Research in Complementary and Alternative Medicine (CAM) has been seriously hampered by a lack of research infrastructure and funding, lack of research expertise among CAM practitioners, lack of appropriate research models and strategies, as well as the scepticism of the conventional scientific community. The Wellcome Trust (Wellcome 2011) is aware of the limited research capacity within the field of CAM, which the House of Lords (2000) inquiry addressed, namely that the majority of CAM practitioners have a number of constraints that make it difficult for them to pursue a research career. Many CAM practitioners do not have time to undertake research, due to the demands of running a practice. Furthermore, there are currently few career development opportunities in CAM research; more is needed to attract people into this field.

Manual therapy has a long history of use in the healing of body ailments. Manual techniques pre-date the organized pharmaceutical industry by centuries, having been in medical literature since Greek and Roman writings (Lederman *et al.* 2005). Willard (2005) states that how manual therapy approaches could alter psychological problems as well as improve the general health of the individual, was not appreciated until a better understanding of the emotional (limbic) system and its relationship to the neuroendocrine system was developed.

Many researchers have often struggled with the challenge of identifying appropriate comparison or control interventions in CAM pain research. It is of fundamental importance in the design of rigorous CAM research to create 'true' controls that do not appear to cause beneficial or harmful effects in a research trial. Placebo controls are a critical component throughout scientific research, and necessitate appropriate sham controls. The development of placebo procedures and interventions is therefore crucial to the development of scientifically rigorous pain research in CAM.

In many instances, particularly in CAM research, shams are designed to control for psychological effects in an attempt to examine what is believed to be the active part of an intervention (Lund, Naslund and Lundeburg 2009). The goal of using a sham protocol is to control for the potentially therapeutic effects of touch and belief, which are components of the placebo effect. When participants are blinded to group assignment, the placebo effect can be controlled. However, it is challenging to design a sham protocol that is both ineffective (carries little or no therapeutic effect) and plausible (Noll *et al.* 2004). When attempting to establish the efficacy of a given procedure, the study design must be crafted in a way that has the potential to provide an unequivocal answer. A sham control has been broadly defined in the Merriam-Webster Dictionary as 'a treatment or procedure that is performed as a control and that is similar to, but omits a key therapeutic element of the treatment or procedure under investigation'. In developing a sham control, it is important to aim to create something that is realistic and plausible enough for the participant to believe they are receiving the 'proper' treatment, and yet is devoid of any therapeutic effect. Montague (1987) notes that tactile stimulation has profound effects, both physiological and behavioural, upon the organism. In designing a sham control, it is important that touch is a primary factor in both interventions; otherwise the effect of touching/being touched could affect the results. Based upon this, creating a sham control which involved touching the participant was paramount; however, the challenge is in designing a method which still involves contact with the skin (directly or through light clothing) and be a light touch move, but not involve the three elements which make up a Bowen move (skin slack, pressure and a rolling-type move).

However, there are differing opinions in the use of a sham treatment as the control group within a research study. The misuse of sham controls in examining the efficacy or effectiveness of CAM has created numerous problems, according to Horn, Balk and Gold (2010). The theoretical justification for incorporating a sham is questionable. The sham does not improve our control of bias and leads to relativistic data that, in most instances, has no appropriate interpretation with regards to treatment efficacy. However, while the use of sham controls is likely to provide the highest quality and potentially most generalizable clinical trial data, as Sutherland (2007) writes, the use of a sham control must be carefully contemplated in light of its appropriateness and feasibility, and applied within a formalized ethical framework.

Overall, though, sham control arms, such as other placebo control arms in controlled clinical trials, have the potential benefit of reducing the introduction of bias, particularly with regard to three critical areas of experimental design and conduct: treatment allocation, treatment adherence and the assessment of subjective outcomes modified by treatment. Thus, concludes Sutherland (2007), sham controls are particularly useful for trials of devices or procedures with subjective endpoints (e.g. symptoms) and provide a robust means of controlling for the ancillary effects of a procedure, optimizing the ability of the investigator to evaluate for a placebo or procedural effect in an unbiased fashion. According to Birch (2006), for a sham to be seen as effective, it must capture the 'nonspecific' elements of the treatment without containing those that are 'specific' to the research question at hand.

Psychological factors often play a significant role in the development of and adaptation to chronic low back pain (LBP) (Goldberg and Lox 1999). Pre-existing depression, anxiety and stress, together with lack of effective coping skills, may predispose individuals to back pain, for example. Research has shown that having a variety of coping strategies, a person's belief in their ability to control their pain and the level of catastrophizing about their condition are strongly associated with healthy adjustment in chronic pain patients and their families (Simmons, Kumar and Lechelt 1996).

Once LBP has occurred, it will impact on the quality of life of the individual and the family. Often, while this can be a disruptive influence, it can also produce what is termed 'secondary gain'. This describes a situation in which an illness can produce advantages for a patient, such as increased attention and family support or disability from work. Addressing these kinds of reactions to chronic pain is an important part of successful treatment (Stenger 1992).

From clinical experience, there is no 'typical response' following a Bowen treatment, and subjects report changes on various levels, and not necessarily an immediate reduction in pain levels. Often the assessment of outcome means measuring changes in severity of symptoms and assumes that treatment will reduce symptom severity (Ostelo and de Vet 2005). As such, trying to measure any treatment outcome using just one method may prove frivolous – indeed, as Bowen can have an effect on a biopsychosocial level, then a measure, or collection of measures, must be used to capture the correct outcome following treatment. Therefore, the choice of a measure, or set of measures, for assessing LBP should be made based on several factors including the goal of therapy, setting, ease of administration and responsiveness to change. A number of clinical tools designed for evaluating the functional status of patients with LBP have been developed (Grotle, Brox and Vollestad 2005), and in more recent times several score systems have been developed to assess the functional status of patients with LBP (Beurskens *et al.* 1995). A better understanding of the biological component of LBP in relation and, most importantly, in addition to psychosocial factors is important for a more rational approach to management of LBP (Hancock *et al.* 2011).

There is growing evidence to suggest that pain intensity, in combination with its interference with activities, contributes to an underlying construct of global pain severity (Von Korff, Jensen and Karoly 2000). The idea of the subject self-reporting also highlights a more recent idea that back pain has much more of an effect on the person than just the pain or function (or lack of) may suggest.

ᴄᴏ

Conclusion

We all have to start somewhere. If every Bowen practitioner could start by producing some case studies to share with GPs and/or other medical professionals and then join forces with other practitioners to produce larger-scale RCT research, we might find, as Michael Morris suggests, that there is a real way forward to present, document and work towards sufficiently evidence-based Bowen work.

References

Beurskens, A.J., Devet, H.C., Koke, A.J. Vanderheijden, G.J. and Knipschild, P.G. (1995) Measuring the functional status of patients with low-back-pain – assessment of the quality of 4 disease-specific questionnaires. *Spine* 20 (9), 1017–1028.

Birch, S. (2006) A review and analysis of placebo treatments, placebo effects, and placebo controls in trials of medical procedures when sham is not inert. *Journal of Alternative and Complementary Medicine* 12 (3), 303–310.

BTPA (2014) National study to show how complementary therapy can help alleviate RSI. Bowen Therapy Professional Association. Available at www.btpa.co/Bowen/repetitive-strain-injury-bowen-study.asp, accessed on 21 May 2014.

Centre for Reviews and Dissemination, University of York (2012) Systematic Reviews: CRD's guidance for undertaking reviews in health care. Available at www.york.ac.uk/inst/crd/pdf/Systematic_Reviews.pdf, accessed on 26 June 2014.

Duncan, B., McHugh, P., Houghton, F. and Wilson, C. (2011) Improved motor function with Bowen Therapy for rehabilitation in chronic stroke: a pilot study. *Journal of Primary Health Care* 3(1), 53–57.

Ernst, E. (1995) Complementary medicine: common misconceptions. *Journal of the Royal Society of Medicine* 88, 244–247.

Ernst, E. (2000) The role of complementary and alternative medicine. *British Medical Journal* 321, 1133–1135.

Ernst, E., Cohen, M. and Stone, J. (2004) Ethical problems arising in evidence based complementary and alternative medicine. *Journal of Medical Ethics* 30, 156–159.

Frenkel, M. and Borkan, J. (2003) An approach for integrating complementary-alternative medicine into primary care. *Family Practice* 20 (3), 324–332.

Goldberg, R.T.L. and Lox, D.M (1999) The role of the psyche in low back pain: the mind-body connection. *Physical Medicine and Rehabilitation* 13, 411–426.

Grotle, M., Brox, J.I. and Vollestad, N.K. (2005) Functional status and disability questionnaires: What do they assess? A systematic review of back-specific outcome questionnaires. *Spine* 30 (1), 130–140.

Hancock, M., Maher, C., Laslett, M., Hay, E. and Koes, B. (2011) What happened to the 'bio' in the bio-psycho-social model of low back pain? *European Spine Journal* 20 (12), 2105–2110.

Hansen, C. (2011) What is Bowenwork®? A Systematic Review. *The Journal of Alternative and Complementary Medicine* 17 (11), 1001–1006.

Hansen, C.A. (2012) A Pilot Study on Bowenwork® for Symptom Management of Women Breast Cancer Survivors with Lymphedema. PhD thesis, University of Arizona. Available at www.nursing.arizona.edu/Library/Christine%20Hansen%20-%20Dissertation%20March%202012.pdf, accessed on 26 June 2014.

Hipmair, G., Ganser, D., Bohler, N., Schimetta, W. and Polz, W. (2012) Efficacy of Bowen Therapy in postoperative pain management – a single blinded (randomized) controlled trial (translated from German). Available at www.therapy-training.com/research/bowen-pain-research.html, accessed on 19 May 2014.

Horn, B., Balk, J. and Gold, J. (2010) *Revisiting the Sham: Is It all Smoke and Mirrors? Evidence-Based Complementary and Alternative Medicine.* Cairo: Hindawi Publishing Corporation.

House of Lords (2000) Science and Technology – Sixth Report. Available at www.publications. parliament.uk/pa/ld199900/ldselect/ldsctech/123/12301.htm, accessed on 19 May 2014.

Hyland, M. (2003) Methodology for the scientific evaluation of complementary and alternative medicine. *Complementary Therapies in Medicine* 11, 146–153.

Hyland, M., Lewith, G. and Westoby, C. (2003) Developing a measure of attitudes: the holistic complementary and alternative medicine questionnaire. *Complementary Therapies in Medicine* II, 3–38.

Kinnear, H. and J. Baker (1999) Frozen shoulder study: study results. Available at http:// thebowentechnique.com/frozen-shoulder-study, accessed on 26 June 2014.

Lederman, E., Cramer, G.D., Donatelli, R. and Willard, F.H. (2005) *The Science and Practice of Manual Therapy.* London: Elsevier.

Lund, I., Naslund, J. and Lundeburg, T. (2009) Minimal acupuncture is not a valid placebo control in randomised controlled trials of acupuncture: a physiologist's perspective. *Chinese Medicine* 4, 1.

Marr, M., Baker, J., Lambon, N. and Perry, J. (2011) The effects of the Bowen Technique on hamstring flexibility over time: a randomised controlled trial. *Journal of Bodywork Movement Therapy* 15 (3), 281–290.

Mason, S., Tovey, P. and Long, A.F. (2002) Evaluating complementary medicine: methodological challenges of randomised controlled trials. *British Medical Journal* 325 (7368), 832–834

Montagu, A. (1987) *Touching: Human Significance of the Skin.* New York: HarperPerennial.

Morris, M. (2012) The Bowen Technique and Low Back Pain. Bowen Therapy Professional Association. Available at www.btpa.co/Bowen/studies/low_back_pain-study.asp, accessed on 21 May 2014.

Noll, D., Degenhardt, B., Stuart, M., McGovern, R. and Matteson, M. (2004) Effectiveness of a sham protocol and adverse effects. *Journal of the American Osteopathic Association* 104, 107–113.

Ong, C., Peterson, S., Bodeker, G. and Stewart-Brown, S. (2002) Health status of people using complementary and alternative medical practitioner services in 4 English counties. *American Journal of Public Health* 92 (10), 1653–1656.

Ostelo, R.W.J.G. and de Vet, H.C.W. (2005) Clinically important outcomes in low back pain. Best practice and research. *Clinical Rheumatology* 19(4), 593–607.

Pritchard, A.G. (1993) *The Psychophysiological Effects of the Bowen Technique.* Psychophysiology major research project, Swinburne University, Melobourne.

Simmons, M.J., Kumar, S. and Lechelt, E. (1996) Psychological factors in disabling low back pain: causes or consequences? *Disability and Rehabilitation* 18 (4), 161–168.

Stenger, E.M. (1992) Chronic back pain: view from a psychiatrist's office. *Clinical Journal of Pain* 8 (3), 242–246.

Sutherland, E.R. (2007) Sham procedure versus usual care as the control in clinical trials of devices: which is better? *Proceedings of the American Thoracic Society* 4, 574–576.

Vickers, A. (2000) Recent advances in complementary medicine. *British Medical Journal* 321, 683–686.

Von Korff, M., Jensen, M.P. and Karoly, P. (2000) Assessing global pain severity by self-report in clinical and health services research. *Spine* 25 (24), 3140–3151.

Wellcome (2011) *Policy on Complementary and Alternative Medicine.* London: Wellcome Trust.

Whitaker, J.A., Gilliam, P.P. and Seba, D.B. (1997) A gentle hands on healing method that effects autonomic nervous system as measured by heart rate variability and clinical assessment. Paper presented at the American Academy of Medicine 32nd Annual Conference.

Willard, F.H. (2005) *The Science and Practice of Manual Therapy*. London: Elsevier.

Winter, A. and MacAllister, R. (2011) An Evaluation of Health Improvements for Bowen Therapy Clients. Available at www.bowen-technique.co.uk/pdfs/Occupational%20Health%20Report.pdf, accessed on 19 May 2014.

20

The Role of the Bowen Technique in the NHS

Paula Esson

Patient choice has been a priority for successive UK governments since the 1970s. Since 2008 every person has had the right to choose from five providers, including the independent sector. However, the current reality is somewhat different in the UK, where intervention is often slow, incomplete, disjointed and frustrating. This is especially true in the world of musculoskeletal care where the Bowen Technique comes into its own. How many times do we hear of people who have been around the houses, with their treatment being late and loaded towards pharmaceutical intervention together with a reductionist approach?

If a practitioner approaches their local medical practice to offer Bowen as a service, the usual response, with a few exceptions, is one of 'a square peg in a round hole'. Although as therapists we can wholeheartedly see how we can help take the pressures off the NHS, contribute to reduce the high cost of unnecessary hospital care and free up GPs to work with acute scenarios, somehow we hit no end of walls and obstacles.

There are many reasons for this, the main ones being:

- What Bowen is offering as a service is difficult to integrate into the local commissioning service documents. In order to fund Bowen, they will need to de-commission another.

- The non-evidence-based methods and holistic aspects of the Bowen Technique meet with resistance and an inability to sit with the system.

- Bowen is competing against very strong established systems of delivery. Bowen has not yet been fully demonstrated as a stand alone treatment within the seven main pillars of the NHS change model (NHS 2014).

How Has Northern Integrative Health Practice (NIHP) Moved beyond These Obstacles?

General practitioners have recently been handed the budgetary responsibility to deliver primary healthcare in England. They are searching for solutions to the developing pressures of complex health scenarios. Local Clinical Commissioning Group (CCG) commissioning documents can be found at NHS England (2014).

Nationally, the model is now moving in a healthier and more proactive fashion based on Dr John Travis's model *the illness-wellness continuum* from the 1970s (Travis and Ryan 2004), which demonstrates beautifully how dedication to change takes tenacity and pure determination over many decades. A true integrative model works wholeheartedly in prevention and early intervention, leaving acute health care to the hospitals in the case of a medical crisis.

There is now a drive to move 50 per cent of healthcare out of hospitals and into primary care and the community. This is where the Bowen Technique has a huge role to play in the future, as part of an interdisciplinary model of care for the NHS, and one that NIHP is successfully demonstrating. There is a drive to reform the NHS model to include many external providers who are vigilant, professional, capable, measurable and innovative, moving the integrative model to the population as a whole.

In 2012 the Any Qualified Provider (AQP) scheme was released to open up the provision across a number of key areas. In April 2014 this was replaced by 'Contracts Finder' – for more details, see Contracts Finder (2014). Specifically, the NHS is looking for providers who can administer:

- musculoskeletal services for neck and back pain

- primary psychological services

- podiatry services

- diagnostic services closer to home (e.g. respiratory and cardiac services)

- pain management planning such as that offered by the Pain Toolkit (www. paintoolkit.org).

By drawing services together and incorporating the Bowen Technique into a model that includes key services, we have shown that it is possible to deliver all aspects of our work and operate within a therapeutic and clinical team. To achieve this for the public and the awareness of Bowen nationally, all skill bases need to pull together with the client's wellbeing at the centre of every decision, intervention and action we take. As a therapist with a deep passion for excellent outcomes for the client, working in the world of system management, strategy and whole decision-making scenarios is a challenge, and can feel uncomfortable. However, in order to put Bowen firmly on the map and achieve critical mass in terms of awareness, this is exactly what is needed. We need to embrace the process, and challenge the structure with integrity, and solutions that work. The essence and magic of Bowen for the individual is not lost within this process; it provides a great platform to reach thousands who are suffering.

Adding a Robust Approach to Healthcare

Some criticisms made about complementary healthcare are well founded and need to be addressed. To ensure a totally professional and complete service to the client, clinics need to consider the following:

- communicating observations, actions and outcomes to the client's GP by letter or fax

- regular team meetings to discuss action plans for the client

- introducing clinical governance and quality assurance (ISI 1009/CQC)

- measuring the client's progress using a number of tools (see Chapter 19)

- using an expert patient programme to gather testimonials to act as an important compass to your business development

- attending local CCG meetings to share experience and positive progress.

The Dynamic Future for the Bowen Technique inside the NHS

Bowen has the potential to work in Tiers 1–3. The key is to offer solutions to general practitioners and hospitals that make sense financially, strategically and in line with the commissioners' requirements as part of a wider scope model.

References

Contracts Finder (2014) Home page. Available at https://online.contractsfinder.businesslink.gov.uk, accessed on 23 May 2014.

NHS (2014) *NHS Change Model.* Available at www.changemodel.nhs.uk, accessed on 21 May 2014.

NHS England (2014) *CCG Maps.* Available at www.england.nhs.uk/resources/ccg-maps, accessed on 24 May 2014.

Travis, J.W. and Ryan, R.S. (2004) *Wellness Workbook: How to Achieve Enduring Health and Vitality.* Berkeley, CA: Celestial Arts.

Resources

Websites

British Pain Society
www.britishpainsociety.org

Getting Bowen into the National Health Service – What Is AQP? (webinar with Paula Esson)
www.trainings.co.uk/previous-webinars

Northern Integrative Health Practice
www.healthnorth.co.uk

Further Reading

Department of Health (2010) *Equity and Excellence: Liberating the NHS White Paper.* London: Stationery Office. Available at www.gov.uk/government/publications/liberating-the-nhs-white-paper, accessed on 19 May 2014.

NHS England (2013) NHS England launches revolutionary plan to get patients more involved in their care (press release 25 September). Available at www.england.nhs.uk/wp-content/uploads/2013/09/trans-part-pn.pdf, accessed on 19 May 2014.

Appendix 1

Exercise as a Support to Bowen Work

This appendix is a brief overview of some types of exercise that can support Bowen work between sessions. It is by no means designed to be a complete list. There are many types of exercise that can be helpful in repair and in maintenance, but this is a highly individual thing and needs careful individual attention. The key to successful rehabilitation is, above all, good advice, something that is often hard to come by. The following information is for guidance only – it is essential to see a fully qualified specialist instructor to get the full benefit of any exercise regime and, crucially, to avoid making a condition worse, something that is all too common with some clients who do a lot of gym work.

It is also important to understand the impact of shoes on people's health, especially if they walk or run. Some shoes, for example, will have a soft heel, making it equivalent to walking on sand, which will have little if any benefit to their fascial fitness and will also stress their calf muscles. There are many different theories about shoes, but very few (if any) take into account the importance of biotensegrity. Generally, it is good advice for clients to remove their shoes when walking about the house and, if they are doing sport, to vary their footwear.

Tom Bowen advised most clients to walk at least 20 minutes a day. This still remains good advice, as walking increases breathing, gets the lymphatic system moving, increases vascular supply to the limbs and improves cardiovascular fitness. Even for people with low back pain, walking only increases the pressure on the lumbar intervertebral discs by around 15 per cent (Nachemson and Elfstrom 1970). Although bed rest was traditionally recommended for patients with low back pain around the time Bowen was working, it seems he didn't go along with that advice. In fact, bed rest has now been shown clearly to slow recovery from sciatica. The reasons why some clients have a reluctance to exercise is discussed in Chapters 2 and 7 by Kelly Clancy, but it is clear that types of exercise that combine gentle stretching with mobilization can be very helpful for the majority of clients (see Chapter 15 for specific thoughts on stretching). With the list below, we have purposely emphasized approaches that encourage more 'body awareness', or what are called somatic exercises. In fact, it can be helpful to bring a more somatic approach to any exercise regime that we do, as well as encouraging clients to be more body aware when doing everyday activities such as gardening, cycling or even sitting at a desk. Whole meditation practices can be built around simple activities such as walking.

Somatic Practices

Hanna coined the term somatics, which may be defined as an intricate study discussing the body from a first-person perspective. Hanna said that 'Somatics is the field which studies the soma; namely, the body as perceived from within by first-person perception' (Hanna 1986, p.4). Somatics takes a holistic view of a mind–body relationship and integrates them both, and this would make sense in people having control and ownership of their body (Eddy 2002; Green 2002). The value of using the somatic approach with people is an enhanced awareness of their body and how best to care for it, for example, when injured (Brodie and Lobel 2004; Fortin 2003; Knaster 1996). Somatic work supports Bowen work because following a Bowen treatment the body has been subtly introduced into a new way of being that is more efficient, following work on remodelling the fascia and bodily alignment. Somatic practices will take this work further and encourage the body into an even more efficient way of moving and 'being' in the body. Many of us have a very poor awareness of our bodies, so somatics will support this concept along with Bowen work.

What Are Somatic Practices?

Somatic practices encompass Body-Mind Centering (BMC), Feldenkrais Method (FM), Alexander Technique (AT), yoga, the Skinner Releasing Technique and Laban Movement Analysis (Eddy 2002). Somatics is about developing a 'one-ness' with the body and establishing unity within body and mind. Fortin describes this as 'connectedness'. She writes: 'When practising somatics I sometimes get an incredible feeling of being at home (in my body), of being so peaceful…' (Fortin 2003, p.4).

The Feldenkrais Method®

The Feldenkrais Method® (FM) is about increasing the amount and variety of movement a person is capable of (Bober 2003). In Moshe Feldenkrais's words, 'You can't do what you want 'til you know what you are doing, and most of us don't know what we are doing' (Fitt 1996, p.325).

Feldenkrais practitioner Maggy Burrowes writes:

The Feldenkrais Method® (FM) uses movement as a way of developing greater self-awareness: Moshe Feldenkrais was as interested in helping people to free themselves from habitual thinking as he was to free them from habitual action. He designed his work with the intention of integrating thinking, feeling, sensation and action in order to restore and improve proprioception in children and adults. He combined his experience of engineering and judo teaching with his knowledge of child development and came up with a process designed to give people strategies that would enable them to help themselves, through greater sensory-motor (kinaesthetic) awareness and the direct experience of new possibilities… Feldenkrais work focuses on instilling a clear sense of the way a well-organized skeleton moves and the lessons – many hundreds of them – have been carefully designed to make skeletal connections much clearer. (Burrowes in Knight 2013, p.304)

See www.vocaldynamix.com for more details.

Alexander Technique

Somatic practices can address poor postural habits that we frequently develop. With reference to Alexander Technique (AT), Barlow writes that 'The Alexander Principle states that there are ways of using your body which are better than certain other ways.' The phrase 'Use affects functioning' effectively sums up the Alexander Principle in three words (Barlow 1973, pp.17, 18).

The experience of being 'all wound up' is a common one in our culture; but how do we wind ourselves up? The simple answer is that we stiffen our necks and literally throw ourselves off balance in an unconscious response to many aspects of our environment. (Gelb 1987, p.61).

With Alexander, habit is what has to change. Practising the Alexander Technique gently encourages the body into a more correct way of being, and is an excellent adjunct to Bowen work, especially when clients revert to habitual postures that are harmful to their health. It can complement the realignment of the body in a more efficient and organized way, but it is an approach that needs dedication, commitment and a qualified teacher to be worthwhile.

Pilates

cℴ Jessica Moolenaar, London (www.mindfulpilates.co.uk)

The Pilates Method, although not strictly a somatic practice, is a holistic movement programme originally designed by Joe Pilates (1880–1967). We can distinguish 'classic' Pilates, exercises on the mat and on Pilates equipment, closely resembling Pilates' hardcore conditioning regime, from 'evolved' Pilates, a form of Pilates that has developed into being a more person-centred form of movement education, taking into consideration the personal needs of the student and modifying the classic movement repertoire somewhat. The Pilates Method as it is mostly practised in the UK is usually evolved – that is, an intelligent holistic series of movement sequences on both mat and equipment, that allow the body–mind to re-pattern movement habits and allow for a balancing of strength and mobility in the soft tissues. Pilates is inherently 'rehabilitative' in that it rebalances anybody, whether it is a body trained in dance and unbalanced by an injury or a body with a physical condition such as hypermobility. The key is always the person-centred nature of the movement education: everybody needs a different set of movement sequences with a different teaching approach.

Joe Pilates originally coined his technique Contrology (Pilates and Miller 1998) and left us with a body of work consisting of two books, in which he set out the philosophy behind his regime and with the description of the movements themselves. As Pilates was not aware at the time of the way in which the sensory motor system acquires new movement patterns, he has given us little instruction as to *how* to perform or teach his system. However, he uses language that might give us an idea of his philosophy: '… our muscles obeying our will…and our will not being dominated by the reflex action of our muscles' (Pilates and Miller 1998). These phrases imply a programme based on a body–mind connection, whereby our mind is *in control* of our body. The more we listen to the body, that is, the more we are *in* the body with the mind, the more we discover about ourselves and how best to develop. One could say that the body as part of the body–mind is a container of memory and is manifesting that which we need to uncover and develop, through making a conscious connection with it through our mind.

PILATES PRINCIPLES

Friedman *et al.* outlined the principles that are at work in modern use Pilates: breathing, control, precision, flowing movement and centring (Friedman and Eisten 1980). Brooke Siler, 20 years later, names the principles as follows: concentration, control, centring, fluidity, precision, breathing, imagination, intuition and integration (Siler 2000). I have renamed these principles yet again for them to become a reflection of the inherent *holistic* nature of Pilates practice, in which the body–mind connection is central to the efficacy of sensory motor learning and which reflects the learning taking place through movement and embodiment rather than mindless and often boring bio-mechanical 'exercise' (Knight 2013, pp.224–225).

Other Movement and Exercise to Support Bowen

ᘒ *Sharon Levin, South Africa (www.fitnessfanatics.co.za)*

As a Bowen practitioner, it is advisable to encourage clients to participate in exercise that uses the full range of movement and facilitates the use of muscular strength, muscular endurance, cardiovascular fitness, flexibility and functional mobility. There are many forms of movement/dance/exercise and the Bowen therapist requires an understanding of which discipline would be best suited to the client to achieve the best short and long-term benefits. The trouble is that the range of movement/exercise classes available is endless, with many new techniques evolving and old techniques being revisited.

It is not possible to give a full overview here, but it is important to encourage clients and explain why movement/exercise is such an important part of healing. Most clients need guidance and supervision, and a good therapist should be able to direct their clients to the most suitable form of movement (ideally with supervision) which will prevent them becoming dependent. There are many groups that sign people up for 6-week or 12-week programmes. They often have the most amazing successes, with all kinds of benefits in weight loss, mobility, fitness, etc. However, the success can be short-lived.

When the course is over, the participant reverts to either putting on more weight than they lost on the organized programme, or returns to the same fitness level as when they had started the managed programme. The reason for this is because they only trained whilst under the supervision of a class/instructor and never on their own. Therefore, the programme that they successfully participated in was a failure because the participant did not have the motivation or confidence to continue exercising on their own.

Walking

As a Bowen practitioner, it is important to understand the different techniques and styles of walking. These might include casual walking, structured walking, treadmill walking, Nordic walking or hiking. Each of these styles has its own advantages and disadvantages: for example, in treadmill walking, the gait and stride changes on a moving belt, there is considerable variation in cushioning on treadmills, there is a lack of fresh air, the potential to overheat in a closed environment and the fact that many people tend to hold on to the rails of the treadmill thus preventing a natural walking gait and stance.

Nordic walking can be a good recommendation for people who have had knee and hip replacements as well as those with back and neck problems. A study of people suffering from severe stress found that the thought process of learning to coordinate the planting of the poles and correct gait stimulated the release of hormones which assisted in de-stressing them significantly (Tschentscher, Niederseer and Niebauer 2013). Other studies have shown benefits of Nordic walking in lowering blood pressure, Parkinson's, obesity, fibromyalgia, diabetes and COPD (Nordic Walking UK 2014; Breyer *et al.* 2010). A Bowen practitioner should research their area for a Certified Nordic Walking Coach or Instructor before recommending it to a client.

Gyrokinesis

The Gyrotonic Expansion system is a holistic approach to movement that works on the entire body through seven natural elements of spinal movement: forward, backward, left side, right side, left twist, right twist and circular, as well as all other joint articulations. This approach systematically and gently works the joints and muscles through rhythmic and undulating movements, which stimulate the body's internal organs while different corresponding breathing patterns are integrated along with the movements. The exercises offer complete freedom of movement. The exercises are synchronized with corresponding breathing patterns, thus enhancing aerobic and cardiovascular stimulation and promoting neuromuscular rejuvenation. The classes can be performed on Gyrokinesis equipment or floor classes held in groups or individually. The instructor must be trained, qualified and certified as a Gyrokinesis Instructor. I believe that this technique is very beneficial because it adds additional dimension and rotation to Pilates. Therefore, I would recommend using both techniques when designing a programme.

Aqua-Aerobics

Aqua-aerobic programmes/classes have grown rapidly. The popularity has grown from people requiring anything from rehabilitation to general fitness. Unfortunately, due to the lack of understanding and knowledge of sound water principles, it has attracted many people who are actually high risk (i.e. injuries, heart conditions, overweight, pregnant, etc.). Water offers greater resistance against the movement of the body than does air. Therefore, the body gets a 'harder' workout with no stress. However, depending on the activity, depth of the pool, person's body type, it was assumed that there is little strain on the body because the resistance slows down movements and the water lessens the effect of gravity on the body. But this is a myth and the scientific principles of water must be understood.

When recommending a client to participate in aqua-aerobics, it is most important to send them to a qualified and certified aqua-aerobic instructor. There are many aerobic instructors and personal trainers who are not qualified aqua-aerobic instructors, who teach aqua-aerobics with no understanding of the scientific principles of water and how to design a safe and effective aqua-aerobic class. This can create further risk to your client.

Considering the major forces acting on the body when it is immersed in water, either when stationary or in motion, it is very different to exercising on land. A well-designed aqua-aerobic programme should use, correctly, the effects of the various forces created in the water.

CASE STUDY

A client had a water skiing accident. He dislocated his shoulder and also ruptured his hamstring. He had surgery to the shoulder and physiotherapy on the hamstring. He was referred to me. After assessment, I designed a land-based programme which incorporated mobility, flexibility and building up his cardiovascular fitness as he wanted to stay 'fit' and then I designed an aqua programme. I used Deep Water exercise, jogging with an aqua jogger. This, of course, has to be started very gently because he could not have much movement in the shoulder and small movements in the legs to prevent overuse of legs and hamstring. The buoyancy belt supports the client in a vertical position and therefore the client does not have to stress to keep afloat and therefore stress the shoulders.

The benefit of this training for this client was that he had the opportunity to be able to move again, he felt secure in the buoyancy belt, the hydrostatic pressure encouraged healing, and it was a more controlled way to improve range of movement and cardiovascular fitness.

References

Barlow, W. (1973) *The Alexander Principle*. London: Victor Gollancz.

Bober, J. (2003) Theoretical Principles of the Feldenkrais Method in Relation to Selected Theories of Motor Learning. In M. Hargreaves (ed.) *New Connectivity: Somatic and Creative Practices in Dance Education*. London: Laban.

Breyer, M.K., Breyer-Kohansal, R., Funk, G.C., Dornhofer, N. et al. (2010) Nordic walking improves daily physical activities in COPD: a randomised controlled trial. *Respiratory Research* 11, 112. Available at http://respiratory-research.com/content/pdf/1465-9921-11-112.pdf, accessed on 26 June 2014.

Brodie, J. and Lobel, E. (2004) Integrating fundamental principles underlying somatic practices into the dance technique class. *Journal of Dance Education* 4 (3), 80–87.

Eddy, M. (2002) Dance and somatic inquiry in studios and community dance programs. *Journal of Dance Education* 2 (4), 119–127.

Fitt, S. (1996) *Dance Kinesiology*. New York: Schirmer Books.

Fortin, S. (2003) Dancing on the Mobius Band. In M. Hargreaves (ed.) *New Connectivity: Somatic and Creative Practices in Dance Education*. London: Laban.

Friedman, P. and Eisten, G. (1980) *The Pilates Method of Physical and Mental Conditioning*. New York. Penguin Press.

Gelb, M. (1987) *Body Learning: An Introduction to the Alexander Technique*. London: Aurum Press.

Green, J. (2002) Somatic knowledge – the body as content and methodology in dance education. *Journal of Dance Education* 2 (4), 114–118.

Knaster, M. (1996) *Discovering the Body's Wisdom*. New York: Bantam Books.

Knight, I. (2013) *A Multidisciplinary Approach to the Management of Ehlers-Danlos (type III) Hypermobility Syndrome and Other Chronic Complex Conditions*. London: Singing Dragon Press.

Hanna, T. (1986) What is Somatics? *Somatics* 5 (4), 4–8.

Nachemson, A. and Elfstom, G. (1970) *Intravital Dynamic Pressure Measurements in Lumbar Discs. A Study of Common Movements, Maneuvers and Exercises*. Stockholm: Almqvist and Wiksell.

Nordic Walking UK (2014) See how effective it is. Available at http://nordicwalking.co.uk/?page=see_effect&c=30, accessed on 26 June 2014.

Pilates, J. and Miller, W. (1998) *A Pilates Primer: The Millennium Edition*. Incline Village, NV: Presentation Dynamics.

Siler, N. (2000) *The Pilates Body*. London: Penguin.

Tschentscher, M., Niederseer, D. and Niebauer, J. (2013) Health benefits of Nordic Walking: a systematic review. *American Journal of Preventive Medicine* 44 (1), 76–84.

෴

Appendix 2
Minerals, Diet and Homeopathy

Tom Bowen was adamant that his clients follow any advice about changes to their diet and lifestyle, as well as doing any exercises that he gave them regularly. Bowen practitioners nowadays have access to a much more refined understanding about suitable exercises and a deeper understanding about the role of diet and supplementation. Generally, Bowen would discourage clients from having any other therapy at the same time as receiving Bowen. This still makes good sense, as at best it is difficult to ascertain what approach is working, and at worst the body can become overloaded with the potential for aggravation of symptoms. It is easy for clients to underestimate the powerful changes that go on in the days between Bowen sessions. Other manual therapies such as acupuncture or osteopathy can be counter-productive during this time, in the same way that it would be foolish for someone to take ten aspirin for a headache when one or two would be better.

However, some supporting approaches can be helpful in allowing repair, such as the strapping that Bowen used to support joints (elbow, ankle, knee, wrist, etc), and the dietary advice to eat a more alkalizing diet, which is discussed below. Some of Bowen's advice included soaking inflamed or swollen joints in Epsom salts (magnesium sulphate) or washing soda (sodium carbonate). The important role of magnesium and other minerals is discussed below, along with information on how dietary changes can impact on inflammatory conditions. It is not known if Bowen advised the use of homeopathy, but many practitioners these days find it immensely helpful as a support to Bowen sessions. Some information on its role in helping repair in musculoskeletal problems is given below.

Magnesium and Other Minerals
Alastair McLoughlin
Minerals are absolutely essential to our bodies. We'd die without them. There are two groups of minerals: macro-minerals and trace minerals. The macro-mineral group is made up of calcium, phosphorus, magnesium, potassium, chloride, sodium and sulphur. Trace minerals include iron, manganese, copper, iodine, zinc, chromium, fluoride, copper and selenium. All of these have a vital role in our health and wellbeing.

However, nowadays there has been a significant drop in the mineral content of nearly all our common foods. In a study of the decline in the mineral content in one medium-sized apple over the last 80 years, the loss has been nearly 50 per cent in calcium, 96 per cent in iron, 84 per cent in phosphorus and over 80 per cent in magnesium. It is a similar story with common vegetables such as cabbage, lettuce, tomatoes and spinach (US Department of Agriculture figures 1914 and 1997 (US Department of Agriculture, Agricultural Research Service 2000; Mayer 1997)). But what role do these minerals play in human health? A brief resumé of their roles will suffice for our discussion:

- Calcium: important for healthy bones and teeth; helps muscles relax and contract; important in nerve functioning, blood clotting, blood pressure regulation, immune system health.

- Phosphorus: important for healthy bones and teeth; found in every cell; part of the system that maintains acid-base balance.

- Magnesium: found in bones; needed for making protein, muscle contraction, nerve transmission, immune system health.

- Potassium: needed for proper fluid balance, nerve transmission, muscle contraction.

- Chloride: needed for proper fluid balance, stomach acid.

- Sodium: needed for proper fluid balance, nerve transmission, muscle contraction.

- Sulphur: found in protein molecules.

- Iron: part of a molecule (haemoglobin) found in red blood cells that carries oxygen in the body; needed for energy metabolism.

- Manganese: part of a molecule (haemoglobin) found in red blood cells that carries oxygen in the body; needed for energy metabolism.

- Copper: part of many enzymes; needed for iron metabolism.

- Iodine: found in thyroid hormone, which helps regulate growth, development and metabolism.

- Zinc: part of many enzymes needed for making protein and genetic material; has a function in taste perception, wound healing, normal foetal development, production of sperm, normal growth and sexual maturation, immune system health.

- Chromium: works closely with insulin to regulate blood sugar (glucose) level.

- Fluoride: involved in formation of bones and teeth; helps prevent tooth decay.

- Copper: forms part of many enzymes; needed for iron metabolism.

- Selenium: helps as an antioxidant.

Unfortunately this is only a partial list of the estimated 76 minerals and trace elements vital to maintain human health. The explanation of their vital functions listed here is only intended as an overview. Let's delve into just one vital mineral which is starting to get the recognition it deserves: magnesium.

Magnesium: The Research

Magnesium (Mg) is vital for our health, and lack of it is probably responsible for a multitude of diseases today. Whilst studying this subject I have been astounded at the number of research papers that highlight the need for magnesium and the disastrous consequences of becoming magnesium deficient. These include:

DEPRESSION

The first information on the beneficial effect of magnesium sulphate given hypodermically to patients with agitated depression was published almost 100 years ago. Magnesium is one of the most essential minerals in the human body, connected with brain biochemistry and the fluidity of neuronal membrane. Magnesium preparations seem to be a valuable addition to the pharmacological armamentarium for management of depression (Serefko *et al.* 2013).

OSTEOPOROSIS

Magnesium deficiency contributes to osteoporosis directly by acting on crystal formation and on bone cells and indirectly by impacting on the secretion and the activity of parathyroid hormone, as well as by promoting low-grade inflammation (Castiglioni *et al.* 2013).

PARKINSON'S DISEASE

Systemic and intracellular Mg deficiency has long been suspected to contribute to the development and progress of Parkinson's disease and other neurodegenerative diseases (Kolisek *et al.* 2013).

CARDIAC ARRHYTHMIA

A large percentage of patients with arrhythmias have an intracellular Mg deficiency. Magnesium has benefits as an atrial anti-arrhythmic agent (Ganga *et al.* 2013).

The use of magnesium as single agent or as an adjunct to other therapeutic actions in the prevention and therapy of cardiac arrhythmias can be effective and, in the case of oral administration, very safe (Vierling *et al.* 2013).

Low serum magnesium is moderately associated with the development of atrial fibrillation in individuals without cardiovascular disease (Khan *et al.* 2012).

RESPIRATORY DISEASE

Low magnesium intake is associated with lower lung functions, and hypomagnesaemia was found in 16 per cent of patients with acute pulmonary diseases. Magnesium is used for the treatment of asthmatic attacks (Fridman and Linder 2013).

CATARACTS

Magnesium supplementation may be of therapeutic value in preventing the onset and progression of cataracts in conditions associated with Mg deficiency (Agarwal *et al.* 2012).

BLOOD PRESSURE

Magnesium is an essential element for vascular function and blood pressure regulation. Several studies have demonstrated that Mg concentration is inversely associated with blood pressure, and that Mg supplementation attenuates hypertension (Jin *et al.* 2013).

DIABETES

Hypomagnesaemia is reported in type 2 diabetes; magnesium deficiency may play a role in the development of endothelial dysfunction and altered insulin function (Dasgupta, Sarma and Saikia 2012). It is reported that shortage of oral magnesium intake increases the incidence of diabetes. In addition, magnesium replacement therapy improves insulin resistance and glycemic control (Munekage, Takezaki and Hanazaki 2012). Hypomagnesaemia is a novel predictor of ESRD (end-stage renal disease) in patients with type 2 diabetic nephropathy (Sakaguchi *et al.* 2012).

OXIDATIVE STRESS

Decrease of Mg2+ concentration in tissues and blood is accompanied with elevation of the oxidative stress markers, including products of the oxidative modification of lipids, proteins and DNA. Different mechanisms including systemic reactions (hyper-activation of inflammation and endothelial dysfunction) and cellular changes (mitochondrial dysfunction and excessive production of fatty acids) are supposed to be involved in development and maintenance of the oxidative stress due to Mg2+ deficiency (Spasov, Zheltova and Kharitonov 2012).

MIGRAINE

Magnesium deficiency may be present in up to half of migraine patients, and routine blood tests are not indicative of magnesium status, so empiric treatment with at least oral magnesium is warranted in all migraine sufferers (Mauskop and Varughese 2012).

OTHER HEALTH ISSUES

Low Mg intakes and blood levels have been associated with type 2 diabetes, metabolic syndrome, elevated C-reactive protein (an inflammatory marker), hypertension, atherosclerotic vascular disease, sudden cardiac death, osteoporosis, migraine headache, asthma and colon cancer (Rosanoff, Weaver and Rude 2012).

The studies I've cited are just the tip of the 'magnesium iceberg'. There is no getting away from the fact that the health problems associated with magnesium deficiency are well documented and researched, and the health implications for us are even greater.

How Do We Know If We're Magnesium Deficient?

I'm often asked this question. The answer is quite apparent: in the first instance, having some of the health problems in the aforementioned list is a big indicator of magnesium deficiency. So you probably don't need a test if you experience any of these health problems. It's pretty much assured.

Second, if we consume highly refined foods, then we're almost guaranteed to be magnesium deficient. The food source has to be grown in mineral-rich soil. Even simply adding additional nutrients in the processing stage of food production is no guarantee that you're going to be absorbing the necessary nutrients. As an example, simply taking a calcium supplement for osteoporosis will not add extra calcium into your bones.

Signs and Symptoms of Magnesium Deficiency

If you or your clients experience any of the following, you may already be magnesium deficient: tics, tremors, muscle spasms, cramps, seizures, anxiety, migraine headaches, insomnia, depression, lethargy, chronic fatigue, irregular heart beat, hyperglycaemia.

Medical conditions related to magnesium deficiency include: coronary heart disease, atherosclerosis, previous incidence of cardiac arrest, Parkinson's disease, osteoporosis, ADHD, type 2 diabetes and asthma.

Sources of Magnesium

The following are some of the best food sources for magnesium: almonds, cashews, halibut, mackerel, pumpkin seeds, figs, apricots, dates, spinach, soya beans, lima beans. However, please remember that the food needs to be grown in mineral-rich soil for it to be nutrient dense. In both the USA and UK there has been a significant decline over the years in the magnesium content of fruits and vegetables (Mayer 1997). It is also worth remembering that our ability to absorb nutrients through our digestive system declines with age due to problems with stomach acid, low digestive enzymes and poor absorbability in the gut.

Warning: If you have kidney disease (renal failure), you must not take any magnesium supplements without first consulting your physician.

Efficient Ways of Boosting Magnesium Levels

Ancient peoples such as the Egyptians, Greek and Romans certainly had the right idea of bathing in mineral-rich pools, lakes or baths, and this became ritualized as the health benefits became known. Today, bathing in magnesium salts is probably the most efficient and pleasant method of boosting our magnesium reserves. Simply pouring a cupful of magnesium salts into our bathwater and relaxing for 20–30 minutes allows the magnesium to be absorbed through the skin and transported around the body.

One of Tom Bowen's home remedies was the advice to bathe in Epsom salts (magnesium sulphate). It's great advice. It seems that a better form of magnesium (magnesium chloride) allows for better absorption and storage by the body and if you can locate a source of this form of magnesium, all the better.

If you can't actually get into a bath due to physical limitations, or you don't have a bath (you take a shower instead), then putting a couple of tablespoons of magnesium salts into a bowl of warm water and soaking your feet (or hands if they're stiff and arthritic) will also be of great benefit. Leg cramps will disappear even if you only soak your feet in the magnesium solution.

In addition you can make a concentrated solution of magnesium by adding the salts to a small amount of boiling water to make an 'oil'. (The water thickens with the addition of magnesium salts and takes on the feeling of oil – even though it isn't.) Allow the water to cool and pour into a spray bottle. You can then spray the magnesium 'oil' onto your limbs and massage into the body. Massage therapists can also use the magnesium oil as a medium to use in their clinics. If you're absorbing too much magnesium, your bowel will start be be loose and you may have slight diarrhoea.

Increasing magnesium levels has many potential health benefits. Initially, you may begin sleeping better and you may notice increased energy levels. These simple but highly beneficial effects should encourage you to pursue your goal of better health.

The addition of magnesium to your regular scheduled Bowen treatments is time well spent and will pay many dividends to your overall health for years to come.

References

Agarwal, R., Iezhitsa, I., Agarwal, P. and Spasov, A. (2012) Magnesium deficiency: does it have a role to play in cataractogenesis? *Experimental Eye Research* 101, 82–89.

Castiglioni, S., Cazzaniga, A., Albisetti, W. and Maier, J.A. (2013) Magnesium and osteoporosis: current state of knowledge and future research directions. *Nutrients* 5, 3022–3033.

Dasgupta, A., Sarma, D. and Saikia, U.K. (2012) Hypomagnesemia in type 2 diabetes mellitus. *Indian Journal of Endocrinology and Metabolism* 16 (6), 1000–1003.

Fridman, E. and Linder, N. (2013) Magnesium and bronchopulmonary dysplasia. *Harefuah* 152 (3), 158–161, 182.

Ganga, H.V., Noyes, A., White, C.M. and Kluger, J. (2013) Magnesium adjunctive therapy in atrial arrhythmias. *Pacing and Clinical Electrophysiology*, 36 (10), 1308–1318.

Jin, K., Kim, T.H., Kim, Y.H. and Kim, Y.W. (2013) Additional antihypertensive effect of magnesium supplementation with an angiotensin II receptor blocker in hypomagnesemic rats. *Korean Journal of Internal Medicine* 28 (2), 197.

Khan, A.M., Lubitz, S.A., Sullivan, L.M., Sun, J.X. *et al.* (2012) Low serum magnesium and the development of atrial fibrillation in the community: the Framingham Heart Study. *Circulation* 127 (1), 33–38.

Kolisek, M., Sponder, G., Mastrototaro, L., Smorodchenko, A. *et al.* (2013) Substitution p.A350V in Na+/Mg2+ Exchanger SLC41A1, potentially associated with Parkinson's disease, is a gain-of-function mutation. *PLoS ONE* 8 (8), e71096.

Mauskop, A. and Varughese, J. (2012) Why all migraine patients should be treated with magnesium. *Journal of Neural Transmission* 119 (5), 575–579.

Mayer, A.-M. (1997) Historical changes in the mineral content of fruits and vegetables: a cause for concern? *British Food Journal* 99 (6), 207–211.

Munekage, E., Takezaki, Y. and Hanazaki, K. (2012) Shortage and metabolic disturbance of magnesium in diabetic patients and significance of magnesium replacement therapy. *Clinical Calcium* 22 (8), 1235–1242.

Rosanoff, A., Weaver, C.M. and Rude, R.K. (2012) Suboptimal magnesium status in the United States: are the health consequences underestimated? *Nutrition Reviews* 70 (3), 153–164.

Sakaguchi, Y., Shoji, T., Hayashi, T., Suzuki, A. *et al.* (2012) Hypomagnesemia in type 2 diabetic nephropathy: a novel predictor of end-stage renal disease. *Diabetes Care* 35 (7), 1591–1597.

Serefko, A., Szopa, A., Wlaź, P., Nowak, G. *et al.* (2013) Magnesium in depression. *Pharmacological Reports* 65 (3), 547–554.

Spasov, A., Zheltova, A. and Kharitonov, M. (2012) Magnesium and the oxidative stress. *Rossiiskii fiziologicheskii zhurnal imeni I.M. Sechenova/Rossiiskaia akademiia nauk* 98 (7), 915–923.

US Department of Agriculture, Agricultural Research Service (2000) USDA Nutrient Database for Standard Reference, Release 13.

Vierling, W., Liebscher, D.H., Micke, O., von Ehrlich, B. and Kisters, K. (2013) Magnesium deficiency and therapy in cardiac arrhythmias: recommendations of the German Society for Magnesium Research [in German]. *Deutsche Medizinische Wochenschrift* 138 (22), 1165–1167.

છ૭

Inflammation, Diet and pH

છ૭ *Andrew Johnson*

Researchers have concluded that inflammation may play a significant role in many chronic conditions, including some cardiovascular diseases, diabetes, metabolic syndrome, Alzheimer's, autoimmune disorders, rheumatoid and osteoarthritis, MS, Parkinson's, osteoporosis, obesity, allergies and food intolerance, eczema, asthma, ME and chronic fatigue syndrome, fibromyalgia, inflammatory bowel conditions (such as ulcerative colitis, IBS, etc.) and many other pain-related disorders. Acute inflammation may also relate to an accident or trauma to an area, but this should subside with adequate healing.

What Is Inflammation?

The term 'inflammation' originated in the 1970s. The word comes from the Latin *inflammo* meaning 'ignite' or 'set alight'. Inflammation is an immunological response that affects the area of tissue involved or it may be throughout the system. The inflammatory response is initially helpful as it helps the body to deal with disease-causing pathogens or the effects of an injury. Inflammation is caused by the tissues releasing multiple substances, including histamine, bradykinin, serotonin, prostaglandins, hormonal substances from sensitized T-cells and various other reaction products. Some of them activate the macrophage system, which acts to dispose of the damaged tissue but can also further injure the cells and tissues.

Chronic Inflammation

With chronic inflammation (long-term unresolved inflammation in the body), there is increased free radical or 'oxidative' stress. This is bad because free radicals can damage structural tissues in joints and almost any other part of the body. In chronic inflammation the body tends to become depleted in antioxidants, and therefore the free radicals continue to do more damage which increases inflammation even more. This free radical stress is also a major factor in the process of ageing. The body counteracts free radicals with antioxidants.

The Medical Approach to Inflammation

Anti-inflammatory medical treatments can start with non-steroidal anti-inflammatory drugs (NSAIDs), such as ibuprofen or aspirin, and, if needed, steroid medications are prescribed. Physiotherapy, moderate exercise such as walking, and weight loss, if needed, are also prescribed. NSAIDs tend to irritate the stomach so long-term use may lead to digestive ulcers and other problems. Steroids also have significant side effects with long-term use.

Factors that May Encourage Inflammation

Increased free radical production could play an important role. This may come from excessive exercise or physically overworking the body, accidental injury, environmental pollution (such as contamination from pesticides, heavy metals, toxic chemical overload), radiation and excessive sunlight (sunburn causes free radical stress), food sources such as from excessive consumption of trans and hydrogenated fats made from processing or heating vegetable oils (but coconut and olive oil are OK), and a diet deficient in antioxidants.

Many people in the modern world eat a diet high in calories and lacking in other nutrients, resulting in obesity and poor health. Micro-nutrient deficiencies (including antioxidants) from poor diets may make us more vulnerable to low-grade infections, which can contribute to chronic inflammation in the body. A significant part of the immune system is found in the gut. The gut contains many billions of friendly immune-enhancing bacteria; however, a poor diet and other common triggers may cause bad bacteria to develop and reduce the friendly immune-enhancing bacteria. This is known as gut dysbiosis, which may also contribute to low-grade inflammation throughout the body. A symptom of poor gut health can be food intolerance, which may then also create more inflammation.

Emotional stress can contribute to inflammation partly through influencing gut health and immunity. The effects of stress upon adrenal glands can also reduce cortisol hormone levels, which have a natural regulatory role with inflammation. In obesity, fat cells can behave like immune cells and may then increase the inflammatory immune responses in the body.

Anti-inflammatory Ways of Eating

This is really a matter of reducing foods that may have a pro-inflammatory effect whilst increasing those that may help reduce inflammation. There are several versions of this form of diet available in book form – see below. Some versions are similar to the typical 'Mediterranean diet'. Balancing pH (acidity and alkalinity) can also be helpful, as well as eating a rainbow diet of colours that includes emphasis on eating nutrient-dense plant foods, including a wide variety of different coloured vegetables, salads, legumes, nuts, seeds and fruits, which are all rich in phytonutrients.

FOODS TO REDUCE OR AVOID

- Common allergens – get tested for food intolerances and allergies. These may create chronic pro-inflammatory conditions in the body. Also be cautious of the nightshade family of vegetables (aubergines, tomatoes, potatoes and peppers).

- Sugar (added sugar or sucrose), alcohol, white or refined bakery products and starchy foods, such as potatoes, partly as they may contribute to blood sugar imbalances and can feed bad bacteria in the gut, which can create more inflammation in the body. Strong black tea, coffee and fizzy drinks are also more acid-forming, which may increase inflammation. Green and white teas are often OK in moderation.

- Saturated fats, fatty meat, red meat, processed meats, high-fat hard cheeses and cow's milk can contribute to obesity and chronic inflammation. Have lean red meat less than three times a week. Eggs are also a common allergen so get tested to check.

- Trans and hydrogenated vegetable oils in processed bakery and other products (such as hydrogenated margarine and vegetable fats), cooking with polyunsaturated and vegetable oils (except olive and coconut) – they may increase free radical stress on the body and inflammation.

FOODS TO EMPHASIZE

- Vegetables and salads are even more important than having lots of fruits. Greens such as kale, broccoli, sprouts, cucumbers, carrots, purple cabbage, fennel, fresh herbs are more alkalising and reduce acidity, which may create inflammation and pain.

- Fresh fruits, especially red, purple and blue berries (raspberries, blueberries, blackberries, also cherries, red grapes, etc.), apples, pineapple, oranges, bananas, kiwi, as they contain many antioxidants and alkalising minerals, which can help protect the body against damage from inflammation and acidity.

- Lean organic protein: free-range chicken, turkey, oily fish, fermented organic soy products such as tempeh and miso, grass-fed free-range animal meat (such as lamb, venison, etc. – in moderation) as these can be lower in fat or have a different quality of fat, and protein can help maintain blood sugar balance. Also combine legumes (pulses) with whole grains, nuts and seeds for protein.

- Oils and fats: use coconut oil for cooking (or olive oil if not heated to smoking point); not other vegetable oils as these may create more free radical stress on the body when over-heated. Eat foods high in omega 3 which can be anti-inflammatory: walnuts, also flaxseed oil (use unheated) and seeds, oily fish such as salmon, herring, mackerel, sardines and anchovies. Avoid farmed fish unless organically produced. Eat foods high in omega 6, including most nuts and seeds.

- Eat foods containing vitamin D, as deficiency may contribute to systemic inflammation; foods include cod liver oil, most oily fish (herring, mackerel, tuna, sardines, salmon), free-range egg yolk, organic liver and lean grass-fed organic meats. Or, get appropriate sunshine exposure for your skin type which creates vitamin D synthesis (see below under lifestyle for details).

- Spices and herbs: turmeric, cayenne pepper, fresh ginger and rosemary.

- Drinks: stay hydrated by having plenty of pure water, also herb teas, green and white tea.

Lifestyle and Other Recommendations

- Sunshine: aim to get a suitable level of sun for your skin type, as vitamin D may be important for people with inflammation, but avoid getting burnt as this increases free radical stress and skin cancer risk. Most vitamin D synthesis takes place in the first few minutes of exposure to the sun – more sun does not give more vitamin D synthesis so there is no need to overdo it and risk burning. If you cannot get enough sunshine, get a vitamin D3 blood test to assess your need for supplementation. You are more likely to be low in D3 during late winter (January to February) in the northern hemisphere

- Moderate exercise: for 30–60 minutes may improve joint lubrication and mobility, reducing pain and inflammation, and reduce obesity. If you have specific joint problems, or other structural/mechanical problems get professional advice on the right type of exercise for you.

- Sleep: get at least 7–8 hours of sleep every night. Be asleep by 10–11pm and, if up later, try to sleep in until 9am.

- Stress: reduce stressful situations; take up some form of regular relaxation or stress management system such as meditation, yoga, aromatherapy massage, and if you have ongoing unresolved emotional stress, also consider psychotherapy or EFT.

- Consider earthing (i.e. barefoot walking in suitable places). Earthing is based on the theory that connecting to the ground can encourage health in the body (search online for more on earthing/grounding by Dr Stephen Sinatra and Clint Ober).

- Consider near infra-red saunas as an aid to detoxification (avoid far infra-red type). Search online for information by Dr Lawrence Wilson MD on Sauna Therapy, but get professional advice first on appropriate use.

- Consider other therapies such as craniosacral, Bowen Technique, Alexander Technique or other structural therapies.

- Other information that could be supportive includes: pH (acid alkaline) food charts, the phytonutrient rich food charts (for more of a rainbow-coloured diet), and a low GL (glycaemic load) way of eating.

Supplements and Herbs

This information is for educational purposes and not a specific recommendation, as what is safe and appropriate varies in each case. I recommend that practitioners and individuals seek professional advice first. Here are just a few that have been used.

- Post-trauma: keep in mind that pain management may not be as swift or obvious with alternatives to medical drugs such as NSAIDs.

- Bruising: a topical application of 'homeopathic' arnica cream can be applied to the affected tissues 2–3 times a day. This may initially encourage the bruising to develop more but also helps its dispersion, reducing tissue congestion and tension. *Do not use on broken skin.*

- Proteolytic enzymes such as bromelain or animal-derived protease enzymes. This has been used by practitioners involved in musculoskeletal therapies and sports therapists to assist recovery from trauma. Proteolytic enzymes may help regulate inflammation by a variety of mechanisms.

- Herbs with natural anti-inflammatory properties, including turmeric and Boswellia.

- Antioxidants including vitamins and trace elements such as vitamins A, C, E, selenium, also antioxidant enzymes.

- Collagen supplements may assist the repair of connective tissues.

- Omega 3 fatty acids (EPA) from fish oil.

References and Further Reading

Akhtar, N.M., Naseer, R., Farooqi, A.Z., Aziz, W. and Nazir, M. (2004) Oral enzyme combination versus diclofenac in the treatment of osteoarthritis of the knee – a double-blind prospective randomized study. *Clinical Rheumatology* 23 (5), 410–415.

Appleton, N. (2005) *Stopping Inflammation: Relieving the Cause of Degenerative Diseases*. Square One Publishers.

Baumuller, M. (1990) The application of hydrolytic enzymes in blunt wounds to the soft tissue and distortion of the ankle joint: a double-blind clinical trial [trans. from German]. *Allgemeinmedizin* 19, 178–182.

Challem, J. (2010) *The Inflammation Syndrome: Your Nutrition Plan for Great Health, Weight Loss, and Pain Free Living*. John Wiley and Sons.

Deitrick, R.E. (1965) Oral proteolytic enzymes in the treatment of athletic injuries: a double-blind study. *Pennsylvania Medicine* 68 (10), 35–37.

Ebrahimi, M., Ghayour-Mobarhan, M., Rezaiean, S., Hoseini, M. *et al.* (2009) Omega-3 fatty acid supplements improve the cardiovascular risk profile of subjects with metabolic syndrome, including markers of inflammation and auto-immunity. *Acta Cardiological* 64 (3), 321–327.

Kamenícek, V., Holán, P. and Franěk, P. (2001) Systemic enzyme therapy in the treatment and prevention of post-traumatic and postoperative swelling. *Acta Chirurgiaw Orthopaedicae et Traumatologiae Cechoslovaca* 68 (1), 45–49.

Kerkhoffs, G.M., Struijs, P.A., De Wit, C. *et al.* (2004) A double blind, randomised, parallel group study on the efficacy and safety of treating acute lateral ankle sprain with oral hydrolytic enzymes. *British Journal of Sports Medicine* 38, 431–435.

Lopez-Garcia, E., Schulze, M.B., Fung, T.T., Meigs, J.B. *et al.* (2004) Major dietary patterns are related to plasma concentrations of markers of inflammation and endothelial dysfunction. *American Journal of Clinical Nutrition* 80 (4), 1029–1035.

Wall, R., Ross, R.P., Fitzgerald, G.F. and Stanton, C. (2010) Fatty acids from fish: the anti-inflammatory potential of long-chain omega-3 fatty acids. *Nutrition Reviews* 68 (5), 280–289.

> *Disclaimer: This information is for educational purposes only and is not designed for treating a specific disease or symptom. Please consult a suitably qualified practitioner before significantly changing your diet or taking supplements and herbs. If you are receiving medical treatment or prescription medicines, pregnant, trying to conceive or breast-feeding, please consult your doctor before significantly changing your diet or taking supplements and herbs.*

ೋ

Bowen Treatment and Homeopathy

ೋ *Tim Robinson*

The musculoskeletal system is a complex interaction of living tissues that provides stability, support and movement to the body. These functions are compromised when there is breakdown of the musculoskeletal system due to trauma, poor posture, strain or unbalanced forces and tensions. These result in the symptoms and signs of musculoskeletal breakdown, namely pain, tenderness and stiffness of the affected joint, muscle or ligament, along with impairment of function. Manipulative techniques effectively assist the restoration and resolution of musculoskeletal breakdown. Further assistance may be achieved by the use of homeopathic medicines in conjunction with Bowen treatments.

Homeopathy is the system of medicine that stimulates natural healing that is safe, effective and without side effects. Homeopathy will not reverse advanced degenerative disease but it can ease symptoms as well as help the reparative processes and restore normal tissue function. Homeopathic medicines are derived from plant, mineral and animal materials, and are prepared by the process of serial dilution to standardized strengths or potencies. The most frequently used potencies are 6c and 30c ('c' denotes centesimal or one-hundredth dilution). As a rough guide, for conditions that have occurred recently, particularly if they show signs of acute inflammation, 30c potency taken three times daily is needed. For conditions that are low-grade, grumbling and long-term, 6c potency taken twice daily is needed. The medicine should be taken before a meal as it is absorbed from the mouth; food and drink will interfere with its absorption. Tip a tablet into the mouth, suck it and wait for it to dissolve. The medicine should be taken while the symptoms are present; as soon as the symptoms are settling the medicine should be stopped but restarted if the symptoms return.

The principle that underlies homeopathic prescribing is to match a medicine to the condition or symptom the patient is experiencing, the so-called 'like with like' concept. Thus, full understanding and appreciation of the symptoms by the practitioner is important in order to find the medicine whose features are most like the symptoms. External factors that modify those symptoms, improving or worsening them, are also very important in deciding which medicine to choose. In the context of a musculoskeletal condition affecting joints, muscles and tendons, the most relevant factors would be the reaction to temperature and movement of the affected part – for example, a painful joint may be better when warmed but worse in the cold and damp. The prescription is based on these factors that modify the symptoms along with the symptoms themselves.

There are three homeopathic medicines that are especially helpful in musculoskeletal conditions because of their specific 'modifying' features and tissue affinities; these are Rhus Tox, Ruta and Bryonia.

Rhus Tox is the most important musculoskeletal medicine that is indicated for joint or tissue conditions in which the pain and stiffness is worse in the cold and damp but better in the warmth. The pain and stiffness is also worse upon first movement of the affected part but better with continued movement. An example would be an arthritic hip joint that is worse in the winter months, very painful and stiff upon getting up from sitting but improves with walking.

Ruta has many features and modifying factors similar to Rhus Tox and is often used if Rhus Tox has not been successful. However, Ruta also has a special affinity for tendons, particularly at their point of attachment to bone.

Bryonia is different to Rhus Tox and Ruta; this is indicated for severe tearing joint or tissue pain that is made worse by the slightest movement. The patient will resist examination and guard the affected part. The relieving and worsening temperature features are the same as for Rhus Tox and Ruta.

As an aide memoire, the modifying features for these three medicines are summarized as follows:

- better for warmth – Rhus Tox, Ruta, Bryonia

- better for movement – Rhus Tox, Ruta

- worse for cold – Rhus Tox, Ruta, Bryonia

- worse for movement – Bryonia.

For simplicity's sake, only the three most commonly used homeopathic medicines for musculoskeletal conditions have been mentioned, based on the commonest modifying factors. However, there are many other less common but well-recognized modifying factors in musculoskeletal conditions for which there are specific medicines relevant to those features. A number of these will be mentioned in the following sections depending on which tissues and condition they are helpful for.

Osteoarthritis or degenerative joint disease occurs due to joint space narrowing, bone thickening and remodelling, along with cartilage catabolism and reduced synthesis. This results in joint stiffness, pain, swelling and reduced range of movement. This occurs in large load-bearing joints such as hip, knee, lumbar vertebrae as well as smaller joints of the fingers, thumbs, sacroiliac, jaw and cervical vertebral joints. The homeopathic medicines most indicated in osteoarthritis are Rhus Tox, Ruta and Bryonia, depending on the associated modifying features of the joint symptoms. Other medicines that are relevant are Calc Carb if the joint pain is much worse in the damp or wet weather, Pulsatilla if the pains seem to wander around from joint to joint, and Guaiacum, which is especially good for pain of the thumb joint at the wrist. As osteoarthritis is a low-grade chronic grumbling condition, 6c potency of the medicine should be taken twice daily and stopped when the symptoms are relieved, as outlined previously.

Tendon and ligament inflammation or strain may be due to injury or overuse. This results in symptoms such as pain, inflammation, tenderness. In bicipital and Achilles tendonitis, these symptoms are usually worse upon first movement but better as the patient moves it, and so Rhus Tox and Ruta are most helpful. For de Quervain's tendonitis, all movement aggravates and so Bryonia is best suited. In tennis or golfer's elbow, Ruta is especially effective as the pain occurs at the point of tendon attachment to the bone (periosteum). In addition to treatment with tablets, application of Ruta cream to the area of maximal tenderness will further assist in pain relief in this and other cases of tendonitis and ligament inflammation. The same medicines should be used for painful conditions of the heel including plantar fasciitis; typically the patient experiences extreme pain under the calcaneum upon getting out of bed in the morning. The pain is especially severe for the first few steps, making the patient hobble around the bedroom. Calc Fluor should be considered along with Ruta; this medicine has an action on the calcaneal spur if this is the main source of the pain. In Osgood Schlatters there is tenderness at the front of the tibia due to pulling of the infra-patella tendon and micro-fractures at the tibial tubercle; to assist healing of those fractures, the medicine Symphytum should be taken at 6c potency twice daily along with Ruta. Pain in the coccyx, known as coccydynia, may be due to a fall directly on to it or following childbirth. As this is a nerve-rich area where the sympathetic and parasympathetic chains lie, the medicine Hypericum 30c is useful, three times daily along with Rhus Tox or Bryonia depending on the type of pain and its modifying features.

Bursitis is the inflammation of a synovial fluid filled sack that lies over a bony prominence such as in trochanteric bursitis of the hip and ischial tuberosity bursitis of the pelvic 'sitting' bone. The the pain is similar in nature to other musculoskeletal conditions and so Rhus Tox, Ruta and Bryonia should be tried, at 6c potency, taken twice daily. Other forms of this condition such as pre-patella (housemaid's knee) and olecranon (student's elbow) bursitis present with red hot swelling. In this instance, two other medicines should be considered as long as infection has been excluded. Apis Mel is indicated if the area is pink and swollen with a burning, stinging pain which is relieved by gentle application of cold and worsened by warmth. Belladonna is indicated if the area is red and swollen, with a throbbing pain that is worse for movement or jarring.

Muscle strain and sprain due to over-strenuous or unaccustomed exercise leads to microscopic tears of individual muscle fibres and blood leakage; this initiates tissue inflammation and internal bruising. As a result, the muscle feels sore, tender, bruised and swollen. As before, our familiar musculoskeletal homeopathic medicines Rhus Tox, Ruta and Bryonia should be considered based on the type of pain and its modifying factors. As there is bruising present, Arnica should be taken, especially if trauma or an accident has occurred. For severe tissue damage, take one dose hourly throughout the day of the trauma; then four times daily thereafter until the bruising has resolved and the muscle returns to normal. Another medicine, Bellis Per, is useful for bruising, especially if it is in deep tissues. This should be taken four times daily following childbirth until the bruised feeling in the perineum settles.

Muscle spasm such as in torticollis (wry neck) is an extremely painful sudden-onset condition. The neck is usually twisted and held in a fixed position with the head tilted. All movement is excruciatingly painful and the patient resists attempts to turn the head; Bryonia is especially indicated for this. Another medicine, Causticum, must also be considered, especially if there is some relief from warmth and aggravation by cold or a draft. Both medicines should be given at 30c potency, two-hourly when the pain is at its worst; as it eases, reduce the dosage to 4–6 hourly and stop when the pain settles.

Muscle cramp in any of the muscle groups such as calves and thigh, or in smaller individual muscles such as in the feet or hands, is effectively treated homoeopathically. Cuprum Met is the most successful medicine for cramp, taken twice daily at 6c potency. If this is unsuccessful, increase to 30c and continue until the bout of cramp settles. Stop the medicine but restart if a further bout occurs. Other medicines for cramp are Mag Phos if the cramp muscle is better for pressure on it and Colchicum for cramp in the feet. Take either of these in the same regime as outlined for Cuprum Met.

Another troublesome condition involving the limbs is restless leg syndrome. Instead of using conventional medicine such as Ropinirole, there are a number of homeopathic medicines that can be tried. Tarantula is indicated for twitching, jerking leg movement in which there is an irresistible urge to move them, Zinc for a trembling feeling in the muscles, Arsenicum Alb if there is a general restlessness and Sepia if the restlessness is better with exercise. As this is a low-grade condition, take the medicine at 6c potency twice daily until the restlessness settles.

Bone fracture must be treated conventionally by an orthopaedic surgeon; management may be by immobilization, manipulation or operative internal fixation depending on the fracture. Having restored the bony anatomy, the fracture then unites and heals through bone growth and remodelling. To aid bone union and promote bone healing processes, Symphytum, a homeopathic medicine derived from the herb Comfrey, commonly known as Knitbone, should be taken twice daily at 6c potency. As there has been significant trauma at the time of the injury, along with escape of blood from the bone marrow and cortex, Arnica 30c should be taken three times daily over the first few weeks. Rib fracture is managed conventionally with simple analgesics and anti-inflammatories but homeopathy should be considered in this condition. As the pain is continuous and worse for the slightest movement, Bryonia 30c three times daily should be taken along with Symphytum to promote bone union.

Another bone condition in which homeopathy should be considered is childhood growing pains. This is a condition, of unknown cause and no proven conventional treatment, which wakes the child each night with pain that improves with rubbing. This responds well to Calc Phos 6c twice daily; increase to 30c if needed and continue until the pains settle.

The use of homeopathic medicine is safe alongside Bowen treatment. The combined effects of these two therapeutic strategies have a complementary and mutually beneficial effect. They will enhance their respective healing processes, enabling restoration and more rapid resolution of the musculoskeletal condition. As always, it is essential and our professional obligation to our patient to treat responsibly, within the bounds of our training and expertise. To be sure that this is the case, full assessment of the patient and the symptoms is necessary to diagnose the condition. If there is any doubt or uncertainty in the diagnosis, the patient should be referred to their doctor. The patient should follow the instructions as previously outlined; this is to continue the medicine until the patient notices a change, better or worse. If worse, the clinical picture may have changed and so advice from a doctor is needed. If better, stop the medicine at that point as the problem is cured and the patient has been restored to health.

Patient Instruction Sheet for Homeopathic Medicines:
How to Take Homeopathic Tablets

- Do not swallow tablets.

- Homeopathic medicines are absorbed from the mouth.

- Food/drink in the mouth will interfere with their absorption. Therefore take the medicine just before a meal/drink as the mouth is clean at that time.

- Tip tablet/pill into cap of bottle. Then tip into mouth. Do not handle.

- Chew tablet or place under tongue and wait for it to dissolve.

- Absorption occurs within a few minutes. If you are taking the medicine near a meal time, wait approximately five minutes before eating/drinking.

General Notes on Homeopathic Medicine

- Homeopathic medicine is a natural system of treatment which stimulates the body's own healing mechanisms.

- Homeopathic medicines are completely safe and will not interact with conventional/orthodox medicines.

- Homeopathic medicines cannot be taken in excess/overdose. The effect of the medicine is due to the frequency of dose rather than the size of dose.

- For children, homeopathic medicines can be crushed between two teaspoons and tipped on to the tongue or mixed into half a glass of water and sipped at the frequency recommended.

- Homeopathic medicines can occasionally cause an 'aggravation' reaction – that is, the illness symptoms may become slightly worse initially. This is an encouraging sign as it indicates that the medicine is correct for the condition. The reaction is usually brief and self-limitings but if it continues or becomes severe, stop the medicine and consult your practitioner.

- Homeopathic medicines should be stopped once the symptoms settle. You do not have to finish the supply of medicines. Restart the medicine if the problem/symptoms return.

ↁ

The Contributors

Joanne Avison met Tom Myers in 1998 and became one of his early teachers at KMI, pioneering the application of Anatomy Trains in motion for movement practitioners. In 2006 she co-founded a Yoga Teacher Training programme awarding a worldwide two-year Diploma in the Art of Contemporary Yoga and the Science of Body Architecture. Jo has spent recent years working with Robert Schleip and is a licensed Fascial Fitness teacher. After years of human dissection and her long fascination with moving structure and *applying* anatomy, through experience, she has developed a series of talks and roadshows with Nicola Brooks at BodyworkCPD. She is based in Brighton, West Sussex, UK.

Maggie Chambers is a qualified naturopath and homeopath who graduated from the College of Naturopathic Medicine in 2006. She runs a clinic in London where she practises holistic treatments with a combination of nutrition, homeopathy, iridology, herbs, Traditional Chinese Medicine, cupping, aromatherapy and flower essences. She has written health articles for various publications and runs a website of natural health tips (vinegarbrownpaper.com).

Kelly Clancy OTR/L CHT SMS RBI is the founder and owner of the Seattle Center for Structural Medicine. She graduated from Colorado State University's school of Occupational Therapy in 1987 and completed her sub-speciality training in Hand Therapy in 1994. Kelly became a registered Bowen instructor in 2010 and completed a three-year Structural Medicine degree through the Institute of Structural Medicine. Kelly holds a certificate in holistic health counselling from the Institute for Integrative Nutrition, and is also on the clinical faculty of the University of Washington's rehabilitation department. She teaches nationally and internationally on topics related to manual therapy and fascia. For more information, visit her website at www.scfsm.com.

Lina Clerke is a registered midwife, Doula (birth attendant), Bowen practitioner and Childbirth Educator, specializing in pregnancy and postnatal relaxation. She was a contributor to the Childbirth Education Teacher Training programme for midwives and health workers at Melbourne's Royal Women's Hospital and did an Active Birth teacher training in London with Janet Balaskas. She is based in Brighton, West Sussex, UK.

John Coleman was suffering severe symptoms of stage IV Parkinson's disease and early-stage Multi-System Atrophy in 1995 when he decided to pursue alternative approaches to recovery. By 1998 he was symptom-free. His book, *Stop Parkin' and Start Livin': Reversing the Symptoms of Parkinson's Disease*, was published in 2005. (www. returntostillness.com.au)

Nickatie DiMarco BSc Hons Applied Health Sciences, Diploma in Palliative Care, has five years' experience working in a specialist palliative care setting in a hospice in Herefordshire. She is currently training to teach Bowen.

Paula Esson BSc is clinic director of the Northern Integrative Health Practice (www. healthnorth.co.uk). Following a training in Sport Science, specializing in Exercise Physiology, she is now focused on contributing to and changing health care in the North East of the UK by integrating Bowen into the NHS.

Titus Foster MBAcC BTAA trained as an acupuncturist in the UK and Shanghai and has practised Bowen for over 15 years. He trained in the Manaka and Kiko Matsumoto styles of Japanese acupuncture as well as TCM. He works in Shoreham-by-Sea in West Sussex, UK.

Dr Carolyn Goh is a medically qualified doctor with a Bachelors in Engineering, a Masters in Bioengineering and a PhD in Bioengineering. She is currently a research associate at Imperial College London and runs a private Bowen Therapy practice in St John's Wood, London. She is also author of the self-help e-books *Baby Bowen – Natural Colic Relief* and *Stop Wheezing and Start Breathing – The Bowen Technique for Asthma* (with Alastair Rattray).

Sandra Gustafson MHS BSN RN has a healthcare career spanning 30 years, working in integrative medicine as a registered nurse and as a holistic healthcare practitioner. She has been a Bowen practitioner for 23 years and has taught the technique for 20 years. She is based in Santa Rosa, California.

Andrew Johnson has been working as a nutritional therapist since 1984 and works at clinics in Somerset and Dorset. He is also a qualified Herbalist and Kinesiologist. (http://andrewjohnson.info)

Isobel Knight MSc BTAA Isobel studied for her Bowen Diploma under the Bowen Academy of Australia (Bowtech), qualifying in 2003, and has two busy clinics in central London. Isobel has a particular interest in treating chronic fatigue and chronic pain, fibromyalgia and clients who have Ehlers-Danlos (Hypermobility-Type) (EDS-HT) syndrome. She is also very interested in working with dancers, especially classical ballet dancers. Isobel completed an MSc in Dance Science at Trinity Laban which has enhanced her skill base in working with and treating injured dancers. Isobel is an internationally published author on EDS-HT. Her first book on the topic, *A Guide to Living with Hypermobility Syndrome, Bending without Breaking*, was published in 2011 (Singing Dragon Press). Her next, *A Multi-Disciplinary Approach to Managing Ehlers-*

Danlos (Type III) Hypermobility Syndrome – Working with the Chronic Complex Patient, was published in March 2013. Isobel is now lecturing in the UK and internationally on the topics of both Bowen and EDS-HT. For further information please visit www. bowenworks.org.

Sharon Levin is a Bowen practitioner, specializing in assessment and body alignment. She has developed aerobic, aqua-aerobic, sports specific and wellness programmes in South Africa and abroad since the early 1980s and has been an integral part of the transformation of the fitness industry in South Africa. She is an official master presenter of workshops and courses for Virgin Active South Africa and is certified with the Register of Exercise Professionals South Africa and the UK, the International and British Nordic Walking Federations, Exercise Teachers Association South Africa and the American Council for Exercise.

Rosemary MacAllister was a nurse for 50 years and an occupational health advisor for 25 years before learning the Bowen Technique in her retirement. Along with seven colleagues, she helped set up a project within the occupational health service in Lanarkshire, using Bowen to help people back to work after sickness.

Alastair McLoughlin is an honorary member of the London and Counties Society of Physiologists and gained a Diploma in Remedial Massage from the Northern Institute of Massage. Alastair became a registered instructor for the Bowen Therapy Academy of Australia in 1997 and initiated Bowen training in Italy, Norway, Cyprus and Spain. He wrote an e-book in 2012 entitled *The Bowen Technique – A New Perspective* and now teaches Bowen as an independent instructor in the UK and abroad.

Vicki Mechner has been a Bowenwork practitioner since 1996 and an instructor for the Bowen Therapy Academy of Australia since 2001. She teaches primarily in the area around Washington, DC, and maintains a private practice in Springfield, Virginia. Vicki was an early advisor to the Tom Bowen Legacy Trust Fund, an Australian charity that benefits children with disabilities. Her current focus is coaching practitioners in getting their Bowenwork research published in peer-reviewed journals.

Charlotte Meerman Dip BT, Dip DA, AMBAA, AMBTAA is a Bowen practitioner in Bundaberg, Australia, having been introduced to Bowen in 2007. She has worked in rheumatology, dental and obstetric clinics in Holland and Australia.

Michael Morris MSc BSc (Hons) LCSP(Phys) MBTPA began his training in Sports Massage in 1996, and later studied Remedial Massage and Manipulative Therapy with the Northern Institute of Massage. He is currently completing a Masters by Research degree with the University of Warwick, looking into the effectiveness of the Bowen Technique for non-specific chronic low back pain. Michael started teaching for the European College of Bowen Studies in 2007.

Jean Nortje is a former registered nurse and midwife based in Cape Town, with over 40 years of practical nursing experience. She became an instructor with Bowtech in 2006 and teaches all over South Africa.

Michael Quinlivan is the founder of the Border College of Natural Therapies, Wodonga, Victoria, Australia (http://bowen.bcnt.net.au/) with his partner Karen Hedrick and developed the Certificate IV in Bowen Therapy and Diploma of Bowen Therapy in 2005, providing an opportunity for hundreds of Bowen Therapists to undertake a Nationally Recognised Training (Government approved) course in Australia. He has a background in athletics and learned Bowen Therapy in 1994.

Alastair Rattray acquired the Football Association Treatment of Injury Certificate in 1972 and spent many years as physiotherapist to a semi-professional football club. He has taught for the European College of Bowen Studies and practises Bowen in the southeast of the UK. Following some remarkable successes with child asthma, he was asked to appear on Discovery Health Channel in the series Complementary Kids, broadcast in 2002. His work has also featured in both *The Sunday Times* and *Allergy Magazine*. Alastair is an associate member of the Royal Society of Medicine and secretary of the FA Medical Society.

Dr Tim Robinson MB BS MSc MRCGP DRCOG MFHom is a GP who has been practising in Dorset, UK, for almost 25 years. He has been providing homeopathy to his patients over the last 15 years. He lectures in homeopathy both in the UK and abroad and is a former examiner for the Faculty of Homeopathy. (www.doctorTWRobinson.com)

Anne Schubert DipBT was one of the original Bowen students from 1987 and has a particular interest in the release of memory to facilitate mind–body integration. She is a Bowtech Senior Instructor based in Australia but teaches all over the world.

Margaret Spicer BPharm ND DipBT is a senior Bowtech instructor. She has been a Bowen practitioner for 20 years and involved in complementary health for well over 25 years. With Anne Schubert, she developed the Mind Body Bowen approach. She is based in Sydney, Australia.

John Wilks MA RCST BTAA has been practising the Bowen Technique and craniosacral therapy full time since 1995, and works at three clinics in the southwest of England. He has taught Bowen since 1998 in many countries throughout the world including the UK, USA, South Africa, New Zealand, Germany, Denmark, Portugal, Norway, Israel, Australia, Central America, Ireland, Austria and France. He is the author of four books on Bowen and craniosacral therapy, a contributing author to a recent book on hypermobility syndromes and is currently completing a commission for a new book on choices in pregnancy and childbirth for Jessica Kingsley Publishers. In 2005 he set up a two-year practitioner training for midwives in craniosacral therapy, the first of its kind to be accredited by the Royal College of Midwives and has also been involved in setting up a number of charitable projects organizing therapeutic work overseas. (www.cyma.org.uk)

Ann Winter worked for over 30 years in nursing within the NHS, part of that time in a respiratory intensive care unit, before taking on a nursing officer post with the Scottish Heart Health Study. After obtaining a BSc in Occupational Health, she now works with the West of Scotland Bowen Therapy Team.

Jo Wortley has been a practising Bowen practitioner since 2003, and is also the BTPA Children's Clinics Coordinator. During 2014, Jo will be working closely with Howard Plummer with the aim of becoming a Fascia Bowen teacher. She is based in Bury St Edmunds, Suffolk, UK.

Recommended Reading

Avison, J. (2014) *Yoga: Fascia, Anatomy and Movement.* Fountainhall: Handspring Publishing.

Baker, J. (2001) *The Bowen Technique: Principles and Practice.* Chichester: Corpus.

Baker, J. (2013) *Bowen Unravelled – a Journey into the Fascial Understanding of the Bowen Technique.* Chichester: Lotus Publishing.

Balaskas, J. (1991) *New Active Birth: A Concise Guide to Natural Childbirth.* London: Thorsons.

Balch, P.A. (2010) *Prescription for Nutritional Healing: A Practical A-to-Z Reference to Drug-Free Remedies Using Vitamins, Minerals, Herbs and Food Supplements.* New York: Avery.

Bartholomew, A. (2003) *Hidden Nature: The Startling Insights of Viktor Schauberger.* Edinburgh: Floris.

Becker, R.O. and Selden, G. (1985) *The Body Electric: Electromagnetism and the Foundation of Life.* New York: Morrow.

Biel, A. and Dorn, R. (2010) *Trail Guide to the Body: A Hands-on Guide to Locating Muscles, Bones, and More.* Boulder, CO: Books of Discovery.

Butler, D. and Matheson, J. (2000) *The Sensitive Nervous System.* Adelaide: NOI Group Publications.

Campbell-McBride, N. (2010) *Gut and Psychology Syndrome: Natural Treatment for Dyspraxia, Autism, A.D.D. Dyslexia. A.D.H.D., Depression, Schizophrenia*: Cambridge: Medinform Publishing.

Carter, R. (2010) *Mapping the Mind.* London: Phoenix.

Chaitow, L. (2001) *Fibromyalgia and Muscle Pain: Your Self-Treatment Guide: What Causes It, How It Feels and What to Do about It.* London: Thorsons.

Chamberlain, D.B. (1998) *The Mind of Your Newborn Baby.* Berkeley, CA: North Atlantic Books.

Chamberlain, D.B. (2013) *Windows to the Womb: Revealing the Conscious Baby from Conception to Birth.* Berkeley, CA: North Atlantic Books.

Dalton, E. (2012) *Dynamic Body.* Oklahoma City: Freedom from Pain Institute.

Dooley, M.M. (2007) *Fit for Fertility.* London: Hodder Mobius.

Flanagan, M.D.C. (2010) *The Downside of Upright Posture: The Anatomical Causes of Alzheimers, Parkinsons, and Multiple Sclerosis.* Minneapolis, MN: Two Harbors Press.

Fox, S. (2005) *Practical Pathology for the Massage Therapist.* Lydney: Corpus.

Fox, S. (2008) *Relating to Clients: The Therapeutic Relationship for Complementary Therapists.* London: Jessica Kingsley Publishers.

Gerhardt, S. (2004) *Why Love Matters: How Affection Shapes a Baby's Brain.* Hove and New York: Brunner-Routledge.

Gibb, T. and Wilks, J. (2008) *Applying the Bowen Technique* DVD. Sherborne: Cyma Ltd.

Gintis, B. (2007) *Engaging the Movement of Life: Exploring Health and Embodiment through Osteopathy and Continuum.* Berkeley, CA: North Atlantic Books.

Goddard, S. (2005) *Reflexes, Learning and Behavior: A Window into the Child's Mind.* Eugene, OR: Fern Ridge Press.

Gokhale, E. (2013) *8 Steps to a Pain-Free Back: Natural Posture Solutions for Pain in the Back, Neck, Shoulder; Hip, Knee, and Foot* Chichester: Lotus Publishing.

Gordon, Y. (2002) *Birth and Beyond: Pregnancy, Birth, Your Baby and Family: The Definitive Guide.* London: Vermilion.

Ho, M.-W. (2008) *The Rainbow and the Worm: The Physics of Organisms.* Singapore and Hackensack, NJ: World Scientific.

Juhan, D. (2003) *Job's Body: A Handbook for Bodywork.* Barrytown, NY: Barrytown/Station Hill.

Keltner, D. (2009) *Born to Be Good: the Science of a Meaningful Life.* New York: W.W. Norton.

Kern, M. (2005) *Wisdom in the Body: the Craniosacral Approach to Essential Health.* Berkeley, CA: North Atlantic Books.

Knight, I. (2011) *A Guide to Living with Hypermobility Syndrome: Bending without Breaking.* London: Singing Dragon Press.

Knight, I. (2013) *A Multi-Disciplinary Approach to Managing Ehlers-Danlos (type III) – Hypermobility Syndrome: Working with the Chronic Complex Patient.* London: Singing Dragon Press.

Koch, L. (1997) *The Psoas Book.* Felton, CA: Guinea Pig Publications.

LeDoux, J.E. (1999) *The Emotional Brain: The Mysterious Underpinnings of Emotional Life.* London: Phoenix.

Levine, P.A. (1997) *Waking the Tiger: Healing Trauma – The Innate Capacity to Transform Overwhelming Experiences.* Berkeley, CA: North Atlantic Books.

Levine, P.A. (2010) *In an Unspoken Voice: How the Body Releases Trauma and Restores Goodness.* Berkeley, CA: North Atlantic Books.

Magee, D.J. (2008) *Orthopedic Physical Assessment.* St Louis, MO: Saunders Elsevier.

McCarty, W.A. (2009) *Welcoming Consciousness: Supporting Babies' Wholeness from the Beginning of Life – An Integrated Model of Early Development.* Santa Barbara, CA: Wondrous Beginnings.

Myers, T.W. (2013) *Anatomy Trains: Myofascial Meridians for Manual and Movement Therapists.* London: Elsevier.

Oschman, J.L. (2000) *Energy Medicine: The Scientific Basis.* Edinburgh and New York: Churchill Livingstone.

Oschman, J.L. (2003) *Energy Medicine in Therapeutics and Human Performance.* Amsterdam and Boston, MA: Butterworth Heinemann.

Pennington, G. (2012) *A Textbook of Bowen Technique.* Victoria: Barker Deane Publishing.

Pert, C.B. (1999) *Molecules of Emotion: Why You Feel the Way You Feel.* London: Pocket Books.

Peterson, L. and Renström, P. (2001) *Sports Injuries: Their Prevention and Treatment.* London: Martin Dunitz.

Porges, S. (2013) *Clinical Insights from the Polyvagal Theory The Transformative Power of Feeling Safe.* New York: W.W. Norton.

Reinagel, M. and Torelli, J. (2007) *The Inflammation-Free Diet Plan: The Scientific Way to Lose Weight, Banish Pain, Prevent Disease, and Slow Aging.* New York and London: McGraw-Hill.

Sapolsky, R.M. (2004) *Why Zebras Don't Get Ulcers: An Updated Guide to Stress, Stress-Related Diseases, and Coping.* New York: Owl.

Schleip, R., Findley, T.W., Chaitow, L. and Huijing, P. (2012) *Fascia: the Tensional Network of the Human Body: the Science and Clinical Applications in Manual and Movement Therapy.* Edinburgh, New York: Churchill Livingstone.

Schleip, R. (2014) *Fascia in Sport and Movement.* Fountainhall: Handspring Publishing.

Tremblay, L. (2007) *The Little Bowen Book*. Available at www.miraclepainrelief.com/THE%20 LITTLE%20BOWEN%20BOOK.pdf, accessed on 23 May 2014.

Walsh, D. (2007) *Evidence-Based Care for Normal Labour and Birth: A Guide for Midwives*. London and New York: Routledge.

Wilks, J. (2004) *Understanding the Bowen Technique*. Lydney: First Stone Publishing.

Wilks, J. (2004) *Understanding Craniosacral Therapy*. Lydney: First Stone Publishing.

Wilks, J. (2007) *The Bowen Technique: The inside Story*. Sherborne: CYMA.

Wilson-Pauwels, L., Stewart, P.A. and Akesson, E.J. (1997) *Autonomic Nerves: Basic Science, Clinical Aspects, Case Studies*. Malden, MA: Blackwell Science.

Yates, S. (2008) *Beautiful Birth: Practical Techniques That Can Help You Achieve a Happier and More Natural Labour and Delivery*. London: Carroll and Brown.

Young, R.O. and Young, S.R. (2009) *The pH Miracle: Balance Your Diet, Reclaim Your Health*. London: Piatkus.

Zainzinger, M. (2007) *BOWTECH – The Original Bowen Technique*. Books on Demand.

Contacts and Resources

Author: John Wilks

Books and DVDs: www.cyma.org.uk
Training courses: www.therapy-training.com
Webinars: www.ehealthlearning.tv
Worldwide: www.bowenprofessionals.com
Email: john@ehealthlearning.tv

Author: Isobel Knight

www.bowenworks.org
Email: bowtherapy@gmail.com

Author: Kelly Clancy

www.scfsm.com
Email: kellyclancy@balanceot.com

Training Organizations

International: Bowtech: www.bowtech.com
UK: Bowen Training UK: www.bowentraining.co.uk
European College of Bowen Studies: www.thebowentechnique.com
Europe: Bowen Akademie Europe: www.bowen-akademie.com
Bowen Europe: www.boweneurope.com
Germany: www.bowtech.de
Italy: www.bowenitalia.org
Canada and Europe: www.techniquebowen.com and www.boweninstitute.ca
Holland and Belgium: www.bowned.nl
USA: Bowenwork Academy USA: www.bowenworkacademyusa.com
Australia: Bowen Training Australia: www.bowentraining.com.au

Practitioner Associations and Directories

Bowen Association UK: www.bowen-technique.co.uk

Bowen Therapy Professional Association: www.bowentherapy.org.uk

American Association of Bowenwork Practitioners: www.bowenworkamerica.com

Canada: www.ibowen.ca and www.cbbg.ca

Australia: www.bowen.org.au and www.bowen.asn.au

Germany, Austria, Switzerland: www.bowen-akademie.com/cms

Holland: www.bowned.nl

New Zealand: www.bowtech.org.nz

Bulgaria: www.bowen.bg

Romania: www.bowtech.ro

Poland: /www.bowenpolska.pl/

Cyprus, Serbia: www.bowtech.ro/en

Croatia: http://bowen.ergovita.hr

Portugal: http://apt-bowen.pt

Ireland: http://ibowen.ie

Switzerland: www.bowtech.ch

Turkey: www.bowen.web.tr

France/Canada: www.techniquebowen.com/Louise/Louise-fr.htm

International Practitioner Directories

iBowen: available from the Apple Store and www.ibowen.ca

Bowen Therapy Worldwide: www.allbowentherapyworldwide.com

Bowen Supplies (UK)

www.bowensuppliesbyhelen.com/index.asp

Subject Index

Sub-headings in *italics* indicate figures and
illustrations.

Author Index